Cardiovascular Disease

Cardiovascular Disease
New Concepts in Diagnosis and Therapy

Edited by
Henry I. Russek

UNIVERSITY PARK PRESS
Baltimore · London · Tokyo

UNIVERSITY PARK PRESS
International Publishers in Science and Medicine
Chamber of Commerce Building
Baltimore, Maryland 21202

Copyright © 1974 by University Park Press

Printed in the United States of America

Library of Congress Cataloging in Publication Data
Main entry under title:

Cardiovascular disease.

"Edited proceedings of the American College of Cardiology-St. Barnabas Hospital symposium, 'Paths of progress in cardiovascular disease,' " held in New York City, Dec. 8-10, 1972.
  1. Cardiovascular system–Diseases–Congresses. I. Russek, Henry I., 1911-   ed. II. American College of Cardiology. III. New York. St. Barnabas Hospital for Chronic diseases. [DNLM: 1. Cardiovascular diseases–Congresses. WG100 A497c 1972]
RC667.C39   616.1   73-12297
ISBN 0-8391-0719-6

CONTENTS

Advancing Frontiers in Surgical Treatment
for Cardiovascular Disease

Valve Replacement or Repair?

Coronary Bypass Grafts – Artery
or Vein?

Cardiac Transplantation or the Mechanical Heart?

CONTRIBUTING AUTHORS

William B. Abrams, M.D., Vice-President and Director of Clinical Research, Ayerst Laboratories, Inc., New York, New York; Clinical Associate Professor of Medicine, New Jersey College of Medicine and Dentistry, Newark, New Jersey

Ezra A. Amsterdam, M.D., Assistant Professor of Medicine, Assistant Professor of Physiology, and Director, Coronary Care Unit, Section of Cardiovascular Medicine, University of California, School of Medicine, Davis, California

Charles P. Bailey, M.D., Director of Thoracic and Cardiovascular Surgery, St. Barnabas Hospital, New York, New York

Murray G. Baron, M.D., Associate Professor of Radiology and Associate Attending Radiologist, Mount Sinai School of Medicine of the City University of New York, New York, New York

John E. Batchelder, M.D., Trainee in Cardiology, United States Public Health Service Hospital, Indianapolis, Indiana

Sol Bernstein, M.D., Associate Professor of Medicine, University of Southern California, School of Medicine; Medical Director and Head, Infective Endocarditis Research Team, Los Angeles County/USC Medical Center, Los Angeles, California

Eugene Braunwald, M.D., Physician-in-Chief, Peter Bent Brigham Hospital; Hersey Professor of the Theory and Practice of Physic, Harvard Medical School, Boston, Massachusetts

Henry Buchwald, M.D., Ph.D., Associate Professor of Surgery, The University of Minnesota Medical School, Minneapolis, Minnesota

George E. Burch, M.D., Henderson Professor and Chairman, Department of Medicine, Tulane University School of Medicine, New Orleans, Louisiana

Kanu Chatterjee, M.B., Associate Cardiologist and Clinical Director, Myocardial Infarction Research Unit, Cedars-Sinai Medical Center, Los Angeles, California

Roy H. Clauss, M.D., Professor of Surgery, New York Medical College, New York, New York

Jacques J. Col, M.D., University of Louvain; Former Fellow in Cardiology, Good Samaritan Hospital, Dayton, Ohio

James S. Cole, M.D., Assistant Professor of Medicine, Department of Medicine, Baylor College of Medicine, Houston, Texas

Eliot Corday, M.D., Clinical Professor of Medicine, the UCLA School of Medicine; Senior Attending Physician and Chairman, Cardiac Care Committee, Cedars of Lebanon Hospital Division of Cedars-Sinai Medical Center, Los Angeles, California

Costantino Costantini, M.D., Research Fellow, Cedars-Sinai Medical Center, Los Angeles, California

Marina Dalmastro, M.D., Research Fellow, Cedars-Sinai Medical Center, Los Angeles, California

Irany M. deAzevedo, M.D., Research Associate, Division of Cardiology, Hahnemann Medical College and Hospital, Philadelphia, Pennsylvania

Eugene Dong, Jr., M.D., Associate Professor of Surgery, Stanford University School of Medicine, Stanford, California

Leonard S. Dreifus, M.D., Associate Clinical Professor of Medicine and Research Associate Professor of Physiology, Hahnemann Medical College and Hospital, Philadelphia, Pennsylvania

Stephen E. Epstein, M.D., Chief, Cardiology Branch, National Heart and Lung Institute, National Institutes of Health, Bethesda, Maryland; Clinical Associate Professor of Medicine, Georgetown University School of Medicine, Washington, D. C.

Charles Fisch, M.D., Professor of Medicine and Director, Cardiovascular Division, Indiana University School of Medicine; Director, Krannert Institute of Cardiology, Marion County General Hospital, Indianapolis, Indiana

Frank S. Folk, M.D., Associate Attending Thoracic and Cardiovascular Surgeon, St. Barnabas Hospital, New York, New York

Peter L. Frommer, M.D., Chief, Myocardial Infarction Branch, National Heart and Lung Institute, National Institutes of Health, Bethesda, Maryland

William Ganz, M.D., Senior Research Scientist, Department of Cardiology, Cedars-Sinai Medical Center and Professor of Medicine, University of California, Los Angeles, California

Thomas Davis Giles, M.D., Associate Professor of Medicine, Tulane University School of Medicine, New Orleans, Louisiana

Donald H. Glaeser, D.Sc., Assistant Professor of Experimental Medicine, Departments of Surgery and Medicine, Baylor College of Medicine, Houston, Texas

Herbert Gold, M.D., F.A.C.C., Associate Clinical Professor of Medicine, University of California School of Medicine, Los Angeles, California

Robert E. Goldstein, M.D., Senior Investigator, Cardiology Branch, National Heart and Lung Institute, National Institutes of Health, Bethesda, Maryland

George E. Green, M.D., Associate Attending Surgeon, St. Luke's Hospital; Assistant Professor of Surgery, New York University School of Medicine, New York, New York

George C. Griffith, M.D., D.Sc. (Hon.), Emeritus Professor of Medicine (Cardiology), University of Southern California School of Medicine, Los Angeles, California

Dwight E. Harken, M.D., Clinical Professor of Surgery, Emeritus, Harvard Medical School, Boston, Massachusetts

Sansern Hastanan, M.D., Associate Attending Thoracic and Cardiovascular Surgeon, St. Barnabas Hospital, Bronx, New York

Shigeru Hirose, M.D., Staff Surgeon, Department of Cardiovascular Surgery, Nagoya University Hospital, Nagoya, Japan

Teruo Hirose, M.D., Senior Attending in Thoracic and Cardiovascular Surgery, and Director, Cardiovascular Laboratory, St. Barnabas Hospital, New York, New York

Fred N. Huffman, M.D., Senior Research Associate, Harvard Medical School, Boston, Massachusetts

Huascar E. Jessen, M.D., Fellow in Cardiology, Good Samaritan Hospital, Dayton, Ohio

W. Dudley Johnson, M.D., Associate Clinical Professor of Surgery, The Medical College of Wisconsin; Chief of Cardiovascular Surgery, St. Luke's Hospital, Milwaukee, Wisconsin

Michael R. Katz, M.D., Associate Professor of Medicine, Hahnemann Medical College and Hospital, Philadelphia, Pennsylvania

John D. Keith, M.D., Professor of Surgery, Hospital for Sick Children, Toronto, Canada

Kenneth M. Kent, M.D., Senior Investigator, Cardiology Branch, National Heart and Lung Institute, National Institutes of Health, Bethesda, Maryland

Demetrios Kimbiris, M.D., Assistant Professor of Medicine, Hahnemann Medical College and Hospital, Philadelphia, Pennsylvania

Peter T. Kuo, M.D., Professor of Medicine, University of Pennsylvania School of Medicine, Philadelphia, Pennsylvania

Tzu-Wang Lang, M.D., F.A.C.C., Senior Research Scientist, Cedars-Sinai Medical Center, Los Angeles, California

John H. Laragh, M.D., Professor of Clinical Medicine, Columbia University College of Physicians and Surgeons, New York, New York

William Likoff, M.D., Clinical Professor of Medicine, Hahnemann Medical College and Hospital, Philadelphia, Pennsylvania; Chairman, National Program Committee for Continuing Medical Education, American College of Cardiology

Dean T. Mason, M.D., Professor of Medicine, Professor of Physiology, and Chief, Section of Cardiovascular Medicine, University of California, School of Medicine, Davis, California

Rashid A. Massumi, M.D., Professor of Medicine, Director, Electrophysiology, Section of Cardiovascular Medicine, University of California, School of Medicine, Davis, California

Arthur M. Master, M.D.,[1] Emeritus Clinical Professor of Medicine, The Mount Sinai School of Medicine; Consulting Cardiologist, The Mount Sinai Hospital, New York, New York

Thomas W. Mattingly, M.D., Clinical Professor of Medicine, Georgetown University School of Medicine and George Washington University School of Medicine, and Consultant in Cardiology, U. S. Department of State, Washington, D. C.

Henry D. McIntosh, M.D., The Bob and Vivian Smith Professor and Chief of Medical Service, The Methodist Hospital, and Chairman, Department of Medicine, Baylor College of Medicine, Houston, Texas

Samuel Meerbaum, Ph.D., F.A.C.C., Senior Research Scientist, Cedars-Sinai Medical Center, Los Angeles, California

Richard R. Miller, M.D., Assistant Professor of Medicine, Assistant Director, Coronary Care Unit, Section of Cardiovascular Medicine, University of California School of Medicine, Davis, California

John H. Moyer, III, M.D., Professor and Chairman, Department of Medicine, Hahnemann Medical College and Hospital, Philadelphia, Pennsylvania

John C. Norman, M.D., Associate Professor of Surgery, Harvard Medical School, Boston, Massachusetts

Oglesby Paul, M.D., Professor of Medicine, Northwestern University Medical School, and Attending Physician, Passavant Memorial Hospital, Chicago, Illinois

Osler L. Peterson, M.D., Professor of Preventive Medicine, Harvard Medical School, Boston, Massachusetts

---

[1] Now deceased.

Walter Redisch, M.D., Visiting Professor of Medicine and Research Surgery, New York Medical College, New York, New York

David R. Redwood, M.D., Head, Section on Cardiovascular Diagnosis, Cardiology Branch, National Heart and Lung Institute, National Institutes of Health, Bethesda, Maryland

Steven Rubins, M.D., Assistant Clinical Professor of Medicine, University of California School of Medicine, Los Angeles, California

Henry I. Russek, M.D., Research Professor of Cardiovascular Disease and Clinical Professor of Medicine, New York Medical College, New York, New York

Takio Shimamoto, M.D., Professor and Chairman, Department of Medicine, Institute for Cardiovascular Diseases, Tokyo Ika-Shika National University Medical School, Tokyo, Japan

Eldon R. Smith, M.D., Department of Medicine, Victoria General Hospital, Halifax, Nova Scotia, Canada

F. Mason Sones, Jr., M.D., Head, Department of Cardiovascular Diseases and Cardiac Laboratory, Cleveland Clinic Foundation, Cleveland, Ohio

H. J. C. Swan, M.D., Ph.D., Professor of Medicine, The UCLA School of Medicine; Director of Cardiology, Cedars-Sinai Medical Center, Los Angeles, California; President-Elect, American College of Cardiology

Erwin N. Terry, M.D., Research Associate Professor of Surgery, New York Medical College, New York, New York

Sylvan L. Weinberg, M.D., Chairman, Cardiovascular Center, and Director, Coronary Care Unit, Good Samaritan Hospital, Dayton, Ohio

Stewart Wolf, M.D., Director, The Marine Biomedical Institute, University of Texas Medical Branch of Galveston, Galveston, Texas

Kinsman E. Wright, Jr., M.D., Assistant Professor of Medicine, Department of Medicine, Baylor College of Medicine, Houston, Texas

Robert Zelis, M.D., Associate Professor of Medicine, Associate Professor of Physiology, and Director, Cardiac Catheterization and Clinical Physiology Laboratories, Section of Cardiovascular Medicine, University of California, School of Medicine, Davis, California

PREFACE

> I shall be telling this with a sigh
> Somewhere ages and ages hence:
> Two roads diverged in a wood and I—
> I took the one less traveled by,
> And that has made all the difference.
> ROBERT FROST

As in other fields of science, the paths of progress in cardiovascular disease have been blazed by pioneers with vision, imagination, determination, and courage. Through their efforts, the practicing physician has seen many of the "radical" innovations of yesterday become the accepted routines of today. Progress in medicine, however, frequently places increasing demands upon clinical skill, judgment, and understanding. Thus, while aggressive techniques in the diagnosis and therapy of cardiovascular disease frequently are attended by spectacular success, their use, unfortunately, is not without hazard. Indeed, the calculated risk from the application of such methods, even when they seem indicated and are skillfully applied, requires that clinical decisions be rooted in adequate knowledge and sound judgment. To achieve such perspective, much may be gained from the experiences of the eminent authorities who have contributed to this volume. Within its pages, some of the best-informed experts of our time traverse the paths of recent progress and critically appraise concepts both old and new; they debate current controversial issues, define with candor the bounds of present-day knowledge, and survey prophetically horizons for future achievement.

This publication represents the edited proceedings of the American College of Cardiology-St. Barnabas Hospital Symposium, "Paths of Progress in Cardiovascular Disease," held at the Americana Hotel in New York City, December 8–10, 1972. Like each of the four previous annual meetings in this series, the Symposium was attended by approximately 1,000 physicians representing every state in the Union. The eagerness of these doctors to improve their knowledge of cardiovascular disease and to elevate the standard of medical care in the communities in which they live and practice is not only a tribute to their own dedication but an affirmation of the nobility of medicine as a career.

The American College of Cardiology and St. Barnabas Hospital wish to express their sincere thanks to the members of the faculty of this Symposium who not only served without remuneration but who also provided manuscripts of their work so that by means of this volume their valuable contributions could be made available to an ever wider audience. Such sharing of scientific knowledge has always been in the highest tradition of the medical profession. In the fulfillment of this ideal, the investigator, the teacher, and the clinician have brought into clear focus the historical continuity of all medical progress.

We wish to extend our deep appreciation to Dr. William Likoff and the members of the National Program Committee for Continuing Medical Education of the American College of Cardiology for the confidence expressed in the warm support of our efforts. In providing faultless administrative management, Mr. William Nelligan, Executive Director of the American College of Cardiology, and his able associates Mary Anne McInerny and Patrick Ziarnik, contributed greatly to the success of this meeting. The Russek Foundation, Inc., served as a co-sponsor of the program and provided valuable administrative assistance.

Finally, we wish to express our thanks to the following organizations for educational grants in partial support of this Symposium:

Ives Laboratories   E. R. Squibb & Sons, Inc.
Ayerst Laboratories   USV Pharmaceutical Corporation
William S. Merrell Company   McNeil Laboratories
Warner-Chilcott Laboratories   Parke, Davis & Company
Abbott Laboratories   The Purdue Frederick Company
Ciba Pharmaceutical Company   Schering Corporation
Hoffman-LaRoche, Inc.   Hoechst Pharmaceutical Company
Eli Lilly and Company   Sandoz Pharmaceuticals
Marion Laboratories, Inc.   Burroughs Wellcome Company
Merck Sharp & Dohme   Endo Laboratories, Inc.
Pfizer Laboratories   Knoll Pharmaceutical Company
G. D. Searle & Company

The assistance provided by these organizations in helping to elevate the standards of medical care demonstrates once again their sensitivity and dedication to the public interest.

HENRY I. RUSSEK, M.D.

DEDICATION

With this presentation of recent advances in cardiovascular disease, we honor the late Dr. Arthur M. Master for his long and productive career in cardiology.

Before his death on September 4, 1973, Dr. Master achieved renown for his fundamental contribution in standardizing a relatively simple stress test and investigating its effects on the electrocardiograms of normal individuals and of those with coronary arterial disease. The concept of detecting coronary disease in people with normal electrocardiograms by subjecting them to standard, tolerable, safe stress has proved valid over the years, and extension of this concept has assumed increasing importance in evaluating indications and results in the burgeoning field of coronary arterial surgery. Dr. Master was, of course, best known for the Master Test, but his other contributions have been considerable.

Arthur Master was born in New York City in 1895. In the day of the "work ethic," he worked his way through high school, College of the City of New York, and Cornell University Medical College. After graduation from Cornell at the top of his class in 1921, he began his long career with Mt. Sinai Hospital, New York, serving as an intern from 1921 to 1923. He manifested an early interest in cardiology, and in 1923, he published two important papers ("Electrocardiogram and Heart Muscle Disease" with Dr. H. E. Pardee and "Fatty Degeneration of the Heart" by himself). He then studied under Sir Thomas Lewis in London, and in 1924, he published work on experimental heart block and the influence of atrial rate on atrioventricular conduction. It is of interest that the observations made in these studies are still valid 50 years later.

Subsequently, he devoted his major efforts to the emerging field of electrocardiography, and he became Chief of the Cardiographic Laboratory at Mt. Sinai in 1934. He had an active career in teaching, investigation, and patient care, and vigorously pursued these three interests until his death. He published 438 articles and five textbooks, and his contributions to cardiology have been recognized internationally.

In this small space we cannot include all of his contributions, but in many instances he gave initial direction to ideas which are well accepted today. In 1923, he abolished the accepted concept of "fatty degeneration" of the heart as a clinical entity by showing that equal amounts of fat could be found in normal and diseased hearts. He was among the first to advocate weight reduction in cardiac patients, having investigated some of the hemodynamic and electro-

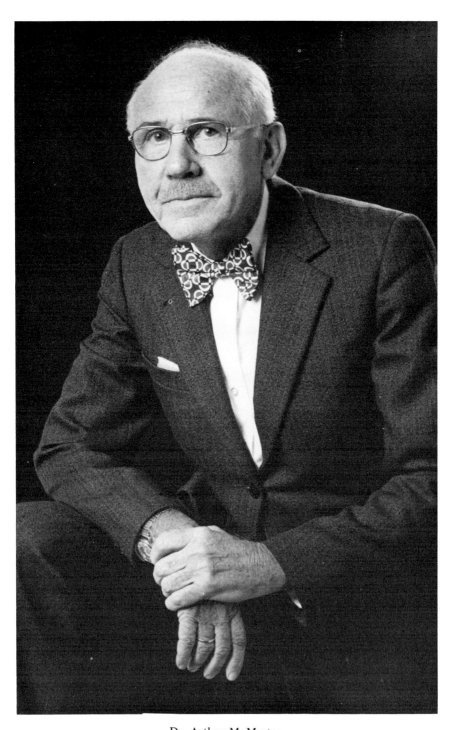

Dr. Arthur M. Master

cardiographic effects of obesity. He initiated the concept that patients often made complete recoveries from acute myocardial infarction and that they should be urged to return to work and to resume reasonable physical activity, a concept widely opposed at that time within the profession and by patients. He pioneered the concept that coronary occlusion with transmural infarction often was not associated with physical effort. He put an end to the high-calorie diet as a treatment of acute myocardial infarction, establishing the routine of not over-feeding or overmedicating such patients. Early and persistently, he pointed out the frequency of clinically "silent" coronary arterial disease, an observation which is well appreciated today.

Another of Dr. Master's important contributions to clinical cardiology was the concept of "acute coronary insufficiency" as a clinical entity, a notion which stressed noncardiac causes of diminished coronary blood flow, such as hemorrhage, anemia, and hypotension. Dr. Master detailed the characteristic clinical and electrocardiographic features and emphasized the differentiation between acute coronary insufficiency and transmural infarction. In addition, Dr. Master was among the first to describe fluoroscopic evidence of akinesia or dyskinesia of the heart following acute myocardial infarction. Moreover, he made major contributions in a prodigious study of the blood pressures of 74,000 apparently normal individuals in different age groups, 20 to 106 years, in an effort to delineate normal values.

Arthur Master achieved civic distinction apart from his efforts in medicine. He served in the U. S. Navy in both World Wars. He served as President of the New York County Medical Society and of the American College of Chest Physicians and occupied executive posts in the New York Academy of Medicine and the New York Heart Association. He was the recipient of numerous honors and citations from lay and medical organizations and governmental bodies. He remained very much a "humanist," devoted in a very special way to his patients, his close family, and his many friends. Perhaps none of his many awards and accomplishments honors him as well as the respect of his peers in recognizing his contributions with the publication of this volume.

LESLIE A. KUHN, M.D.

CORONARY ARTERIES IN THE CHILDHOOD YEARS

JOHN D. KEITH

Atherosclerosis in the aorta or in the coronary, cerebral, or other peripheral arteries is now entrenched as a major cause of morbidity and mortality in most countries around the world, particularly the more affluent ones. Although death usually occurs in the middle-aged or the elderly, concern has recently been directed to the vessels in childhood or early adult life. An increasing number of studies in this age group are being reported (1–4). These authors found evidence of early atherosclerosis in approximately half of the young men examined, whose average age was in the mid-twenties.

It has now become obvious that vascular changes take place over many years, leading to significant pathology in middle age. It is not yet clear how early in childhood the original pathologic alterations begin to evolve, but histologic investigation of arteries from infants and children or adolescents dying in the first two decades of life suggests that this is a pediatric problem initially.

Recently, Neufeld (5) and Jaffe (6) and co-workers have reviewed the literature and added to our knowledge in this field. The former have studied the coronary arteries in infants and children of different cultural origins in Israel, represented by three groups, the Ashkenazis, the Yemenites, and the Bedouins. The prevalence of coronary atherosclerosis in adult Yemenite Jews and Bedouins is low, both as an absolute rate and in comparison with other ethnic groups in Israel. It is considerably higher in the Ashkenazis. The authors found that after birth the intima in the Ashkenazi males gradually became thicker than that of the other groups studied and this continued on through childhood. They also presented evidence that early changes were accelerated by higher pressure in the systemic arteries in those children with coarctation of the aorta.

Obviously children rarely have strokes, myocardial infarction, gangrene, or aortic aneurysms. Calcification of the arteries is rare, and even atheromatous plaques are uncommon in the childhood groups. Thus one must try to identify the very early stages of change in the coronary arteries and the aorta; such an investigation leads to fatty streaks and endothelial thickening, minimum lipid necrosis, cellular infiltration, musculoelastic layering, and similar conditions. There is some difference of opinion regarding the significance of the fatty streaks that may appear in the endothelium of the aorta in infants in the first year of life. They occur in the population of all countries studied and at all ages.

1

Although they may develop ultimately into atherosclerotic plaques, they may at times remain unchanged or possibly disappear entirely. When such streaks are associated with disintegrating cells of lipid debris, they appear more likely to evolve into atherosclerotic plaques.

Myocardial infarction in childhood is an uncommon event that may occur in such rare conditions as progeria or in diabetes mellitus, or in anomalous origin of coronary arteries from the pulmonary artery. Occasionally one may find embolism or coronary thrombosis in such unusual conditions as lupus erythematosus, polyarteritis nodosum, and interstitial myocarditis. Such rare situations have been summarized by Seganti (7) and Bohr (8).

As is well known, the factors involved in atherosclerosis in the human include hypertension, hyperlipidemia, diabetes mellitus, obesity, a diet rich in saturated fats, cholesterol, and sucrose, cigarette smoking, habitual physical inactivity, and family history. Males appear to be more susceptible than females. All of these factors may be relevant to some degree in studying the pediatric group.

In childhood, an attempt is made to control overweight. In diabetic clinics metabolic control is emphasized. Hypertension may be alleviated or controlled. Physical inactivity is relatively uncommon in the first two decades of life. Cigarette smoking may be a problem in certain age groups in some countries.

Hyperlipidemia, as a possible cause of atherosclerosis, appears to be a factor in early life in some cases. Recent evidence from the Framingham study suggests that at least in young and middle-aged adults the risk of coronary heart disease is reflected, to some degree, by the presence of an elevated serum cholesterol level (9). Proof that its control through primary prevention diet will improve the prognosis in later decades is still lacking or is incomplete, but there is sufficient evidence to suggest that a study should be undertaken in the pediatric group to help clarify this problem. Numerous investigations are in progress in adults to determine whether, after a coronary episode, life may be prolonged or further episodes prevented by the use of a low-fat or polyunsaturated fat diet. It is difficult or impossible to control or change the eating habits of a population of a country, especially when the evidence is not clear that such changes will be universally beneficial.

In childhood it is possible to identify hyperlipoproteinemia Type II, even in very early life and probably by cord blood studies. This type of biochemical response appears to occur in about 1 in 200 members of the population. It is, therefore, a relatively common occurrence. It is frequently a familial abnormality, transmitted as a dominant gene in the heterozygous form. However, occasionally this response is found in the homozygous situation and in such cases there is accelerated atherosclerosis in childhood with a high serum cholesterol leading to atherosclerotic episodes in the teenage years or early twenties. In the heterozygous form, Slack and Nevin (10) have shown that the first degree relatives of the heterozygous Type II cases stand a 10—20 times greater chance of developing ischemic heart disease than the rest of the population.

Clinical investigations are now underway in the pediatric field to see if one can control the serum cholesterol by dietary means in different age groups. At the present time this approach is chiefly limited to a study of the problem of controlling serum cholesterol in children who have familial Type II hyperlipo-proteinemia, since more knowledge is needed in this particular group regarding the possible beneficial effects of diet. The advantages of such diets hopefully will be clarified in a few years as far as the blood chemistry is concerned, but the effect on the final end point, that of coronary or other atherosclerotic episodes, will take 30, 40, or 50 years to evaluate in children being treated at the present time. However, investigations being made in the adult field at the moment may lead to more concrete knowledge in this area in the next few years, which will guide us in how best to manage children as they advance in age.

Preliminary studies in childhood suggest that the serum cholesterol level can be gradually reduced by dietary means in the majority of infants with hyperlipo-proteinemia. In older children the problem appears to be more difficult and may require the additional use of drugs.

REFERENCES CITED

1. Enos, W. F., Holmes, R. H., and Beyer, J. 1953. Coronary disease among United States soldiers killed in action in Korea. J.A.M.A. 152:1090.
2. Rigal, R. D., Lovell, F. W., and Townsend, F. M. 1960. Pathologic findings in the cardiovascular systems of military flying personnel. Amer. J. Cardiol. 6:19.
3. Mason, J. K. 1963. Asymptomatic disease of coronary arteries in young men. Brit. Med. J. 2:1234.
4. McNamara, J. J., Molot, M. A., Stremple, J. F., and Cutting, R. T. 1971. Coronary artery disease in combat casualties in Vietnam. J.A.M.A. 216:1185.
5. Neufeld, H. N., and Vlodaver, Z. 1968. Structural changes in the coronary arteries of infants. Proc. Assoc. Europ. Paediat. Cardiol. 4:35.
6. Jaffe, D., Hartroft, W. S., and Manning, M. et al. 1971. Coronary arteries in newborn children. Acta Paediat. Scand. Suppl. 219.
7. Seganti, A. 1968. Myocardial infarction in children. Proc. Assoc. Europ. Paediat. Cardiol. 4:43.
8. Bohr, I. 1969. Myocardial infarction and ischaemic heart disease in infants and children. Arch. Dis. Child. 44:268.
9. Kannel, W. B., Castelli, W. P., Gordon, T., and McNamara, P. M. 1971. Serum cholesterol, lipoproteins and the risk of coronary heart disease. Ann. Intern. Med. 74:1.
10. Slack, J., and Nevin, N. C. 1968. Hyperlipidaemic xanthomatosis. J. Med. Genet. 4:4.

Congestive Heart Failure

CONSIDERATIONS OF SELECTED ASPECTS OF PHYSICAL SIGNS OF HEART FAILURE

G. E. BURCH and T. D. GILES

Too many physicians, and patients as well, equate modern cardiology with "gadgets," computers, techniques, and procedures. The accuracy, simplicity, and quantitative nature of bedside medicine, as practiced by a well-trained and master clinician, are rarely appreciated by patients and many physicians. The physician who has a thorough knowledge of the fundamentals of physiology, anatomy, biochemistry, pathology, pharmacology, and other branches of medicine and chemical disciplines, and who has followed patients to autopsy, does not require complex and expensive procedures to study and evaluate adequately the pathophysiology of disease and to outline therapy for his patients. Furthermore, many complex procedures are frequently dangerous. In fact, those physicians who employ these complex and dangerous diagnostic procedures have recently classified them as "invasive." In addition, the data obtained from such procedures are certainly not as accurate, reliable, and quantitative as popularly believed. The shortcomings of the truly invasive, complex, hazardous, expensive and painful procedures are never adequately stressed in the literature and rarely in teaching sessions.

The rather indiscriminate use of cardiac catheterization and hemodynamic recordings and other complex, expensive, and unnecessary procedures unfortunately tends to create an inferiority complex among well-trained bedside doctors. The impression is created that the bedside clinician is not studying the patient adequately even though he arrives at the correct diagnosis. Nevertheless, the well-trained clinician can evaluate his patients adequately by bedside medicine without resorting to such procedures. For clinical purposes, techniques other than history taking, physical examination, electrocardiography, teleoroentgenography, and a few laboratory examinations are rarely indicated for evaluating patients with acquired heart disease. Furthermore, if training programs in cardiology are not built around such clinical bedside approaches to diagnosis, cardiologists will be produced who, limited by their training, will be unable to evaluate patients at the bedside by history and physical examination.

Supported by grant HL-06769 from the National Heart and Lung Institute of the U.S. Public Health Service, the Rudolph Matas Memorial Fund for the Kate Prewitt Hess Laboratory, the Rowell A. Billups Fund for Research in Heart Disease, and the Feazel Laboratory.

7

Displaying a graph, chart, or recording may impress the layman or novice, but merely doing so does not verify the quantitative accuracy of the recording of the physiologic state at the site under study. For example, any recording obtained with a pressure transducer on the external end of a cardiac catheter, unless corrections are made at least for blood viscosity, length and bore of the catheter, rate of change in pressure, and fidelity of the electronic recorder (1,2), cannot be accepted as quantitatively accurate in reflecting the time course of pressure at the site under study. So, why make an issue of the recording or of the need for it if the recording is not quantitatively accurate anyway? Furthermore, with such recordings allowances cannot be made in interpretation for the state of the patient, underlying unusual circumstances, and drugs which influence the physiologic state at any given moment and in an unknown fashion and degree. Thus, physiologic recordings, even if quantitatively accurate, only indicate the situation and conditions for a brief time in the patient's life and may not be readily repeatable for learning progress or change in the health of the patient. The use of drugs and medication for the catheterization procedure independently alters the physiologic state of the patient.

The good clinician has learned, primarily from experience and the more generally accepted clinical literature, how much information is useful and necessary for accurate diagnosis and excellent management of his patients. He compromises cost, time, suffering, physical and psychic stress, and other sacrifices that the patient and he must make to establish a diagnosis and to achieve proper management. He also knows when he needs (and this is rare) to employ special procedures and when the data obtained are reliable. The astute physician can merely look at his patient and obtain more information than any mathematician, engineer or physiologist can program on a computer. The master clinician has learned to evaluate qualitatively signs and symptoms which he feeds into his own computer, the brain, for analysis and decision making. For example, the doctor at the bedside can estimate cardiac output from palpation of the pulse with sufficient accuracy to satisfy his needs for diagnosis and excellent treatment. It is not important to him whether the cardiac output is 2.1 liters per minute or 1.9 or 2.2 in an elaborate catheterization laboratory with the patient frightened, under the influence of many drugs, surrounded by nurses, doctors, technicians, buzzing apparatus, flashing lights, and clicking noises, with a surgical procedure being performed on his arms and legs, a catheter being inserted through one or more vessels, painful needles in place, and with premature contractions and even more complex arrhythmias occurring. Cardiac output can be estimated satisfactorily from physical examination. A weak, thready, fast pulse reflects low cardiac output, whereas a full, slow pulse reflects a good cardiac output. This is all the information concerning cardiac output that is necessary since the doctor at the bedside is only concerned with whether or not the cardiac function is satisfactory. The physician can readily make quantitative allowances for psychic stress, effects of drugs, the disease of the heart as well as associated diseases, effects of environmental temperature and relative humidity and other factors too numerous to mention, all of which influence the cardiovascular system at any given moment. Even more importantly, the physician at the bedside can repeat his evaluation from minute to minute, hour to hour, or day to day without subjecting his patient to painful and stressful, expensive, hazardous, and inaccurate "invasive" procedures. Furthermore, determination of cardiac output by either the Fick method or by indicator dilution technique is subject to large errors even under ideal circumstances and does not correlate well with the presence or degree of heart failure (3). In addition, the measurement of surface area of the body from body weight and height is based on extremely little data and the extent of the *error* is never known in any given patient (4). It is true that cardiac catheterization is required in congenital cardiac disease, but not for acquired heart disease.

Many of the ideas and concepts discussed above apply also to ballistocardiography, vectorcardiography, phonocardiography, apex cardiography, and other procedures commonly employed today in medical centers. Although not painful and hazardous, these techniques are expensive, time consuming, and unnecessary for adequate service to the patient. Such procedures are largely responsible for the tremendous expense of medical care today. Certainly, when accurately obtained, these studies can be justified for clinical research, but they are rarely needed for excellent service to the sick. Obviously, exceptions exist. For example, if one is interested in the heart sounds of an astronaut on his voyage to the moon, the telemetered phonocardiogram displaces the stethoscope. The physician with an impairment in hearing is extremely handicapped and, therefore, needs the phonocardiograph. However, the physician well trained in auscultation can obtain more information with the stethoscope than anyone can with a phonocardiograph. The splitting of heart sounds, origin, site, intensity, quality and significance of murmurs are more readily appreciated by the well-trained doctor using his stethoscope. The problem of obtaining accurate and satisfactory recordings of phonocardiograms can only be appreciated by those who have tried to record them. Not only is the phonocardiograph unable to quantitate heart sounds, but it also cannot correct for the influence of emphysema, pleural effusion, breast size, obesity, and other factors. However, the physician with his stethoscope can do this extremely well at the bedside for diagnostic and therapeutic purposes. The above example is not intended to imply that phonocardiography used in clinical research has not imparted knowledge; however, its contributions have been much less than commonly believed.

Catheterization of the left ventricle to learn, for purely clinical service, if a patient is in left ventricular congestive heart failure is not only unnecessary but it is unfair to the patient as well. A *careful history* suffices. The physical examination and the x-ray examination may or may not provide significant additional information. For example, the patient who becomes dyspneic during an episode of angina pectoris caused by congestive failure of the left ventricle at the moment of the anginal episode usually does have good cardiac function at other times. His heart can be small and the left ventricular end-diastolic pressure elevated only during the time of the episode of angina pectoris. Furthermore, it is unlikely that the patient would be catheterized during an episode of angina pectoris. And, if by chance it were done, the data would at any rate serve no clinical purpose. Clinicians should also be aware that the left ventricular end-diastolic pressure can only be interpreted correctly if left ventricular "tone" is known (5). This function cannot be calculated from an isolated measurement of left ventricular end-diastolic pressure and, thus, statements about left ventricular function based on such a measurement are not accurate.

Also, the insertion of catheters only for the measurement of central venous pressure is rarely indicated. The hazards of this widespread practice are well documented (6,7,8) and the information derived can be easily obtained from a physical examination (9). At times such isolated measurements of central venous pressure are misleading and may result in improper therapeutic measures (10).

It would be folly to attempt to review in a few pages the symptoms and signs that are of value clinically in the study of a patient with heart disease. They are all important. The importance of each varies with the patient and his illness. The absence of certain symptoms and signs is often as important as their presence. The time of onset, time course of magnitude alone as integrated with other symptoms and signs of heart disease, as well as those of associated diseases, are extremely important. A great deal of time is required to obtain and evaluate these data. The physician is responsible for the evaluation of these relationships which are time dependent. Satisfactory clinical evaluation cannot be done with computer methods. The attitude of the patient, his expressions, his voice, reactions, and rate and nature of response to questions are all among the many extremely important factors which influence the interpretation, value, and reliability of the data obtained. The physician must train and learn to use his senses as clinical sensors to detect data from his patient. These data are channeled into his brain, the indisputably greatest computer of them all, for analysis and finally to render decisions for the benefit of his patient.

For successful practice of clinical cardiology the physician must possess an adequate knowledge of facts and have the ability to use them in logical clinical thinking. These attributes develop only as the result of hard, diligent, and highly motivated work. The well-trained physician possesses the ability to think logically and even extremely rapidly in emergency situations. He knows what questions are relevant and must be asked and he also knows how to evaluate the answers and use them in diagnosis, prognosis, and management.

Such knowledge and training is particularly important for proper care of elderly patients since elderly patients never have heart disease only. Many diseases of variable importance and intensity are usually responsible for the entire clinical picture of the old patient. Emphysema, chronic bronchitis, anemia, diabetes, arteriosclerosis, renal disease, hypertension, cerebral arteriosclerosis, the aging process itself, prostatism, cholelithiasis, hiatus hernia, otosclerosis, impairment of vision, diverticulosis of the colon with or without diverticulitis, family, marital, domestic, and financial problems, loneliness, and dental difficulties are among the associated problems which are the sources simultaneously of symptoms and signs responsible for the elderly patient's clinical state. The well-trained clinician has no difficulties with proper evaluation of each and all of these at the bedside.

A detailed analysis of chest pain or discomfort is usually sufficient in practically all patients to establish or discard the diagnosis of angina pectoris and in turn ischemic heart disease. Coronary angiography, a hazardous and inadequate method for visualizing the coronary arteries, is not nearly as effective in diagnosis and evaluation of ischemic heart disease as are a careful history, physical examination, electrocardiogram, and cardiac fluoroscopy. Only an extremely few vessels are seen with coronary angiography and only the large vessels can be studied, with considerable cost and stress to the patient. The myriads of main branches and small arteries are not displayed. But normal patterns of the large arteries do not rule out disease of the smaller arteries, and narrowing of large vessels does not necessarily establish the precise source of difficulties. Furthermore, left ventriculography, to record disturbances in contractility or contraction, is also expensive, hazardous, and unnecessary. Surely, the information that would be obtained is available from ordinary clinical data, electrocardiography, and roentgenology. The present trend in cardiology to expose patients to expensive and hazardous procedures is not justifiable. The fact that such procedures are obtained in the research laboratory or from research on patients does not imply that they are needed in clinical practice (14,15). The practicing physician must differentiate clinical research from clinical practice with service to patients. For practical clinical purposes the information necessary for proper care of patients is readily available from the usual office or bedside study. The physician who does not have the resources to employ or interest in employing these complex procedures but who is an astute clinician and bedside doctor should not lose confidence in himself and feel inferior. The better the clinician the less special procedures he requires and uses for the study and management of his patients.

In an attempt to illustrate the value of physical signs in diagnosis and care of the patient, the simple, readily recognized signs of heart failure are selected for brief discussion. Heart failure must be approached in an organized manner for accurate diagnosis at the bedside and for therapy, especially for proper digitalization (11).

HEART FAILURE

As previously indicated (12,13), heart failure is easy to detect at the bedside once the physician is aware of the manifestations. A basic understanding of the pathophysiology of heart failure is essential for the physician to evaluate the patient properly and to know how to interrogate and examine him. The required information must be well organized in the mind of the physician in a simple and readily available fashion for rapid recall or retrieval of the manifestations of heart failure when approaching the patient.

There are only two types of heart failure:

    1) anginal, and
    2) congestive.

These two types of failure may exist independently or together. The degree of each in any given patient is simple to determine at the bedside, and it can be determined with greater accuracy and clinical applicability than in any catheterization laboratory. To achieve accurate evaluation of the heart failure requires only a few minutes, patience, and a deliberate, methodical, and knowledgeable approach to the patient (13).

Anginal Heart Failure

Anginal failure may be defined as the failure of cardiac function because of impairment of coronary blood flow. Thus, the clinical manifestations of anginal failure are the symptoms and simple laboratory findings of ischemic heart disease. These are angina pectoris, acute coronary insufficiency, coronary occlusion, myocardial infarction, and ischemic cardiomyopathy. These manifestations are well known (13) but can be extremely subtle at times. Coronary arteriosclerosis is usually present but not necessarily so. Coronary angiography is certainly not necessary to establish a diagnosis; and, even when the main arteries are found to be normal by angiography, the diagnosis is not excluded. Disease of the small vessels or angiospasm of any segment of the coronary arterial system may be the cause of the ischemia. It behooves the physician, therefore, to obtain a detailed, reliable, and objective history, physical examination, routine laboratory data, electrocardiogram, and simple and ordinary roentgenologic information before he diagnoses with certainty the presence or absence of anginal heart failure or coronary or ischemic heart disease.

Anginal heart failure caused by an episode of angina pectoris, acute coronary insufficiency, or myocardial infarction can result in ischemic cardiomyopathy and congestive heart failure, as indicated below. Anginal failure itself is the clinical expression of failure of the coronary arterial circulation to meet the circulatory needs of the myocardium.

Congestive Heart Failure

Congestive failure is the pathophysiologic state which results from failure of the myocardium to pump blood adequately to the tissues of the body to meet their needs (12,13). "Pump failure," as it is often called, results in clinical manifestations readily recognized at the bedside by any competent clinician. The physician not only can recognize the presence of the congestive heart failure (CHF) but can determine the ventricle that is involved and can quantitate the degree of failure to satisfy clinical needs.

Congestive heart failure can be:

1) left ventricular,
2) right ventricular, or
3) both left and right ventricular.

The pathophysiology of CHF must be understood to approximate and recognize the clinical manifestations of congestive heart failure, for the physiologic changes are responsible for the clinical manifestations. Once the physiologic changes responsible for CHF are clearly understood, the physician is better able to elicit and recognize CHF at the bedside, and certainly without the need for the expensive, hazardous, and stressful procedure of cardiac catheterization.

All of the physiologic phenomena are unknown which are set into motion and, in turn, lead to the clinical manifestations of CHF when the myocardium fails to meet the pumping needs of the body. The concepts of "forward" and "backward" failure do not explain the pathophysiologic changes and clinical manifestations of CHF. However, some physiologic phenomena are known and their clinical manifestations are definitely recognizable at the bedside or in the physician's office. Moreover, the degree of CHF is estimable, and the response to proper treatment is dramatic most of the time. It is not possible to detect adequately, if at all, early CHF by cardiac catheterization. It is certainly impossible to quantitate CHF, measure temporal changes in its severity, or regulate the therapy of patients with CHF by using this procedure. However, all of this can be accomplished elegantly by the well-trained cardiologist at the bedside, and improvement in cardiac function can be assured by instituting conventional therapy wisely, in spite of the fact that not all aspects of the pathophysiology of CHF are known.

RELIABLE SIGNS OF CONGESTIVE HEART FAILURE

The reliability of each sign listed below varies. The combination, however, is pathognomonic, with rare exceptions (12,13). It is only possible to list the signs here. Since some can be produced by other disease states, a complete medical inventory is always essential for satisfactory evaluation of the patient's health and for proper management.

Reliable Signs of Left Ventricular Congestive Heart Failure

1. Cardiac dyspnea
   a. Dyspnea on exertion
   b. Orthopnea
   c. Paroxysmal nocturnal dyspnea
   d. Acute cardiac dyspnea or cardiac asthma
   e. Cheyne-Stokes respiration
2. Decrease in vital capacity
3. Accentuated pulmonic second sound
4. Roentgenologic abnormalities
5. Crepitant râles at both lung bases
6. Protodiastolic gallop rhythm
7. Pulsus alternans

These symptoms and signs are readily detected at the bedside or in the physician's office. Early manifestations must be sought, for the earlier the treatment the better the response and the better the overall prognosis. Furthermore, early therapy, when properly instituted and religiously followed by the patient, may prevent serious and advanced or intractable CHF. The signs listed above have been discussed elsewhere (12,13) and have been indicated to vary in intensity and reliability. Furthermore, associated conditions, such as pulmonary disease, can produce some of these signs, but the able clinician readily differentiates the organ source of the various clinical manifestations. Patients with heart disease, especially old people, rarely have only disease of the heart.

Reliable Signs of Right Ventricular Congestive Heart Failure

Congestive failure of the right ventricle has one fundamental manifestation, and that is *generalized symmetrical and proportional venous hypertension.* In fact, except for extremely rare and unusual circumstances, venous hypertension of this nature is always caused by disease of the heart, and usually by right ventricular congestive heart failure. Therefore, the physician need only to establish generalized systemic venous hypertension in order to diagnose right ventricular CHF. In association with this venous hypertension, but not necessarily caused by it alone, other signs develop which are readily noted at the bedside or in the physician's office. Thus, the signs of right ventricular congestive heart failure are:

1. Generalized and symmetric venous hypertension
2. Increase in blood volume (not always)
3. Dependent edema
4. Hepatomegaly

5. Pleural effusion and/or ascites
6. Anascarca.

When all of these signs are present, the patient has heart disease and it is usually attributable to right ventricular congestive failure. The rare exceptions are pericarditis, persistence of the network of Chiari, tricuspid valve orifice obstruction, and the like. Mediastinal masses or venous thrombosis which might equally obstruct the superior and inferior vena cavae to produce a symmetric systemic venous hypertension are extremely rare. The listed manifestations of right ventricular congestive heart failure have also been discussed in detail elsewhere (12,13).

Thus, from the clinical symptoms and signs of heart failure the physician can detect heart disease readily and without the use of gadgets and expensive and hazardous procedures. He must be willing to devote the time required to study his patient adequately and he must understand and know heart disease.

The fine subtleties of anginal and congestive heart failure become known to the cardiologist only from careful and meticulous history taking and physical examination. Furthermore, the other symptoms and signs of heart disease assist in establishing the background of heart disease upon which heart failure develops. It is also common for anginal failure to result in congestive heart failure. Congestive heart failure can follow the various types of anginal failure, either as acute CHF or as chronic CHF. The congestive failure can be brief, prolonged, or intractable depending upon the pathologic and physiologic state of the myocardium and the cardiac mechanism. A discussion of these relationships is beyond the scope of this presentation.

One of the most important problems in cardiology is congestive heart failure associated with ischemic heart disease or anginal failure. The temporal relationships, degree, importance, and management can only be determined from symptoms and signs observed by physicians; these will never be displaced by cardiac catheterization, computers, or other forms of complex gadgetry.

REFERENCES CITED

1. Cronvich, J. A., and Burch, G. E. 1969. Frequency characteristics of some pressure transducer systems. Amer. Heart J. 77: 792–797.
2. Fry, D. L. 1960. Physiologic recording by modern instruments with particular reference to pressure recording. Physiol. Rev. 40:753–788.
3. Wade, O. L., and Bishop, J. M. 1962. Cardiac output and regional blood flow. Blackwell, Oxford.
4. Burch, G. E., and Giles, T. D. 1971. A critique of the cardiac index. Amer. Heart J. 82:424–425.
5. Burch, G. E., and Giles, T. D. 1970. Heart tone. Amer. Heart J. 79:283–285.
6. Fenn, J. E., and Stansel, H. C., Jr. 1969. Certain hazards of the central venous catheter. Angiology 20:38–43.

7. Schapira, M., and Stern, W. Z. 1967. Hazards of subclavian vein cannulation for central venous pressure monitoring. J.A.M.A. 201:327–329.
8. Walters, M. B., Stanger, A. D., and Rotem, E. C. 1972. Complications with percutaneous central venous catheters. J.A.M.A. 220:1455–1457.
9. Forrester, J. S., and Swan, H. J. C. 1971. Letter to the editor, correspondence section. New Engl. J. Med. 285:1088–1089.
10. Rubin, L. R., and Bongiovi, J., Jr. 1970. Central venous pressure: an unreliable guide to fluid therapy in burns. Arch. Surg. 100:269–274.
11. Burch, G. E. 1972. Elegant digitalization for congestive heart failure. Amer. Heart J. 83:543–551.
12. Burch, G. E. 1972. A primer of venous pressure. Charles C Thomas, Springfield, Ill.
13. Burch, G. E., and Reaser, P. 1963. A primer of cardiology. Lea & Febiger, Philadelphia.
14. Pollack, G. H. 1970. Maximum velocity as an index of contractility in cardiac muscle. A critical evaluation. Circ. Res. 26:111–127.
15. Noble, M. I. 1972. Problems concerning the application of concepts of muscle mechanics to the determination of the contractile state of the heart. Circulation 45:252–255.

RATIONAL APPROACH TO DIURETIC THERAPY
IN REFRACTORY CARDIAC FAILURE

JOHN H. LARAGH

The basic "lesion" in congestive heart failure is a consequence of an inappropriate compensation. The sequence, of course, begins with degenerative changes in the myocardium leading to incompetence of the cardiac pump. It can then be traced to the decreased mean arterial pressure generated during cardiac contraction which provides the energy for glomerular filtration and for delivery of blood to the kidney. In some manner, not yet fully understood, this reduction of renal blood flow is associated with a signal to the kidney to conserve sodium, and this conservation underlies the fluid retention that produces congestion in the lungs, liver, abdomen, and peripheral tissues. Thus, ultimately, the compensation reaction produces a congested situation which leads to further embarrassment of the already compromised pump.

As long as one keeps in mind that the original failure is myocardial, it is completely appropriate, and clinically quite pragmatic, to regard congestive heart failure as secondarily but predominantly a disease for which the major determinant is the kidney. Equally, diuretics can be discussed as the key to any regimen for the management of congestive heart failure. Not that a theoretical basis is needed for assigning such primacy to the diuretics. Every clinician is aware of the revolutionary improvement in our ability to manage and to understand disorders characterized by abnormal fluid accumulation and/or elevated blood pressure that has resulted from the development of effective oral diuretic agents, starting with the introduction of chlorothiazide in 1958. Now, physicians treating congestive heart failure have available at least five different classes of diuretic agents, each of which is capable of selectively interfering in a different way with the active transport mechanisms involved in tubular reabsorption and thereby promoting natriuresis and diuresis.

RENAL TRANSPORT MECHANISMS

A brief review of the mechanisms of salt and water transport in the kidney is appropriate here as a basis for subsequent discussion of the selective action of different diuretics. The glomerular filtration rate in man is approximately 100 ml/min, with the resulting filtrate containing concentrations of sodium and other electrolytes equal to those found in plasma. Tubular reabsorption returns at least

99% of the filtrate to the circulation, the remaining 1% being excreted. Normally, about 70% of the filtrate is returned to the circulation by the proximal tubule in the form of an isotonic solution containing equivalent amounts of sodium and water (Fig. 1). In other words, there is no dilution or concentration in conjunction with reabsorption from the proximal tubule, and water absorption in this region is secondary to activation of sodium reabsorption. The permeability of the proximal tubular membrane to water permits passive isotonic reabsorption of water first into the interstitium and from there into the circulation. Two qualitatively different transport processes operate in the proximal tubule. Via one mechanism, actively reabsorbed sodium is accompanied by chloride and isosmotic amounts of water. Via the other mechanism, sodium is reabsorbed in exchange for the hydrogen ions generated within the proximal tubular cells by the hydration of CO_2 —a reaction catalyzed by the enzyme carbonic anhydrase. The hydrogen ions elaborated into proximal tubular fluid in exchange for sodium combine there with filtered bicarbonate ions to form CO_2 and H_2O, a reaction facilitated by the presence of carbonic anhydrase in the proximal tubular cells. The reabsorbed sodium ions are returned to the peritubular blood along with an amount of newly generated HCO_2 equivalent to approximately 90% of the bicarbonate which was filtered at the glomerulus.

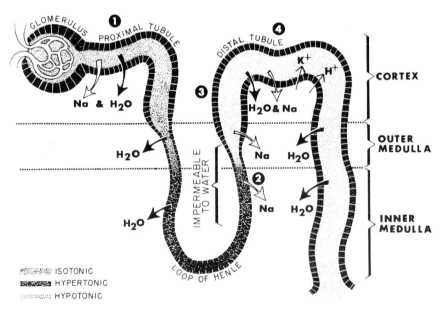

Fig. 1. Schematic diagram of renal transport.

The other major changes in composition occur distally in the nephron, where the remaining 30% of the filtrate is acted upon. The next reabsorption site is the renal medullary portion of the ascending limb of the loop of Henle. This portion of the nephron is impermeable to water. So, although active sodium reabsorption takes place, returning anywhere from 15% to 30% of the filtered sodium to the body, an equivalent amount of water is not removed. The fluid remaining in the lumen becomes dilute in terms of its concentration of sodium, chloride, and other electrolytes. Conversely, fluid on the interstitial side of the nephron, in the renal medulla, becomes hypertonic to plasma, generating the driving force for the eventual production of concentrated urine when the filtrate passes by again in the collecting ducts. The process of dilution continues as the dilute tubular fluid passes back into the renal cortex and as sodium reabsorption continues without equivalent water movement in the next portion of the nephron, still within the ascending limb of the loop of Henle. The passage of fluid through the distal convolution and the collecting duct then continues without osmotic equilibration with the hypertonic medullary interstitium unless the kidney is under stress to retain water mediated by antidiuretic hormone (ADH), which acts to increase the water permeability of the descending limb and collecting ducts. ADH activity can result in a concentrated urine with approximately a 1,200 milliosmolal concentration of solutes, about four times the osmolality of plasma. In this way, small volumes of water with high concentrations of sodium are excreted. On the other hand, under stress of water ingestion, dilution can occur that will produce urine with one-sixth or less of the normal osmolality. Thus, large volumes of water with low concentrations of sodium are excreted.

Essentially, all diuretic agents function by affecting the processes of tubular reabsorption, either directly or by inhibiting those hormones that regulate these processes. Because different agents affect different steps in the sequence, the physician has not only a choice that may be governed by definable physiologic needs but also the opportunity to design a diuretic regimen that is rationally tailored to specific clinical problems. This will be discussed in terms of the specific diuretic agents now available. First, however, let us return to the concept that congestive heart failure represents an inappropriate compensation in response to derangement of the normal interactions between the heart and the kidney.

The obvious premise is that the initial fluid overload in congestive failure results from the failure of the heart as a pump, a failure that relates back to a basically mechanical defect, albeit one that probably has a biochemical basis, faulty performance by the muscle fibrils. Cardiac output is reduced as is the delivery of blood to the kidneys. This, in turn, reduces the kidney's capacity to excrete salt and therefore leads to the accumulation of water and to congestion, which then increases the demands on a cardiac pump that, to start with, lacked the ability to handle even normal demands.

Physical and Hormonal Factors in Renal Sodium Excretion

The first question to be asked is why the reduction of blood flow in the kidney should lead to retention of salt and water. There is evidence suggesting that the kidney's functional incompetence is not simply the product of underperfusion. It has been shown that the renal tubules are actually hyperactive, that they reabsorb proportionally more of the filtered sodium than does the normal kidney. In a sense, the kidney is responding as if there were a shortage of electrolytes in the circulation. It is not altogether clear why this should be so, but it now appears that changes in intrarenal physical factors in the postglomerular circulation, especially reduced hydrostatic pressure and an increased oncotic pressure, work to promote increased sodium reabsorption in the proximal tubules.

Over and above this, the reduced effective blood volume or reduced arterial "filling" consequent to prior cardiac pumping induces an increased renin secretion by the kidneys. This is induced either by a baroreceptor signal at the afferent arterioles or by a reduced delivery of sodium to the distal tubular macula densa cells which may have a natriastat which modulates renin secretion by the adjacent juxtaglomerular cells of the afferent arterioles.

By whichever mechanism, renin via angiotensin generation elicits the secretion of aldosterone. Aldosterone in turn further amplifies sodium reabsorption. However, the retained sodium continues to "leak" from the effective circulation into the edema spaces so that a signal for inexorable and continued sodium excretion persists, leading to the congested and edematous state.

THE BASIS FOR DIURETIC THERAPY

How can this vicious cycle of cardiac incompetence, decreased output and perfusion, salt exacerbated cardiac incompetence be broken? Certainly one could rationally concentrate on the underlying pathophysiologic flaw by seeking to increase cardiac contractility and output. And indeed this is what is done, whenever possible, with digitalis and other inotropic drugs. However, we have learned in the past dozen years that in patients whose cardiac failure is clinically manifested most conspicuously by edema, more consistent and often more dramatic results can be achieved by addressing our therapeutic attentions to the kidney disturbance—thus the remarkably successful role played by diuretics.

Depending on the taxonomic criteria one uses, the different diuretic agents now available for the management of congestive heart failure and other edematous states can be subdivided in varied ways (Fig. 2). Based on differences in their physiologic effects it is convenient to discuss them as five different groups: the organomercurials; the sulfonamide-carbonic anhydrase inhibitors; the chloruretic sulfonamide compounds, among which the thiazides were the first, and remain the foremost, representatives; ethacrynic acid and furosemide; and the potassium-retaining diuretics, notably aldosterone antagonists (see below). For each of these groups, current concepts of their site and mode of action will be discussed, thus laying the groundwork for a subsequent discussion of the rational design of diuretic regimens.

Organomercurials

For close to half a century from the discovery of their diuretic potential in the early 1900's, the organomercurials served as the only available and effective compounds for removal of excessive body fluid. This property of the mercurials was happened upon by physicians who used them in the treatment of syphilis and observed the profound diuretic effect on some patients. The organomer-

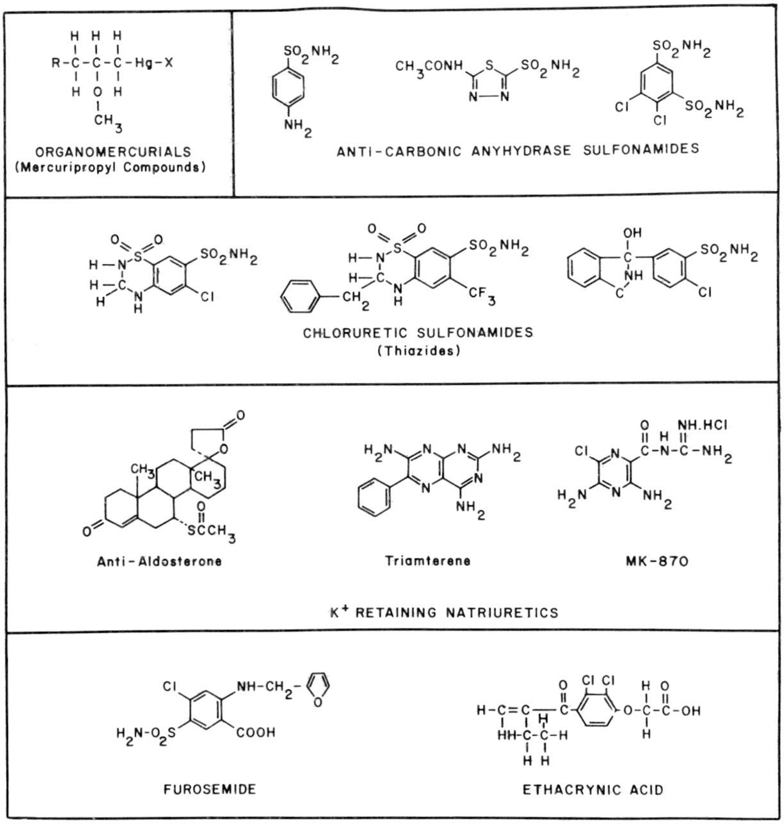

Fig. 2. Diuretic species presently available for management of congestive heart failure and other edematous states.

curials remain among the most effective of diuretic agents, but their use is, of course, severely limited by the need for parenteral administration. In terms of the site of action, there is still no clear evidence as to whether the mercurials act by distal tubular blockade or by proximal tubular blockade, but it has been established that at either site they function primarily by inhibition of an isosmotic reabsorptive process. Mercurial agents do not significantly inhibit either urinary concentrating or diluting mechanisms.

Carbonic Anhydrase Inhibitors

The discovery of the diuretic value of carbonic anhydrase inhibitors in one sense ushered in the new age of diuretic therapy. These drugs were harbingers of the far more important things to come only a year or so after. Once again, progress came in the form of fortuitous fallout from another branch of chemotherapy. It was noted that patients with congestive heart disease receiving sulfanilamide for pneumonia often had impressive diuresis. It was known that sulfanilamide was a carbonic anhydrase inhibitor and that the process of hydrogen ion secretion by the kidney was dependent on the carbonic anhydrase system. From these premises, it was decided to seek sulfonamide compounds more specifically tailored for their carbonic anhydrase inhibition, and these were developed. Although the carbonic anhydrase inhibitor diuretic drugs are still in use, their role has been somewhat limited by the rapid development of tolerance to them. They are generally effective for a day or two and then lose their potency in the person being treated. For this reason, the carbonic anhydrase inhibitors are best used intermittently and as adjuvants to other diuretics. Used in this way they can produce striking diuresis in refractory patients.

The mode and site of action has been suggested above in the observation that the carbonic anhydrase inhibitors act by blocking an enzyme system that is necessary for the secretion of hydrogen ions by the kidney. These drugs act all along the nephron, primarily in the proximal tubule, by inhibiting the acidification of the urine. This serves to produce natriuresis and diuresis because the secretion of hydrogen ions into the tubular urine is accomplished by an exchange with sodium ions, which are then reabsorbed. By blocking acidification, sodium reabsorption is prevented.

Thiazides (Chloruretic Sulfonamides)

If the discovery of the carbonic anhydrase inhibitors was the forerunner of the revolution in management of congestive heart failure, then that revolution came into full force with the discovery and introduction of chlorothiazide. Here at last was an oral drug that could produce a potent diuresis. Nor were any problems of refractoriness apparent with chlorothiazide. Now, of course, there are probably a score or more thiazide drugs on the market. Basically, none of these analogs differs significantly from chlorothiazide. One may need a different number of milligrams of one analog to achieve an equipotent dose with another, and there may be some differences in duration of action, but essentially all the thiazides are closely similar in their therapeutic capacity.

The sites of action of the thiazides have been quite well pinpointed as being in the proximal tubule (Site 1) and in the more cortical diluting segment of the distal tubule (Site 3). These drugs do not interfere with urinary concentration (Site 2). The result, of course, includes the inhibition of free water formation and the excretion of not only sodium and water but also of chloride, potassium, and other ions. The kaliuretic effect of the thiazides constitutes one of the problems in their use. Before discussing this, however, let us turn to the newer compounds, ethacrynic acid and furosemide, which resemble the thiazides in terms of their diuretic and electrolytic effects but are more powerful.

Ethacrynic Acid and Furosemide

Quantitatively, both ethacrynic acid and furosemide exert a much greater effect than do the thiazides, probably because in addition to their thiazide-like interference with diluting mechanisms in the distal cortical tubules they also block sodium transport in the loop or early ascending limb (Site 2). Therefore, they depress urinary concentrating activity as well as urinary diluting activity. For this reason the potent agents are often referred to as "loop diuretics."

Aldosterone Antagonists

The two basic effects of the adrenal hormone aldosterone on electrolytes are the promotion of sodium retention and potassium excretion. It is this combination that tends to make the aldosterone antagonists more ideal diuretics in a clinical context, where the physician is most likely to be seeking sodium excretion and potassium retention. Three pharmacologic agents have proved capable of effective aldosterone antagonism—spironolactone, the most widely used; triamterene; and amiloride (MK-870). The last is the most powerful of the three but although widely used abroad it has not received Food and Drug Administration approval for clinical use. All three of these agents act by competing for receptor sites at the distal renal tubule where the aldosterone-catalyzed exchange between sodium and potassium ions takes place. These compounds are therefore especially valuable in correcting potassium loss produced by the thiazides or other diuretic species. Spironolactone is a true competitive inhibitor of endogenous aldosterone and has no action in the absence of this hormone. On the other hand, triamterene and amiloride can block the aldosterone-directed transport mechanism even in the absence of the hormone and therefore have the properties of a noncompetitive inhibitor. This means that the latter two drugs can still be effective even when endogenous aldosterone secretion is enormous.

In an important sense, spironolactone and other diuretics in its class approach the ideal in their mode of action and in their effects. It is true that they are not as powerful acutely as the thiazides or ethacrynic acid and furosemide as natriuretic agents. This is because aldosterone has only a minor influence on the total bulk of electrolyte reabsorption by the tubule. But practically, a minor effect steadily maintained over a sufficient time becomes a major effect. By administering spironolactone over, say, a period of three or four weeks, one may actually induce a greater sodium and water loss than with more powerful natriuretic agents—even with ethacrynic acid or furosemide. With these latter two drugs there is a tendency in the patient to develop resistance and on cessation of the drug, to experience a rebound from the violence of its action. The consequent fluid retention may annul the diuretic benefits. There is something to be said therefore, for gradual, smooth diuresis, and in many cases the physician's or patient's impatience to see tangible results quickly may cause an inappropriate turning away from the aldosterone antagonists as the first diuretic to be tried.

DESIGN OF DIURETIC REGIMENS

What is an ideal diuretic regimen? Obviously there is no single answer to this question. What should be stressed is the fact that different classes of diuretics act at least in part on different sites in the renal tubules, thus affecting qualitatively different transport mechanisms. By taking advantage of this selectivity, the clinician may choose a particular diuretic to correct any particular derangement in the blood electrolytes of the patient. There are many practical illustrations of combined use of diuretics to achieve maximum efficacy. In fact, the only two classes that cannot be used effectively in combination are the organomercurials and the carbonic anhydrase inhibitors, since the latter may block the effects of the mercurials by preventing acidification of the urine.

In designing a regimen, one must also take into account the fact that with thiazides, ethacrynic acid, and furosemide there is a tendency to develop some degree of refractoriness. These drugs tend to be most powerful in the first few days of administration, then to lose some efficacy.

This is one of the reasons why many of us have advocated intermittent programs in which "resting periods" are allowed. Not only will this provide recovery time for the drug action but it also will permit restoration of the electrolyte imbalance that commonly occurs with diuretics. For example, if a patient is receiving thiazides there will be some potassium loss and therefore some danger of hypokalemia. If, on the other hand, a three-day period of taking the drug followed by three days of rest is prescribed, the patient may replenish his potassium from natural food sources such as fruit and meat, which are abundant in ionic potassium.

The two main arguments against intermittent therapy are that such regimens are inconvenient for the patient and the physician (an argument which I think can be dismissed) and that a smooth, even diuretic effect is lost. It is true that with intermittent regimens, the patient's weight may fluctuate to a greater extent, climbing during off periods, then dropping sharply when the drug is reintroduced. And I would agree that this is not as desirable as a daily blockade, but on balance I believe the advantages of intermittent therapy outweigh the disadvantages.

One major exception to this evaluation would apply to the aldosterone antagonists. These can only be effective on a continuous basis, since one must strive for high enough blood levels to create a chronic blockade of potassium loss. For this reason we are beginning to feel increasingly that to treat any difficult patient, the best approach is to start with spironolactone or tri-amterene, then add one of the thiazides or ethacrynic acid or furosemide intermittently. In this way one can maintain an even baseline effect while preventing potassium depletion.

In many patients, of course, thiazides alone will do the diuretic job when administered on an intermittent basis. If we start with thiazides and they prove inadequate, our next step is to add an aldosterone antagonist, which we give chronically while using the thiazides intermittently. If this still fails to produce adequate diuresis, we substitute one of the two more powerful agents, etha-crynic acid or furosemide, for the thiazide. In rare cases, with very sick patients, none of these regimens may be effective. As a last resort in such cases we give volume expanders such as hypertonic mannitol (2 liters of a 10% solution given slowly over 10 hours while watching cardiac reserve) or albumin together with cortisone. The purpose of these maneuvers is to correct the poor forward delivery from the heart and consequent underperfusion of the arterial tree that may occur in serious congestive heart failure. By increasing the perfusion of the kidney, the physician may provide a more favorable environment for the action of the diuretics and can thereby increase their efficacy. Cortisone and particular-ly those glucocorticoid analogs with less sodium-retaining action seem to make a specific contribution to the enhancement of renal blood flow. Aminophylline may also be useful for this. Obviously, such combined approaches should not be used on an outpatient basis and, in fact, by definition, are appropriate only to a desperately ill, hospitalized individual.

Illogic and Dangers of K⁺ Replacement

It should be noted that in describing these various regimens no mention is made of using potassium supplementation in the form of potassium salts. We have never advocated such supplementation for ambulatory patients because the amounts of potassium chloride required for correction can be dangerous by virtue of toxicity to the heart and because of their tendency to cause ileal ulceration. We believe that hyperkalemia is far more threatening to the cardiac patient than is hypokalemia. Potassium salts are far more potent physiologic and pharmacologic agents than is generally recognized, even by those who are aware that these salts can be and have been used to induce cardiac arrest. Accordingly, potassium supplementation is best carried out only as a hospital procedure under close supervision.

The best approach to potassium depletion involves 1) intermittent therapy, and 2) use of baseline therapy with an aldosterone antagonist. This is because potassium depletion is most likely to occur in more severely ill patients who exhibit marked secondary aldosteronism. Indeed, our studies indicate that even the most potent loop diuretics will not induce any potassium loss in either adrenalectomized or spironolactone-treated patients. Accordingly, if time is allowed for restoration of effective plasma volume, or when possible if dietary salt is liberalized, the diuretic-induced aldosterone response will abate. If intermittent therapy does not eliminate the problem, therapy with spirono-lactone, triamterene, or amiloride is indicated.

CONCLUSIONS

In looking at the present and the future in any review of a field which has exploded as rapidly as has that of diuretic therapy, one must be concerned with the physiologic implications as well as with the therapeutic criteria. It is significant, therefore, that in the dozen or more years in which oral diuretics have been available, we have used these agents not only for their primary purposes, the dissipation of edema and the control of hypertension, but also as an extremely valuable tool for the dissection of renal tubular transport mecha-nisms. Many of the facts given to explain the sites and mechanisms of action of the various classes of diuretics have actually been learned from observing these drugs in action and then reasoning backwards. We have also made a substantial beginning toward understanding the intrarenal transport mechanisms for regula-tion of sodium reabsorption at a perhaps more basic level, that is to say, in terms of control by signals arising extrarenally. The effects of chlorothiazide and other diuretics on the release of renin and on aldosterone secretion might also involve extrarenal signals. Solution of the problem of how diuretic-induced depletion of electrolytes and fluid triggers increased renin and then aldosterone secretion could, for example, go a long way toward unraveling the delicately entwined mechanisms for sodium and blood pressure homeostasis.

These are but examples of the type of problem that can be productively approached through close study of the roles being played by diuretics. We are in the particularly happy position of being able to pursue such studies while providing our patients with the immense and often lifesaving benefits of the very agents through which increased knowledge will come.

REFERENCES

1. Laragh, J. H., Heinemann, H. O., and Demartini, F. E. 1958. Effect of chlorothiazide on electrolyte transport in man. Its use in the treatment of edema of congestive heart failure, nephrosis, and cirrhosis. J.A.M.A. 166:145.
2. Heinemann, H. O., Demartini, F. E., and Laragh, J. H. 1959. The mode of action and use of chlorothiazide on renal excretion of electrolytes and free water. Amer. J. Med. 26:843.
3. Laragh, J. H. 1962. Hormones and the pathogenesis of congestive heart failure: vasopressin, aldosterone, and angiotensin II. Further evidence for renal-adrenal interaction from studies in hypertension and in cirrhosis. Circulation 25:1015.
4. Cannon, P. J., Heinemann, H. O., Stason, W. B., and Laragh, J. H. 1965. Ethacrynic acid. Effectiveness and mode of diuretic action in man. Circulation 31:5.
5. Stason, W. B., Cannon, P. J., Heinemann, H. O., and Laragh, J. H. 1966. Furosemide, a clinical evaluation of its diuretic action. Circulation 34:910.
6. Laragh, J. H. 1967. The proper use of newer diuretics: diagnosis and treatment. Ann. Internal Med. 67:3.

PANEL DISCUSSION

HEART FAILURE: IS IT REVERSIBLE?

GEORGE E. BURCH, CHAIRMAN,
MURRAY G. BARON, EUGENE BRAUNWALD, JOHN LARAGH,
WILLIAM LIKOFF, and F. MASON SONES, JR.

BARON: I have been asked to comment on distension of upper lobe vessels as an early radiologic sign of heart failure.

This is a valid sign with mitral stenosis, when the first sign in the lungs in congestive failure is dilation of the upper lobe veins and relative constriction of the lower lobe veins.

However, in diagnosing patients with myocardial infarction, this sign is of relatively little use, because a supine x-ray in a normal person will show distension of the upper lobe veins. Since most of the patients are in the reclining position, this sign has relatively little significance.

The second part of this question is concerned with other causes of distended vessels. There is either obstruction, which is venous obstruction, or increased flow. If there is any kind of a left-to-right shunt, the vessels become distended. With obstruction from noncardiac causes, we see localized distention of vessels from a tumor that is blocking a vein or from venous stenoses.

BURCH: Dr. Laragh, by producing hydrogen diuresis, could ethacrynic acid or furosemide interfere with the breathing mechanism?

LARAGH: I think that the respiratory failure problem requires that the diuretics have a secondary priority to the treatment involved in the respiratory failure. Most diuretics will work, and I do not think there is a particular advantage in using one or the other. The goal of treatment will be to monitor the changes induced in the pH and to correct them by using the appropriate agents, as I indicated.

BURCH: Are you talking about the treatment of patients with massive congestive heart failure in the hospital, or are you talking about the average patient seen in an office? I ask this because of the problem of digitalis intoxication that arises when those diuretics are used and alter the electrolyte balance.

LARAGH: I think digitalis intoxication is rather closely related to diuretics; rather closely related to the degree of potassium depletion that is induced. Such depletion, excluding patients who are so sick they are unable to eat, is directly related first to the continued use of diuretics and second to the degree of severity of the heart failure.

29

It is only the very severely ill patient with congestive heart failure who has activated his aldosterone mechanism who loses any significant amount of potassium with diuretics. But in such patients, that is, the very ill ones, I think it is now almost a rule of therapy that you give them either spirolactone, dyrrhenium, or amiloride as a base line medication before you start any thiazide. On the other hand, they are very sensitive to drugs such as spirolactone if they are azotemic, and you may not be able to administer a full dose without hyperkalemia resulting.

However, the way to control potassium loss and cardiac arrhythmia is by attendance to these problems, and I think that the best way to do this is with an anti-aldosterone drug.

BURCH: Isn't the best way to do this, to measure the loss the day before and replace it the next day?

LARAGH: Yes, that would be the best way. The problem is in the very sick patient. In the hospital, I think that potassium repletion is the best way, but that requires computing this balance and giving potassium intravenously. This is hazardous. Even giving it orally is very risky in such patients.

LIKOFF: There is a question concerning the frequency of heart failure with normal-sized heart. It is axiomatic, or has been axiomatic over the years, to teach that congestive heart failure does not occur except in the presence of some alteration in cardiac size. And, although for the most part this still holds true, there are exceptions, aside from pericardial disease, with which we are all familiar; under such circumstances, congestive heart failure can appear and the heart size remains normal.

We have estimated that approximately 10% of heart failure can be encountered in the presence of a normal-sized heart. There are those extreme circumstances in which myocardial ischemia and fibrosis have taken place to a point where there is no effective contractile tissue left, and yet the heart does not dilate and heart failure results. Metabolically, for example, there are those circumstances in extreme hyperthyroidism in association with an antecedent or some subtle form of coronary heart disease in which failure may transpire with normal heart size.

So, in the main, the axiom is somewhat threatened. The percentage of occurrences in which heart failure develops with normal-sized heart is small, but this problem is encountered.

BARON: I agree with Dr. Likoff. I think that another circumstance in which a normal-sized heart develops failure is in the acute failures. A patient with myocardial infarction may develop frank pulmonary edema and all the signs of congestive heart failure in the first 24 or 48 hours before there is evidence of dilation of the heart. So you should not exclude the presence of congestive failure because the heart is normal in size.

BURCH: It is true that if a patient has a small heart, the chances of his having chronic congestive heart failure are unlikely. On the other hand, with acute coronary disease with acute angina or acute infarction, the heart can be small and still the patient can develop acute left-ventricular failure. I think that the reason for this is that the heart muscle of the left ventricle is unable to pump the blood that is being delivered from the right ventricle, and the blood accumulates in the lung. Whenever the heart is small and you think you are dealing with chronic congestive heart failure, you had better check your data carefully to be sure the diagnosis is correct.

BRAUNWALD: I have been given the following question: "In patients with mild or moderate heart failure without atrial fibrillation, what about the use of diuretics alone, that is, diuretics without cardiac glycosides in the treatment?"

A number of years ago we were particularly interested in this question and explored it experimentally. We floated a polyethelene catheter into the pulmonary artery of patients, measured their cardiac outputs at rest and during exercise on a treadmill, and then treated them. These were patients with mild to moderate congestive heart failure. After measuring pulmonary artery pressure and cardiac output during exercise, we treated them with diuretics, so that they lost on the average 8–10 pounds without digitalis; after the weight loss we repeated the studies.

What we observed was interesting. The patients all felt better; they had less pulmonary congestion with this degree of weight loss; they were able to walk further on the treadmill without experiencing dyspnea and without having to stop because of shortness of breath. However, their cardiac outputs during exercise were significantly lower.

In other words, they were not able to elevate their cardiac outputs to the same extent as before. This indicates that while perhaps we helped the patients from a symptomatic point of view by relieving congestion (and this points out again that the primary problem that stops a patient with left-ventricular failure during exertion is pulmonary venous congestion), the oxygen delivery to the tissue was, if anything, impaired. For this reason I think diuretics alone offer a rather superficial approach to treatment in patients with congestive heart failure. I would prefer the time-honored use of cardiac glycoside and then, if necessary, a diuretic, because under those circumstances the oxygen delivery to the tissues during exercise is greatly augmented rather than actually reduced.

BURCH: I have received the following question: "What are the main indications for echocardiography and what are its uses?" I discussed this topic briefly during my presentation. I think that echocardiography will not replace history-taking or physical examination or the usual bedside study, but it can be of extreme value if it is understood. For example, we had a patient at Charity Hospital who had ruptured chordae tendineae. Not only was the rupture of the chordae tendineae detected in the echocardiographic recordings, but it was noted to be at the papillary muscle tip rather than at the attachment to the valves.

Echocardiography can be useful in subaortic hypertrophic stenosis. Dr. Braunwald may want to comment on that because he has worked a great deal with this disease, probably more than anyone else. It is very easy to pick up a myxoma of the heart and also to follow it as it moves from ventricle to atrium.

You can measure the thickness of the ventricular walls and detect pericardial effusion and similar conditions. Echocardiography is very useful. Unfortunately, the equipment is expensive. This does not mean you should use an echocardiograph on every patient seen.

BRAUNWALD: I agree with Dr. Burch's comments. I think it is fair to say that echocardiography ought to be considered to be a major advance in cardiology. It is interesting that Dr. Joiner, who is one of the pioneers, worked with this technique for a number of years, but it still did not become popular. It makes us wonder how many other very, very important things are around that we are not appreciating.

Only in the last three or four years has this technique blossomed. One of the things that has interested me a great deal about echocardiography, and this is an aspect we are examining, is the possibility of using this technique as a noninvasive but very precise method of evaluating cardiac function and myocardial contractility, because one can now measure with a considerable degree of reliability the velocity of myocardial fiber shortening, wall shortening, the rate at which contraction occurs, and the rate at which the posterior wall of the ventricle approaches the ventricular septum. This, I think, is an extremely powerful tool and will become even more useful in the next couple of years.

BURCH: It is a matter of history, since Dr. Braunwald brought this up, that echocardiography was introduced in cardiology back in 1956 in Sweden.

SONES: I have been asked, "Some cardiologists advocate the use of the transvenous pacemaker catheter in the right ventricle as a 'prophylactic' measure during coronary artery cineangiography. Do you use this approach in the Cleveland Clinic? Do you recommend it?"

The reason for this advocacy is that most contrast media, as they pass through the myocardial capillary bed, cause transient, sometimes not transient, profound bradycardia in certain patients. This can progress to asystole and actual arrest. This sort of thing has stimulated the desire of some laboratory directors to use a transvenous or a right-ventricular pacing catheter to maintain the heart rate.

This is totally unnecessary. When the patient develops this type of bradycardia, simply ask him to make a few little explosive coughs after being given a transfusion of about 300 cc of blood in the aortic root. Since the aortic valve is closed during the diastolic phase of the heart cycle, if he makes a few little explosive coughs with a short breath between each cough he simply pushes blood through the capillary bed, pushes the contrast media through the capillary bed, and off he goes again with a good beat. We have never used a transvenous pacemaker of this sort in any of more than 29,500 studies. We find it totally unnecessary.

LIKOFF: Here is the time-honored question of whether the use of digitalis with myocardial infarction, cardiomegaly, and congestive heart failure is indicated and whether it is harmful. Information for the proper answer to this question obviously resides in the work that Dr. Braunwald and his associates and others have done regarding the characteristics of congestive failure, myocardial kinetics, etc.

I am going to answer it from a very practical standpoint. The decision must rest on the balance between possible benefit and possible hazard. The inotropic effects of the drug have been contested against the possible harm that results, and the harm that results obviously is in the production of dysrhythmias in an ischemic environment in which dysrhythmias are quite common to begin. But there are certainly many indications for the use of digitalis in heart failure and myocardial infarction. For example, one needs only to refer to those potentially disrupting dysrhythmias such as atrial fibrillation which need to be controlled in order for heart failure to be properly controlled.

In the presence of heart failure and sinus tachycardia and the obvious manifestations of difficulty, digitalis still is indicated in myocardial infarction if the two basic laws about the pharmacokinetics of the drug are kept in mind; namely, that the effectiveness of digitalis and its toxic effects reside in the proportion of the dose against the half-life of the drug under the clinical circumstances in which it is used.

Therefore, the likelihood of getting into trouble with renal dysfunction or with gastrointestinal dysfunction obviously is greater than under more normal situations.

So, it would be impossible, under these circumstances, to answer the question categorically in the affirmative. Digitalis is indicated in myocardial infarction under the proper circumstances of the use of the drug and with proper concern for the dose system that is used.

BRAUNWALD: I would like to make one comment on this subject, dealing with some recent experimental work we have done. This work was carried out in experimental animals, I emphasize, and not in patients.

We observed that any inotropic agent, such as digitalis, isoproterenol, dopamine, epinepherine, glucagon, etc., when administered in appropriate doses, that is, certainly subtoxic doses following experimentally induced coronary occlusion in an animal not in heart failure, (*not* in heart failure I emphasize), results in extension of the zone of ischemic injury and ultimately in more myocardial necrosis. I think this serves to underline what Dr. Likoff properly pointed out, namely, that under the proper circumstances, digitalis ought to be employed.

I think the mechanism of this augmentation of ischemia is caused by the fact that it increases myocardial oxygen demands. On the other hand, in the failing heart, particularly in the dilated heart, the cardiac glycoside or other inotropic agent will not augment myocardial oxygen demands and therefore does not extend the ischemic injury.

LARAGH: I have been given the question, "In patients with refractory heart failure and gout, how do you approach the treatment?" Another question related to this is: "Would you please comment on the diuretics and increase in uric acid? Are diuretics contraindicated in gout?"

The increased uric acid levels of diuretic therapy are caused in part by one common mechanism, sodium chloride depletion, which in some way impairs the ability of the tubules to secrete uric acid. I think, contrary to all popular belief, that probably all diuretics and even severe sodium depletion per se can produce a good deal of hyperuricemia.

In addition, thiazide agents, furosemide, and ethacrynic acid diminish urate clearance by the kidney, probably by increasing reabsorption proximally. You cannot change from one method to another to get around the problem. If diuretic therapy is needed, there are two ways that it can be accomplished. One is to combine the drug with Benemid, which blocks tubular absorption of urate, and the second is to combine the drug with allopurinol, which reduces urate synthesis.

BARON: The cardiologists in my institution are becoming quite interested in measuring ejection fraction in patients in whom we perform coronary arteriography. We routinely perform left-ventricular angiograms as part of the coronary artery study. I think you can peruse it and get a pretty good idea of the function.

To do ejection fractions requires additional equipment. We all use a 6-inch intensifier, and many ventricles do not fit on this, so we are going to have to get a larger intensifier. I would like to inquire of Dr. Sones or other members as to the value of measuring the ventricle in diastole and systole in order to estimate ejection fraction, and whether this affects the efficacy of choosing patients for surgery.

BRAUNWALD: I think that if I were on a desert island and had available to me a single hemodynamic measurement for the evaluation of patients' myocardial function, not only patients with coronary disease but also valvular disease, cardiomyopathies, etc., at this moment of time I would choose the ejection fraction; I think that it is an extremely important measurement.

In our own institution, at the Peter Bent Brigham Hospital, we found that the risk of coronary bypass surgery correlates better with ejection fraction than with any other retrospective measurement. I think it is an important determination.

BARON: My point is, do you need the number or can you look at that film and tell from the way the heart is beating? In other words, how much are you gaining by going through all the business of measuring it and getting numbers, in comparison to your accuracy in looking at a ventricle and judging from the way it contracts?

BRAUNWALD: I think that in an institution that estimates ejection fractions on a regular basis, it is necessary to do the computation.

SONES: I am in complete agreement with Dr. Braunwald that the measurement of an ejection fraction is a very useful index of myocardial performance. It has been particularly useful in those situations that he described. I would disagree that this is really as useful as we would like it to be in patients with coronary atherosclerosis, because it does not answer the question to which you are really seeking an answer.

What we want to know about patients with coronary atherosclerosis as it relates to myocardial function is whether there is a scar present? Is it transmural scar or is it subendocardial scar? Where is the scar? We want to try to distinguish this from relative failures in myocardial performance caused by segmental underperfusion of viable myocardium. And I do not think this number computed by an ejection fraction is really important in making those discriminations.

I think that is why it is necessary to look carefully at a ventriculogram to try to determine the areas of segmental undercontractility or paradoxic motion. And you need to look at the thickness of the ventricular wall to compare this not just with a number that you can put into a computer but to study this in relationship to the electrocardiographic findings presented by the patient.

In general, if a patient has Q waves in those leads that reflect the diaphragmatic surface of the left ventricle, and if he has Q waves and S-T segment elevation in the precordial leads and this is associated with poor ventricular contractility, you can be pretty sure that the reason for the poor contractility is that he has very extensive, usually transmural scar tissue replacement in the areas involved.

If, on the other hand, these segmental areas have undercontractility demonstrated by ventriculography, and are not associated with Q waves in the electrocardiogram, you can be pretty sure that what you are dealing with is underperfused myocardium, if the vessel perfusing that segment of the myocardium is obstructed severely.

And it is as simple as that. Some of us have to depend on putting numbers in computers to be happy over a long period of time, others of us do not. I think that the simple answer to your question is that you do not need a nine-inch image amplifier and you do not really have to have the number to make intelligent decisions.

BURCH: I would like to make a comment here, too. It seems that Dr. Sones and I agree on something. I do not think, from the point of view of good cardiology, that you need to know what the ejection fraction is; you can estimate that very well at the bedside by examining your patient. I do not think you have to put it in numbers. All a clinician needs to know is whether the cardiac function is adequate or inadequate.

I think that from the size of the heart upon fluoroscopy, from the feel of the pulse, and from the history, you can tell that a patient is not emptying his heart completely and that the amount of emptying is not as much as normal.

A big, dilated heart in a patient with cardiomyopathy and a weak, thready pulse, even if he has a normal sinus rhythm and not a sinus tachycardia, will determine the status of ejection. If he is not vasoconstricted, if he is not in a cold room, and if other factors are not playing a role, you know that the ejection is minimal; in fact, you can estimate his cardiac output fairly well.

So I do not think from the practical, clinical, or bedside cardiologic point of view that cardiac catheterization is needed. I think that from the electrocardiogram, as Dr. Sones said, you can tell when the scar is transmural or when there is a transmural infarct. Not only can the existence and location of the infarct be detected, but also its extent. We know quite well that a scar has no blood vessels of significance and that a scar is not contracting or pumping blood.

Another mistake, I think, is to depend only on Q waves in the electrocardiogram. Q waves inform you only about the part of the heart that is depolarized initially during the depolarization process of heart muscle electrical activation. But other parts of the hearts are scarred. These parts are depolarized last. These parts produce no deformities in the initial part of the QRS. The deformities are in the terminal part of the QRS complex. We see this with high basal scars or infarcts.

Multiple scars or diffuse myocardial damage can be detected from the electrocardiogram and clinical study. It is not necessary to measure ejection fraction at all for clinical purposes. The cost and the risk associated with the procedure are important considerations. I would advise Dr. Baron not to get his intensifier and the like but to get himself a couple of good cardiologists.

BRAUNWALD: Let me just make a comment on this. I think you misinterpreted my statements, Dr. Sones. All of the things that you pointed out are necessary, and the only point I want to make is that the problems that we face with these patients are very substantial; they are very difficult problems, and I think we need every bit of information that we possibly can get.

I think I have had the opportunity to read recently some discussions when other new techniques were introduced, techniques such as cardiac catheterization in the 1940's and electrocardiography early in the century, and it is remarkable how similar the discussions about the introduction of these methods which we now accept and consider essential in the evaluation of patients sounded to the discussion that I just heard.

BURCH: I would like to say that Dr. Braunwald is absolutely correct, but that we also can list a number of things that have been introduced that are very good that are not used today. So I think that we just have to wait and see, and let Dr. Braunwald and others do what they are doing and encourage it and support them. If it turns out to be worthwhile, why not use it? I agree that we should bring together all the data that we can that do not hurt the patient, but I think that until then we have to be careful with patients. It works both ways, from my experience and from the history of medicine.

LIKOFF: There is a concept underlying this discussion which could, under certain circumstances, get very interestingly heated, and I think it should be pointed out.

We are dealing with a situation in which there is a structural deformity in the cardiovascular mechanism, in coronary heart disease obviously in the coronary arteries. The question is whether or not under the same structural conditions there is the same functional impairment and by what means this functional impairment can be measured. There is the clinician, whose interpretation of the signs gives to him adequate information of the pathophysiology; perhaps the radiologist can make his determination by looking at the ventricular contraction, and perhaps those oriented to physiology do better with physiologic parameters. I think this is entirely understandable.

There is one thought to be considered that is more important than anything else. In our present state of knowledge, the same structural abnormality does not give rise to the same functional abnormality, and I think this is the key point. The fact that there are three coronary arteries obstructed, let us say, does not mean for a curious set of circumstances, many of which we do not understand, that the functional incapacity is the same; therefore, it is incumbent upon us to use those methods that we have at hand and that we best understand to measure the degree of functional impairment. We recently have made a study of the structural impairment in people with overt coronary heart disease who had angina, as opposed to those who have yet to be diagnosed as having coronary heart disease and whose coronary atherosclerosis was found quite accidentally. And the structural changes in both, the totally asymptomatic group and those that were seriously impaired functionally, were surprisingly quite similar. So I think this argument ought to be brought into its proper perspective.

BARON: I have been sent the following question: "How does pulmonary embolism cause bronchial obstruction to produce atelectasis and what percent show Fleischner lines?" The bronchial obstruction probably is caused by a combination of factors. When there is a pulmonary embolism, there is spasm of the adjacent bronchus, frequently a pain with splinting of that part of the lung, and edema locally of the bronchial mucosa. All this leads to mucous plugging in the smaller bronchi, which will result in Fleischner lines.

What percentage have Fleischner lines, I have no idea. Because I do not know, if I see Fleischner lines bilaterally, I think that in most instances the patient has had pulmonary emboli.

I have no idea, no way of knowing, how many patients have pulmonary emboli without this sign. I think most of us in such cases probably do not make the diagnosis.

BURCH: I have a question here. "What percentage of patients with congestive heart failure, left-sided congestive heart failure, will not clinically demonstrate right-sided signs, such as venous distension, pulsatile liver and the like?"

Well, I would like to say that practically all patients start off with left-sided heart failure and later develop right-sided heart failure. Left-sided heart failure is usually the beginning; but unfortunately, the initial phases of left-sided heart failure often are not detected, either because the patients do not visit their doctors or because their doctors do not pay enough attention to the symptoms and signs and do not detect the left-ventricular failure until it is rather far advanced with edema and large liver.

The time to treat patients with left-sided congestive heart failure is when they just begin to have it, with the onset of mild dyspnea. As Dr. White said, if we are going to do anything about heart disease, we have to prevent it, and I think that the time to treat left-ventricular congestive heart failure is before patients develop it. We know that certain diseases of the heart will lead to left-ventricular congestive heart failure. When these things are neglected, congestive failure follows.

So, when you see a patient with right-sided heart failure, the chances are good, particularly with the types of heart diseases that prevail in the United States today, that he had left-ventricular congestive heart failure before he ever had failure of the right ventricle.

SONES: I have received this question: "Are blood dyscrasias such as leukemias, polycythemias, and sickle-cell disease contraindications to coronary arteriography?"

Catheter advocates are sort of like surgeons in some ways; if they get into trouble they love to have some sort of obscure reason, the more obscure the better, for why they got into trouble. And there have been a rash of comments about the embolization occurring in patients with polycythemia and sickle-cell disease.

Mostly, I think these complications are caused by the factors that I tried to describe earlier. If you leave a guide wire in the circulation long enough before you push a catheter over it, you peel off the fibrin coat and produce an embolus. Then, if the patient happens to have polycythemia or a sickle-cell trait, you say that is why you have a complication. And that is a bad practice. We have had no more difficulty with patients with polycythemia and sickle-cell disease or sickle-cell trait than we have had with the general population.

My experience in patients with leukemia has been virtually nil, so I cannot comment on that topic on the basis of personal experience, but I certainly would not hesitate to tackle him if the doctor who was taking care of the leukemia told me the patient had a pretty good chance of surviving another five years with that disease.

BURCH: Active sickle-cell disease patients do not live long enough to develop coronary disease. Patients with sickle-cell trait do live long enough to develop coronary disease. They do not develop anemia. Is that true in your experience, Dr. Sones?

SONES: Yes, it is the sickle-cell trait that has been commented on and used as an excuse for this sort of tragedy, and in my opinion, it is not justifiable.

LARAGH: I am going to comment on the question, "How do you explain the infrequency of potassium depletion in hypertensive subjects not in congestive heart failure?" That can be explained very easily, I think, because the potassium loss of all diuretics, as I indicated, is attributable to secondary aldosteronism induced by the drug in the patient. Most ambulatory hypertension patients have a normal salt intake or nearly normal one. They do not develop secondary hyperaldosteronism or any degree of volume depletion; therefore, as a rule with some exceptions, they do not show much potassium loss.

BRAUNWALD: I have a question that deals with the methods of treatment of cardiogenic shock in addition to cardiotonic agents, such as dopamine and norepinephrine.

I think that in approaching a patient who is said to have cardiogenic shock, the first thing I try to do is hope that he does not have it, and I do not say that facetiously. In going through the maneuver, I try to think about those things that might mimic cardiogenic shock caused by massive myocardial infarction, because those are the things that are reversible.

For example, with a large myocardial infarction with dehydration, oftentimes patients come into the hospital and they have been nauseated and have vomited for a couple of days and have had inadequate fluid intake.

Second, there is the possibility of arrhythmias, particularly atrioventricular dissociation with reasonable normal ventricular rates, which could be responsible for impairment of pump function, and for the presence of metabolic acidosis in patients who have had a low cardiac output.

These are things that ought to be attacked rapidly in the hope that the patient does not have cardiogenic shock. I think that the measurement of central venous pressure, and, more recently, the measurement of pulmonary artery diastolic pressure by means of a Swan-Gantz catheter, is a great advance for the assessment of a problem of fluid overload. In patients who have pulmonary artery diastolic pressures of less than 18 mm Hg, (i.e., of approximately 18 mm Hg plus or minus two), we would increase the circulating blood volume by means of low-molecular weight dextran, and in a significant number of these patients a normal pressure and normal cardiac output can be achieved.

Also, in the care of these patients, I think it is mandatory to have an intra-arterial needle, because the peripheral pressure, as recorded by means of a sphygmomanometer, is notoriously inaccurate with the vasoconstriction that occurs in many of these patients.

If one has paid attention to arrhythmia, if one has paid attention to acidosis, if one has paid particular attention to fluid volume, and the patient still is in cardiogenic shock and he already has been treated with inotropic agents (i.e., cardiac glycosides and dopamine), we are facing an almost hopeless situation.

What is presently available is the use of intra-aortic balloon counterpulsation in our institution, which will relieve what might be considered to be a vicious cycle in a very small number of patients (perhaps 10–15%) who have been appropriately treated medically. An even smaller number of these patients who are not relieved by intra-aortic balloon counterpulsation might be considered for emergency surgery.

BURCH: Dr. Braunwald, of those patients in whom you employed counterpulsation in your regimen, how many do you think you helped? What percentage of them?

BRAUNWALD: I think that the number is of the order of 10%. It is a very, very small number. That is why I said I hope it is not cardiogenic shock—in terms of treatment—because the problem in the vast majority is insufficient remaining viable myocardium, and this is something a balloon is not going to do anything about. Only a very small number will be helped. That very small percentage that is helped is probably a group that still has some potentially reversible myocardium that requires improved coronary perfusion for a brief period of time before it can take over.

BURCH: Another question. How many do you think you made worse?

BRAUNWALD: Well, I think probably none, because I think we are dealing with patients . . . .

BURCH: They are going to die anyway?

BRAUNWALD: Yes, I think we are treating patients concerning whom there is a wealth of experience, that we are dealing with an essentially fatal condition.

BURCH: Dr. Sones, do you wish to comment?

SONES: I think that one of the most exciting techniques that has evolved in the past few years has been counterpulsation in patients with acute myocardial infarction. I disagree that the real utility of this technique has to do with trying to save the patient's life as a modality in itself; but in the early phases of acute infarction, if blood pressure begins to drop, I do not think we should wait to utilize this measure until the patient is anuric for an hour and is in prolonged cardiogenic shock.

Effective utilization of counterpulsation in the early phases of blood pressure drop will certainly give you time to make a diagnosis in the laboratory and get the patient to the operating room and revascularize him before irreversible loss of tissue has occurred.

And I think this is one of the major problems we are going to have to face during the next few years.

BRAUNWALD: Incidentally, I agree with your idea that we will be utilizing counterpulsation earlier and earlier in the treatment. What I addressed my answer to was the question of the treatment of cardiogenic shock rather than the early treatment of infarction.

SONES: The answer to that is to treat them before they go into shock.

BURCH: Dr. Sones, do you think that what you are doing is helping people? I agree with you that there is no doubt the concept is a good one, that you are providing a pump when there is an inadequate pump present, but when you consider the stage of its development and the difficulties involved, and the fact that these people are really sick, as you well know, what benefit can be anticipated?

SONES: Then what you are trying to do is make them "unsick."

BURCH: That is right, and the question I want to ask you is how many patients do you think you have helped? How many would have died if you had not used counterpulsation? Just guess; I realize it is not easy.

SONES: Our own personal experience with counterpulsation at this time is nil; we are carefully embarking in that direction, however, and fully intend to do it.

There is another major logistical consideration here. These efforts are leading many of us, not me, but many of us, to believe that what we should do in the patient is to wait. In the patient with coronary atherosclerosis, some physicians want to wait until he has "unstable angina" or is about to have an infarct, or has actually proceeded to acute occlusion in the early phases of myocardial infarction, and then say "let's perform a miracle."

I hope that we have the intelligence to avoid that approach in relation to revascularization surgery. The time to approach these patients diagnostically and surgically is in the period of peace between storms. Then study them electively, effectively, and find out where their obstructions are and fix them before the heart muscle has been irreversibly damaged. If we do it this way, we can approach a very large number of patients and improve their life expectancy tremendously. If we do not do it this way, we will continue to live in an atmosphere of chaos, fear, and tumult, which is exciting to those among us who are young enough to tolerate it, but is not going to solve the problem.

BARON: I have received the following question: "Can you distinguish pulmonary veins from arteries with certainty on an x-ray? And what is the practical application?"

If you give me a normal chest film I could not distinguish veins from arteries with certainty. If you have tomograms and you can show the vessels, the veins, of course, are more vertical and enter the heart at a lower level than the arteries. With tomography, you probably can distinguish them, but I do not feel that it is worthwhile doing tomography for that purpose. If you have congestive failure and the vessels in the upper lobe are distended, they are going to be veins.

If you are dealing with a shunt, both arteries and veins are going to be distended, so from a practical aspect I do not think it makes too much difference. Since you are working with clinical data, basically you know the diagnosis before you start. In congenital heart disease it is a different story, because you are looking for different things. I do not think it is so important to distinguish the two.

BURCH: I think that is a very important question. In fact, I was going to ask Dr. Baron that same question because we encounter the problem frequently in interpreting chest films. The same film will be read one way by one physician and another by a second and, of course, it does make a difference clinically.

Protection of the Coronary-Prone Subject: What Can Be Believed?

DIET, WEIGHT REDUCTION,
AND USE OF ANTILIPEMIC DRUGS

PETER T. KUO

Epidemiologic studies (1,2) have successfully identified a number of risk factors in the development of coronary heart disease (CHD). In considering the use of diet, weight reduction, and antilipemic drugs, the physician aims to control hyperlipidemia (hypercholesterolemia and hypertriglyceridemia) and body weight as important risk factors in CHD.

BRIEF REVIEW OF HYPERLIPIDEMIA AND HYPERLIPOPROTEINEMIA

Increase of plasma cholesterol or triglycerides or both generally constitutes nonspecific evidence of diverse genetic and metabolic abnormalities. Since in vivo these major plasma lipids are transported in the blood stream chiefly as lipoproteins, Fredrickson, Levy, and Lees have translated clinical hyperlipidemia into five types of hyperlipoproteinemia (3) to obtain information on the different underlying hyperlipidemic mechanisms.

These primary hyperlipoproteinemias, as differentiated by these investigators with the aid of plasma lipoprotein electrophoretic patterns (4), are briefly summarized as follows:

Demonstration of chylomicronemia after a 12–14 hour fast in a child or young adult who suffers from bouts of acute "abdominal crisis" and pancreatitis is suggestive of an inborn deficiency in triglyceride lipase resulting in reduced ability to "clear" dietary fat from the blood stream (5); this is Type I abnormality. In Type II$_a$ abnormality, hyperbetalipoproteinemia, the betalipoprotein (low density lipoprotein or LDL) catabolic rate is reduced (6). Persons with this familial trait, with or without tendinous xanthomatosis, are especially prone to premature CHD (7,8). Sometimes LDL elevation may be complicated by concomitant elevation of the prebeta fraction (very low density lipoprotein or VLDL); this is Type II$_b$ abnormality (9). In this case, the prebeta increase (hypertriglyceridemia) is believed to constitute an independent risk factor. An abnormal form of betalipoprotein ("floating" beta) characterizes the relatively

Supported in part by research grants from U.S. Public Health Service grant HL 08805, National Heart and Lung Institute; grant RR-40 from the General Research Centers Program of Division of Research Resources, National Institutes of Health, Bethesda, Maryland; and Thomas B. McCabe and Jeanette E. Laws McCabe Fund, Philadelphia, Pennsylvania.

rare Type III abnormality. The lipoprotein accumulation appears to be caused by a block in the normal conversion of VLDL to LDL (10). An aggregated experience including our own indicates a close association between Type III abnormality and premature development of CHD and peripheral vascular diseases, with preponderance of the latter condition. Either an increase in the synthetic rate or a decrease in the degradation rate of endogenous glycerides (11) can result in VLDL increase (the common Type IV abnormality, hyperprebetalipoproteinemia). This plasma lipid pattern is frequently demonstrated in middle-aged and older atherosclerotic patients. Many of them may also have overt or covert disturbance in carbohydrate metabolism. In Type V abnormality there is difficulty in handling both endogenously and exogenously derived glycerides, resulting in rather marked increases in both VLDL and chylomicron fractions.

DIET, WEIGHT REDUCTION, AND ANTILIPEMIC DRUGS

The diverse mechanisms involved in different types of hyperlipoproteinemia suggest that a specific diet or drug, or both, should be prescribed for optimal control of each type of hyperlipoproteinemia (12,13).

A 20–30g low fat diet is useful in reducing the exogenous fat load in Type I patients with severe hyperchylomicronemia. The diet may be supplemented by medium chain triglycerides which are absorbed via the portal route and do not contribute significantly to chylomicron formation (14). An effective drug has not yet been developed to rejuvenate the depressed triglyceride lipase activity of these patients.

Plasma cholesterol or LDL is influenced by dietary cholesterol, saturated fats, and polyunsaturated fats. Therefore, in general a diet containing less than 300 mg of cholesterol per day and a polyunsaturated to saturated fat ratio of 1.5 to 2.0 is recommended for partial control of betalipoprotein elevation of Type II patients. A bile acid sequestrant such as Questran (15) or Colestipol (16) is the drug of choice for the condition (Type II_a) although nicotinic acid, D-thyroxine, and Atromid-S have also been prescribed to achieve lesser degrees of antilipemic effect, especially in Type II_b patients.

A low cholesterol, low carbohydrate weight-reducing diet should be prescribed to initiate control of Type III "floating" beta disease. Although Atromid-S is generally regarded as specifically effective in this relatively rare condition (17), there are individual differences in response to the drug. In more obstinate cases, the addition of nicotinic acid may help achieve the desirable antilipemic effect.

VLDL increase (Type IV hyperlipoproteinemia) can best be controlled by dietary measures. The best result is obtained by reducing the patient to his lean body weight by severely restricting the dehydrated and refined carbohydrate intake (18,19). Atromid-S is effective to variable extents in different individuals; D-thyroxine is also helpful, if the patient does not have clinical CHD.

In severe Type V abnormality, both dietary carbohydrate and fat intakes should be reduced. Many Type V patients are overweight, sensitive to alcohol (20), and may exhibit an abnormal insulin mechanism. These associated abnormalities should be taken into consideration in prescribing a diet.

The importance of primary or genetically determined types of hyperlipoproteinemia is generally recognized. Clinically, however, only a relatively small portion of cases (estimated to constitute about 5–10% of hyperlipidemics) would have a pronounced disturbance in lipoprotein transport together with a positive familial trait to indicate the preponderance of a genetic factor. In the majority of instances, lipoprotein abnormalities essentially similar to those of primary origin are contributed by a number of common metabolic and nutritional disturbances, as indicated in Table 1. One should also look for hyperlipoproteinemia secondary to systemic diseases such as diabetes mellitus, hypothyroidism, chronic renal disease, dysproteinemia, and others.

Table 1. Common Causes of Hyperlipidemia Manifested as Varied Types of Hyperlipoproteinemia

1. Improper meal habit

2. Excessive use of alcohol, or sensitivity to alcohol ingestion

3. Overnutrition (need not be obese)

4. Disturbance in carbohydrate metabolism

5. Hormonal imbalance

6. Drugs: corticosterols, thiazide diuretics, contraceptives, and others

TREATMENT OF ENVIRONMENTALLY INDUCED HYPERLIPOPROTEINEMIAS

Treatment of hyperlipoproteinemias caused by chronic drug or hormone administration, and by a number of systemic diseases, is directed at the respective diseased conditions.

The bulk of clinically encountered hyperlipidemic states usually respond to appropriate dietary management with little need for antilipemic drugs.

In our clinic a therapeutic diet has been designed to provide overall control of common metabolic aberrations which lead to production of lipid abnormalities.

The principal features of the diet are:

1) substitution of saturated fats with oils high in linoleic acid content (corn, safflower, and soya),
2) emphasis on weight reduction to maintain lean body weight, if lipemia is severe, through restriction of refined and dehydrated carbohydrates,
3) lowering of daily cholesterol intake to 300 mg or less (attention is called, especially, in this regard to the minimum use of eggs),
4) the sharp reduction in alcohol consumption.

This regimen is designed to curb endogenous lipogenic and hypercholesterolemic effects of saturated short and medium chain triglycerides contained in butter fat and coconut oil. The mere restriction of foods rich in such fats would raise the polyunsaturated/saturated fat ratio in the regular American diet from 0.3 to 1.1 without using vegetable oil supplementation. Principles of such a diet are outlined in Table 2.

Table 2. Principles of "Overall Therapeutic Diet"

1. *Fats*

   (a) Substitute saturated fats with oils high in linoleic acid content (corn, safflower, soya)

   (b) Avoid excessive supplementation

   (c) Avoid oils and fats high in short-medium chain triglyceride content (butterfat and coconut oil)

2. *Carbohydrates*

   (a) Avoid refined carbohydrates (sugars and sugar-containing foods and drinks)

   (b) Avoid dehydrated carbohydrates (snacks and nuts)

3. *Cholesterol*

   Restrict intake to <300 mg/day

4. *Alcohol*

   (a) Sharply reduce

   (b) Avoid daily cocktails

Body Weight and CHD

A strong clinical impression holds that subjects with CHD are generally over-weight, but a number of studies suggest that body weight is not of major importance in the etiology of CHD. Some of the problems in assessing the role of adiposity may lie in:

1) the use of relatively crude and inaccurate methods such as reference to ideal height-weight charts and measurement of skin fold thickness to estimate fatness as emphasized by Hirsch and Gillian (21),
2) the frequent co-existence of hypertension, diabetes, and hyperlipidemia with obesity,
3) the lack of proper differentiation of the specific types of hyperlipoproteinemia in overweight subjects (the atherogenic influence of different hyperlipoproteinemias is quite varied).

Irrespective of the role adiposity may play in the etiology of CHD, it has been shown that weight reduction is accompanied by improvement in a number of hemodynamic parameters with reduction in myocardial oxygen consumption (22).

Provision made in the therapeutic diet to restrict simple carbohydrates and snacks of dehydrated carbohydrates has been effective in dealing with the weight problem.

USE OF DRUGS IN COMMON ENVIRONMENTALLY INDUCED HYPERLIPOPROTEINEMIA

Although in certain cases it has been possible to reduce the plasma lipid levels significantly with drug administration alone while the ad libidum diet was continued, we agree with Dayton (23) that the use of drugs should be limited to individuals with overt atherosclerosis or with genetic hyperlipoproteinemia and greatly increased risk of CHD.

Rather modest doses of Atromid-S, Choloxin, Questran, Colestipol, or nicotinic acid have been used to gain optimal control of specific types of hyperlipoproteinemia in patients whose condition has been stabilized on the therapeutic diet. The ready response of these patients to treatment stands in marked contrast to the obstinate hyperlipemias of genetic origin.

Hyperlipoproteinemias of genetic and environmental origins are presumably included in the recently completed primary and secondary CHD prevention trials with Clofibrate (24–27). Friedewald and Halperin (28) have listed several qualifications in accepting the conclusion drawn from these investigations. Future studies will determine whether differentiation made between the genetic and environmental forms of hyperlipoproteinemia could help to define the value of Clofibrate and other antilipemic drugs in CHD. Some of the outstanding features of genetic and environmental hyperlipoproteinemias are listed for comparison in Table 3.

Table 3. Comparison of Genetically Determined and Environmentally Induced Hyperlipoproteinemias

Features	Genetic	Environmental
Lipoprotein phenotype	I–V	II–V
Frequency distribution among hyperlipidemics	~5–10%	~90–95%
Cutaneous and tendinous xanthomata	~30%	Rare
Vascular disease	Premature atherosclerosis	Atherosclerosis in middle and older ages
Covert disturbance in carbohydrate metabolism including adiposity and dysinsulinemia	Inconsistent	Frequent
Response to therapy	Partial response to "specific" diet and drug (large doses)	Usually respond well to diet alone and to small doses of drugs if needed

SUMMARY OF PRELIMINARY DATA ON RESPONSE TO TREATMENT

We have followed 184 atherosclerotic patients with Types II–V hyperlipoproteinemia for 4.5 to 5.5 years. Careful adherence to the program for more than 6–8 months caused the following changes in their clinical status:

1) Moderate to marked loss in adipose tissue weight, amounting to 16–48 pounds,
2) improvement of cerebral, coronary, and peripheral arterial ischemic symptoms,
3) increase in exercise tolerance,
4) improvement of carbohydrate tolerance,
5) reversion to more normal ranges of high basal serum insulin and abnormal serum insulin response to carbohydrate chellenge,
6) maintenance of relatively low plasma preβ- and β-lipoprotein levels as

reflected in low plasma lipid (cholesterol and triglyceride) concentrations,

7) arrest of further progression of arterial lesions over a 2–3 year interval as documented by serial arteriographic studies (28).

CONCLUSIONS

The development of a plasma lipoprotein phenotyping system to convert hyperlipidemias into five types of hyperlipoproteinemia has helped to provide a better understanding of the hyperlipidemic mechanisms for the application of specific therapeutic measures. Experiences, however, indicate that the more frequently encountered environmentally-induced plasma lipid elevations may exhibit lipoprotein patterns essentially similar to those of hereditary origin yet differing in a number of important aspects. Some of the more apparent differences include:

1) the frequency and age at onset of atherosclerosis and its complications,
2) the presence of other clinical manifestations besides atherosclerosis,
3) the responsiveness to low cholesterol, low saturated fat diet, and
4) the responsiveness to antilipemic drug therapy.

I wish to emphasize the large group of environmentally-induced hyperlipoproteinemias which are characterized by a relatively late onset of ischemic vascular disease, by the rare occurrence of xanthomata and pancreatitis, and by a rather satisfactory response, including weight loss, to a "therapeutic diet" with or without the supplemental use of small to moderate doses of antilipemic drugs.

REFERENCES CITED

1. Kannel, W. B., Castelli, W. P., and McNamara, P. M. 1967. The coronary profile: 12-year follow-up in Framingham Study. J. Occup. Med. 9:611.
2. National Heart and Lung Institute. 1971. Task Force on Arteriosclerosis, Vol. 1, DHEW Publication Number (NIH) 72-137. U.S. Superintendent of Documents, Washington, D.C.
3. Fredrickson, D. S., Levy, R. I., and Lees, R. S. 1967. Fat transport in lipoproteins: An integrated approach to mechanisms and disorders. New Engl. J. Med. 276:34, 94, 148, 215, 273.
4. Lees, R. S., and Hatch, F. T. 1963. Sharper separation of lipoprotein species by paper electrophoresis in albumin-containing buffer. J. Lab. Clin. Med. 61:5.
5. Greten, H., Levy, R. I., and Fredrickson, D. S. 1969. Evidence for separate monoglyceride hydrolase and triglyceride lipose in post-heparin human plasma. J. Lipid Research 10:326.
6. Langer, T., Strober, W., and Levy, R. I. 1972. Familial Type II hyperlipoproteinemia—a defect of beta apoprotein catabolism. J. Clin. Invest. 51:1528.
7. Slack, J. 1969. Risk of ischemic heart disease in familial hyperlipoproteinemic states. Lancet 2:1380.

8. Jensen, J. Blankenhorn, D. H., and Kornerup. 1967. Coronary disease in familial hypercholesterolemia. Circulation 36:77.
9. Beaumont, J. L., Carlson, L. A., Cooper, G. R., et al. 1970. Classification of hyper-lipidemias. Bull. W.H.O. 43:891.
10. Quanfordt, S., Levy, R. I., and Fredrickson, D. S. 1971. On the lipoprotein abnormality in Type III hyperlipoproteinemia. J. Clin. Invest. 50:754.
11. Havel, R. J., Kane, J. P., et al. 1970. Splanchnic metabolism of free fatty acids and production of triglycerides of very low density lipoproteins in normotriglyceridemic and hypertriglyceridemic humans. J. Clin. Invest. 49:2017.
12. Fredrickson, D. S., and Levy, R. I. 1972. Familial hyperlipoproteinemia. In J. B. Stanbury et al., eds. The Metabolic Basis of Inherited Diseases, 3rd ed., pp. 545–614. McGraw-Hill, New York.
13. Levy, R. I., Fredrickson, D. S., Shulman, R., et al. 1972. Diet and drug treatment of primary hyperlipoproteinemia. Ann. Internal Med. 77:267.
14. Furman, R. H., Howard, R. P., Brusco, O. J., et al. 1965. Effects of medium chain length triglycerides (MCT) in serum lipids and lipoproteins in familial hyperchylomicronemia (dietary fat induced lipemia) and dietary carbohydrate accentuated lipemia. J. Lab. Clin. Med. 66:912.
15. Bergen, S. S., Jr., Van Itallic, T. B., Tennent, D. M., et al. 1959. Effect of an anion exchange resin on serum cholesterol in man. Proc. Soc. Exp. Biol. Med. 102:676.
16. Parkinson, T. M., Grundersen, L., and Nelson, N. A. 1970. Effects of Colestipol (U26,597A), a new bile acid sequestrant, on serum lipids in experimental animals and man. Atherosclerosis 11:531.
17. Levy, R. I., and Fredrickson, D. S. 1970. The current status of hypolipidemic drugs. Postgrad. Med. 47:130.
18. Kuo, P. T. 1967. Hypertriglyceridemia in coronary artery disease and its management. J.A.M.A. 201:87.
19. Kuo, P. T. 1970. Hyperlipidemia in atherosclerosis: Dietary and drug treatment. Med. Clin. No. Amer. 54:657.
20. Kudzma, D. J., and Schonfeld, G. 1971. Alcoholic hyperlipidemia: induction by alcohol but not by carbohydrate. J. Lab. Clin. Med. 77:384.
21. Hirsch, J., and Gillian, E. 1968. Methods for the determination of adipose cell size in man and animals. J. Lipid Research 9:110.
22. Alexander, J. K., and Peterson, K. L. 1972. Cardiovascular effects of weight reduction. Circulation 45:310.
23. Dayton, S. 1971. Rationale for use of lipid-lowering drugs. Fed. Proc. 30:849.
24. Krasno, L. R., and Kidera, G. J. 1972. Clofibrate in coronary heart disease; effect on morbidity and mortality. J.A.M.A. 219:845.
25. Group of physicians of the New Castle Upon Tyne Region. Trial of Clofibrate in treatment of ischemic heart disease. Brit. Med. J. 4:767.
26. Dewar, H. A., and Oliver, M. F. 1971. Secondary prevention trials using Clofibrate; a joint commentary on the New Castle and Scottish trials. Brit. Med. J. 4:784.
27. Research Committee of the Scottish Society of Physicians. 1971. Ischemic heart disease; a secondary prevention trial using Clofibrate. Brit. Med. J. 4:775.
28. Friedewald, W. T., and Halperin, M. 1972. Clofibrate in ischemic heart disease. Ann. Internal Med. 76:821.
29. Kuo, P. T., Shelburne, J. C., Roberts, B., Manchester, J. H., and Reif, J. S. 1972. Effect of simple-carbohydrate restriction upon clinical course and mortality of atherosclerosis. Circulation 46(II):179.

PARTIAL ILEAL BYPASS SURGERY IN THE MANAGEMENT OF THE HYPERLIPIDEMIAS

HENRY BUCHWALD

Partial ileal bypass is defined by our group as a bypass of the distal 200 cm of the small intestine, or of one-third of the entire small bowel length, whichever is larger. The proximal end of the bypassed loop is closed and attached to adjacent viscera to prevent future intussusception and bowel continuity is restored by end-to-side anastomosis to the cecum. All mesenteric defects are carefully closed to prevent the possibility of internal hernia.

Primary rationale of this limited one-third small intestinal bypass is to achieve a beneficial degree of malabsorption by interference with the enterohepatic cholesterol and the enterohepatic bile acid cycles. Normally, cholesterol enters the small intestine via the bile, by secretion directly through the intestinal mucosa, and in the ingested food. It is for a large part reabsorbed back into the circulation, primarily from the distal small intestine. The enterohepatic bile acid mechanism is extremely efficient so that essentially the same bile acids are used for breakfast, lunch, and dinner. Following the operation there is interference with these cycles with an increase in the loss of cholesterol and bile acids (the metabolic end-product of cholesterol metabolism) in the stool resulting in 1) a direct loss of cholesterol from the body and 2) an indirect drain on the cholesterol pool by the forced conversion of cholesterol to bile acids. It should be emphasized that the partial ileal bypass procedure is entirely different in its purpose from the far more extensive jejuno-ileal bypass operation designed to produce a caloric deficit and weight reduction; partial ileal bypass affects circulating lipid concentrations only, with no attendant weight loss, protein depletion, electrolyte problems, etc.

We have now had ten years of clinical experience with the partial ileal bypass operation and have operated upon better than 120 patients. The average age of our patients, both males and females, is 41 years; the youngest patient in the group was seven years old at the time of operation and there are eight pre-pubertal youngsters in this series. We have found an average serum cholesterol reduction after partial ileal bypass of 40% from the preoperative but post-type specific dietary baseline, i.e. the 40% reduction is measured against the average cholesterol value after at least three months of management by the diet most appropriate for that patient's lipid abnormality. We were able to study a subgroup of 24 patients prior to dietary management, post-diet and preoperatively, and again after bypass. In this cohort, an 11% cholesterol reduction was achieved by dietary management alone (423 mg% to 377 mg%) and subsequent to bypass the total reduction from the pre-management baseline was 53% (423 mg% to 224 mg%), essentially a halving of the cholesterol level. The average serum triglyceride reduction in the type IV patients, those with the primary triglyceride elevation, was 68% in comparison to their preoperative, but again post-type specific dietary baseline.

Our in-hospital mortality has been less than 1% with one patient dying four days following the operation from an acute myocardial infarction; he had experienced three previous myocardial infarctions. There have been eight late deaths in this series of 120, with six of these eight caused by acute myocardial infarction. Complications related directly to surgery consist of three episodes of bowel obstruction caused by the development of adhesions. We have not had any episodes of obstruction attributable to internal hernia formation or any occurrence of intussusception of the closed end of the bypassed loop. Better than half of the patients have some difficulty with the frequency of bowel evacuation; however, 90% of the patients have less than five stools per day within one year following the procedure. The only supplementation management necessary following surgery is the injection of 1,000 micrograms of vitamin B_{12} intramuscularly every two months.

As our study progressed, we became more and more aware that our patients volunteered they had an improvement in their symptoms of angina pectoris. In fact, 69% of all patients with angina pectoris present prior to surgery experienced some degree of improvement and none of the patients free of angina preceding the procedure developed this symptom complex afterwards. We are currently conducting a rheological and hemodynamic research program to quantify, if possible, increased myocardial oxygen availability to marked lipid reduction.

Our partial ileal bypass study is unique in obtaining serial follow-up coronary and aoro-iliac arteriograms in all patients at two- to three-year time intervals. At approximately three years average follow-up, the coronary arteriography progression rate, combining the number of patients with new lesions or occlusions, is 19% in our series; this compares quite favorably with the 50% progression rate in nonlipid managed patients with comparable disease over the same length of time in another published study. In three patients repeat coronary arteriography revealed radiographic evidence of atherosclerotic disease regression.

Comparison of the average serum cholesterol level of our partial ileal bypass patients with the average cholesterol concentration found in comparably aged and sex matched groups in the United States shows that our patients are in the upper 5–10% of the distribution curve preoperatively and well below the mean postoperatively. Plotting the average preoperative cholesterol concentration on the Cornfield Framingham risk curve, the patients in our series fall well above the 200% risk level (100% = normal risk) preoperatively and are at about 75% of normal risk postoperatively. Only the future and the completion of a randomized study can add statistical validity to these predictions.

At present we conclude that the advantages of partial ileal bypass in management of the hyperlipidemias are: 1) maximum effectiveness, 2) maintenance of lipid reduction, 3) safety, and 4) the obligatory nature of the procedure. The data clearly show that diet and drug therapy, singly or in combination, cannot approach the lipid reduction feasible by partial ileal bypass. Contrary to the results of some drug therapy, the cholesterol lowering effect of partial ileal bypass is lasting; there has been no report of response escapes. Patients may or may not adhere to diet, may or may not take pills; but once the operation is performed its therapeutic effects are maintained and obligatory.

THE PROPHYLACTIC SIGNIFICANCE
OF EMOTIONAL RELAXATION

STEWART WOLF

Samuel Fox has questioned, "To what extent does exercise and physical training induce emotional relaxation and hence cloud the evaluation of either one separately?" There is no doubt that emotional stress can be lessened by plunging into vigorous exercise. For example, a hard game of squash or tennis is a well recognized way of heading off or aborting an attack of migraine headache. Then there is the more subtle sense of well-being and power which goes with being physically fit. Naughton and Bruhn found that postcoronary patients who agreed to participate in an exercise rehabilitation program had fewer depressive and neurotic scores on the Minnesota Multiphasic Personality Inventories (MMPI) than did those patients who declined to participate (1). Furthermore, the participators altered several aspects of their behavior more than did the nonparticipators, including attaining better sleep with less need for sedatives, smoking less, and experiencing fewer emotional conflicts on the job and at home.

By contrast, in more acute situations, emotional relaxation has been sought in physical rest and relative inactivity. Groover (2) presented suggestive evidence that impending myocardial infarction could be aborted by admitting the patient to the hospital and sedating him, thus removing him from his day-to-day stresses and responsibilities. Nixon and associates (3), in an attempt to keep pain and apprehension at a minimum following myocardial infarction, instituted with excellent results a regimen of almost continuous sedative-induced sleep in the coronary care unit for the first three to five days following admission.

Unfortunately there are no firm experimental data that test the effects of emotional relaxation as a prophylactic measure. Assumptions concerning its importance derive from the experience of clinicians, who frequently report the occurrence of myocardial infarction in a setting of mounting troubles and emotional tension. There are a large number of descriptive papers in the literature to this effect. With respect to the timing of a myocardial infarction, Theorell and Rahe (4) found a pile-up of life experiences requiring emotional readjustment during the months leading up to the myocardial infarction. We do know from experimental evidence that the serum concentration of cholesterol may vary with an individual's response to emotionally charged events when diet and exercise are rigidly controlled (5). We do not, however, know the significance of such data to the process of atherogenesis.

In studies of long-term survival from myocardial infarction, Bruhn and co-workers (6) found more evidence of emotional disturbance, especially depression, among those who died within the first six years after myocardial infarction than among those who survived the test period.

Assuming for the moment that emotional relaxation is protective to the coronary-prone subject, what does it actually accomplish in pathophysiologic terms? Does it slow down the process of arteriosclerosis or does it reverse it? We have no evidence one way or the other. Furthermore, the extent of arteriosclerosis does not correlate very closely with the presence or absence of a coronary event. Does emotional relaxation postpone or reduce the likelihood of a myocardial infarction, does it do the same for sudden death without the occurrence of a new infarct, or does it do both?

Evidence along all of these lines is difficult to adduce, and at present is at best fragmentary. The best evidence relates emotional stress to cardiac arrhythmias and, by implication, to sudden death, so although the emotional state may be pertinent to atherosclerosis and the natural history of ischemic heart disease, it would be appropriate for the present to focus only on the potential relevance of emotional stress to ventricular arrhythmias.

Some of the most suggestive evidence that excessive challenges and associated anxiety may adversely affect the coronary prone subject comes from the work of several investigators (7–13) on the serum concentration of free fatty acids and cortisol and of catecholamines in association with anxiety and in turn their relationship to cardiac arrhythmias and sudden death.

Quite clearly factors other than emotionally stressful events may result in similar hormonal alterations, especially following a tissue insult such as a myocardial infarction with impending or actual evidences of shock. Furthermore, as Shillingford (14) points out, anxiety may occur as a *consequence* of high circulating catecholamines. Nevertheless, since elevations of free fatty acids, cortisol, and catecholamines have been clearly documented to occur in healthy subjects under severe emotional stress, and since such hormonal changes as they occur in postmyocardial infarction patients are at least *associated* with a high susceptibility to ventricular arrhythmias, it appears safe to conclude that emotional relaxation would be a rational goal in the management of the coronary prone subject.

Reduction of anxiety and the elimination of certain cardiac arrhythmias may be achieved by a variety of maneuvers, including hypnosis, progressive relaxation, operant conditioning, and transcendental meditation (15). Most recently we have been able to effect similar results simply by getting a subject to concentrate on an absorbing topic (16). In two subjects it was possible greatly to reduce the number of ventricular premature contractions during intense mental concentration. Whether or not such a technique would be applicable in a coronary care unit is a subject for future research, but the relationship of the control of the heart beat to cognitive as well as to emotional processes seems well established.

REFERENCES CITED

1. Naughton, J., Bruhn, J. G., and Lategola, M. T. 1968. Effects of physical training on physiologic and behavioral characteristics of cardiac patients. Arch. Phys. Med. Rehab. 49:131.
2. Groover, M. E. 1957. Clinical evaluation of a public health program to prevent coronary artery disease. Trans. Stud. Coll. Physicians Philad. 24:105–114.
3. Nixon, P. G. F., Taylor, D. J. E., Morton, S. D., and Bromfield, M. 1968. A sleep regimen for acute myocardial infarction. Lancet 1:726–728.
4. Theorell, T., and Rahe, R. H. 1971. Psychosocial factors and myocardial infarction–An inpatient study in Sweden. J. Psychosom. Res. 15:25.
5. McCabe, W. R., Yamamoto, J., Wolf, S., Adsett, C. A., and Schottstaedt, W. W. 1962. Changes in serum lipids in relation to emotional stress during rigid control of diet and exercise. Circulation 26(3):379.
6. Bruhn, J. G., Chandler, B., and Wolf, S. 1969. A psychological study of survivors and non-survivors of myocardial infarction. Psychosom. Med. 31:8.
7. Raab, W. 1968. Correlated cardiovascular adrenergic and adrenocortical responses to sensory and mental annoyances in man–a potential accessory cardiac risk factor. Psychosom. Med. 30:809.
8. Bogdonoff, M. D., Estes, E. H., Jr., and Weissler, A. M. 1960. Studies on fat moblization during acute states of arousal. Southern Med. J. 53:680.
9. Carlson, L. A., Levi, L., and Orö, L. 1968. Plasma lipids and urinary excretion of catecholamines in man during experimentally induced emotional stress, and their modification by nicotinic acid. J. Clin. Invest. 47:1795.
10. Greene, W. A., Moss, A. J., Goldstein, S., Levy, A. L., and Klein, R. F. 1972. Psychosocial, hormonal and arrhythmia precursors of the early pre-hospital phase of myocardial infarction. Presented at the American Psychosomatic Society annual meeting, April 1972, Boston, Massachusetts.
11. Olewine, D. A., Simpson, M. T., Jenkins, C. O., Ramsay, F. H., Zyzanski, S. J., Thomas, G., and Hames, C. G. 1972. Catecholamines, platelet adhesiveness, and the coronary-prone behavior pattern. Presented at the American Psychosomatic Society annual meeting, April 1972, Boston, Massachusetts.
12. Wallace, A. G. 1968. Catecholamine metabolism in patients with acute myocardial infarction. In D. G. Julian and M. F. Oliver, eds. Acute myocardial infarction, p. 237. E. and S. Livingstone, Ltd., Edinburgh and London.
13. Oliver, M. F. 1968. The relationship of serum free fatty acids to arrhythmias and death. In D. G. Julian and M. F. Oliver, eds. Acute myocardial infarction, p. 251. E. and S. Livingstone, Ltd., Edinburgh and London.
14. Shillingford, J. P. 1968. Discussion of the relationship of serum free fatty acids to arrhythmias and death. In D. G. Julian and M. F. Oliver, eds. Acute myocardial infarction, p. 264. E. and S. Livingstone, Ltd., Edinburgh and London.
15. Weiss, T., and Engel, B. T. 1972. Operant conditioning of heart rate in patients with premature ventricular contractions. In T. X. Barber, et al., eds. Biofeedback and self-control, Ch. 36. Aldine, Chicago.
16. Long, J., Ziegner, C., Bynum, T. E., and Wolf, S. The control of sinus arrhythmia in man. Manuscript in preparation.

HYPERTENSION, DIABETES, AND CIGARETTE SMOKING

OGLESBY PAUL

Today, every physician knows that hypertension, diabetes, and cigarette smoking are related to the incidence of coronary heart disease. If this is such familiar material, why write about it? The reason is that we still have many problems that require recognition, discussion, and solution before we can feel comfortable.

There is impressive scientific evidence associating these three factors with coronary atherosclerosis and its complications of sudden death, coronary occlusion, and myocardial infarction. The data from the pooled findings from seven prospective 10-year studies in white middle-aged males (1) have shown more than a three-fold increase in fatal heart attacks in persons with diastolic blood pressures of 105 mm Hg or more, as compared with persons having diastolic blood pressures below 85 mm Hg. Those men who smoked more than 20 cigarettes a day were shown also to have a coronary mortality three times that of nonsmokers. There is also other evidence that among diabetic males, aged 15 to 44 years, the mortality from coronary disease is 4.6 times higher than in nondiabetic males; among female diabetics, the mortality rises to 6.4 times that in nondiabetic females (2).

However, the exact mechanisms of action of these three risk factors and their relation to the progression of the disease remain unclear. We really do not know how cigarette smoking damages coronary arteries. We similarly do not have an adequate insight into what diabetes does to the coronary arterial wall. We believe hypertension may produce physical damage to the intima and the media and alter the passage of lipids and the substances across the arterial wall, but there is still much speculation and a paucity of facts.

Do we have means of intervention of all three factors? Yes, of course the smoking habit can be treated by cessation of cigarette smoking. Hypertension can be treated by any one of a number of available effective drugs. The blood sugar in diabetes may be lowered by insulin, oral agents, and diet.

Is there evidence that the measures are effective? There are data indicating an impressive difference in coronary mortality between ex-smokers and current cigarette smokers. In regard to hypertension it is embarrassing to state that there still is no solid evidence that good treatment lowers the rate of heart attacks, although it does lessen the number of strokes and congestive heart failure. I believe it will soon be shown that coronary attacks are also reduced by treatment of hypertension. As far as diabetes is concerned, most investigators are not convinced that careful treatment of diabetes lessens the atherosclerotic complications.

Are there unfavorable effects of intervention on these three risk factors? For hypertension, we must recognize a relatively small incidence of drug toxicity or serious unfavorable results or effects including polyuria, postural hypotension, hypokalemia, gastrointestinal problems, rashes, and fever. For those individuals who stop smoking there are the issues of weight gain and varied transient complaints of nervousness, irritability, and general state of being "hard to live with." For diabetes, the problem is more serious since it appears that at least two oral agents, tolbutamide and phenformin, may actually increase cardiovascular mortality, perhaps through inotropic actions and increased automaticity (3).

Are there physician-related problems? Yes, clearly. As regards hypertension, it is apparent that either because of a shortage of time or interest or from plain ignorance many doctors do a bad job of recognition, treatment, and follow-up on patients with high blood pressure. The handling of chronic conditions and an emphasis on prevention is frankly boring to many physicians. With cigarette smoking, we still need to remind physicians to emphasize the hazards and to emphasize them forcefully; for the minority of physicians who continue to smoke, we should express a mixture of sympathy, regret, and indignation. With diabetes, the physician is understandably confused and feels that the scientific rug has been pulled out from under him.

There are profound patient-related problems too. The patient who is hypertensive rarely has symptoms and is poorly motivated to spend money for long-term treatment when he feels healthy. This partly explains why only about 25% of hypertensive persons are under therapy. It is also well known that programs to influence patients to stop smoking (or lose weight) have permanent success in only 20–40% of the cases.

This recitation is intended to emphasize my belief that the prevention of coronary disease through control of hypertension, diabetes, and cigarette smoking is a very difficult task. We lack a basic understanding of mechanisms. We do not have satisfactory evidence as yet of benefit of intervention in two of the three factors, and there are major physician- and patient-related problems in undertaking a prevention program. This does not deter me from vigorously stating that on the basis of current evidence and our knowledge of the critical nature of this health problem, we must not only continue to obtain more scientific facts but *also* intervene vigorously now to eliminate cigarette smoking and to control hypertension. Our posture with diabetes should stress the value of diet and insulin while we await further developments.

REFERENCES CITED

1. Stamler, J., and Epstein, F. H. 1972. Coronary heart disease: risk factors as a guide to preventive action. Preventive Med. 1:27–48.
2. Epstein, F. H. 1967. Hyperglycemia: a risk factor in coronary heart disease. Circulation 36:609–619.
3. Editorial. 1972. Tolbutamide and the heart. J.A.M.A. 222: 1179–1180.

Angina Pectoris

Diagnostic Considerations

WHO SHOULD HAVE CORONARY ANGIOGRAPHY?

HENRY D. McINTOSH, DONALD H. GLAESER,
JAMES S. COLE, and KINSMAN E. WRIGHT, JR.

There can be little doubt that coronary artery disease is a national calamity. The disease afflicts an estimated 5% of the adult population in the United States. Therefore 3.1 million Americans between the ages of 18 and 79 years definitely have coronary artery disease; another 2.4 million persons are suspected of having the disease. More than 600,000 persons die each year from this disease in the United States alone.

It is generally accepted that high-quality, selective coronary arteriography can define the presence or absence of significant occlusive disease of the coronary arteries with greater than 90% accuracy. However, coronary arteriograms demonstrate only anatomy and morphology; used alone they do not give direct evidence whether ischemic heart disease is present or whether demonstrated coronary artery disease is symptomatic. Accepting these limitations, which patients who have coronary artery disease or who are suspected of having it should have radiographic visualization of their coronary vessels?

RISKS, CONTROLS, AND COSTS

Since there is a high incidence of death and disability associated with coronary artery disease, one might argue that all patients with or suspected of having occlusions of their coronaries should have coronary arteriograms. This philosophy would be acceptable if:

1) the morbidity and mortality of the procedure were negligible not only in the hands of the expert, but also in those of the relative novice,
2) the procedure were relatively inexpensive, and
3) the results of the study permitted the physician to plan therapy that resulted consistently in an improved prognosis for the patient.

The morbidity and mortality of coronary arteriography in well-run catheterization laboratories are almost negligible (1). Some large series report an overall

This study was supported in part by grants in aid HL-13837-03, HL-05435-13/P15C, and HEW-NIH71-2480 of the National Heart and Lung Institute, National Institutes of Health, Bethesda, Maryland.

mortality as low as 0.1%, yet not all patients enjoy such quality performance.

Selzer reported that the mortality from coronary arteriography in the San Francisco area varied from 0.5% in one hospital that performed 500 studies a year to 8% in a hospital that had 25 cases per year (2). The overall mortality for the total group of 2,025 patients was 1%.

Abrams recently determined the reported morbidity and mortality experienced in 46,900 patients studied in a large number of laboratories (3). There were 209 deaths (0.44%). Individual hospitals doing fewer than 100 cases per year had a mortality as high as 8%; when more than 350 cases were done per year, the mortality was no higher than 0.4%. The details of this important study will soon be reported by Abrams and his associates.

The results of catheterization, the morbidity and mortality, reported in large series of patients is obtained by pooling the results of many small series. The larger the pool, the easier it is to "cover up" the poor results of small subgroups or individuals. Thus, each physician performing coronary catheterizations should report his results individually. One does not accept as meaningful the mortality for appendectomies for a given hospital, but rather scrutinizes the results of the individual surgeon. The surgeon with a high mortality rate soon discovers that he no longer has privileges to operate. Furthermore, the Tissue Committee reviews the histories and the specimens that are removed to determine if the procedure was justified.

The Radiology Study Group of the Inter-Society Commission for Heart Disease Resources in 1971 recommended that 300 coronary arteriography procedures per year be the minimum number "required to maintain the expertise of the professional team engaged in these highly complicated procedures" (4). The Study Group also recommended that centers for angiocardiography should be located only where cardiovascular surgery is regularly performed since the procedure may otherwise have to be repeated before surgery, and also because emergency cardiovascular surgery may be needed for patients who experience complications of arteriography.

Quality control must be instituted before routine use of coronary arteriography can be recommended. This does not mean that the procedure should be carried out only in university centers; however, it should be done only in a limited number of high volume laboratories that are located in hospitals capable of carrying out high quality cardiovascular surgery and that police the results of their staff.

Quality control will be difficult to institute. One reason this is so is because of the economics of the studies; coronary arteriography and surgery are profitable ventures. It is profitable both for the hospital and the physician. Relatively few cardiologists consider the financial rewards when deciding whether to study a given patient; yet to a few, a professional fee of $300 or more for two hours or less of work can be a tremendous temptation to study even the most fleeting and innocuous chest pain.

The total cost required to obtain coronary arteriograms is great. It would appear that to admit a patient for three days for coronary arteriography costs about $1,000 in many hospitals. However, the cost is not a significant consideration if there is a reasonable chance that the therapy that can be planned will result in an improved prognosis for the patient. It is obvious that coronary arteriography is essential for determining if coronary artery bypass surgery is feasible.

BYPASS SURGERY

The precise role of coronary artery bypass surgery is yet to be defined. The long-term results of saphenous vein bypass grafts of coronary vessels are unknown. It is known that if the graft is properly placed in carefully selected patients with angina pectoris, the chest pain is nearly always reduced in severity or relieved completely (5); it is also known that from 10 to 15% of these patients sustain definite myocardial infarctions at the time of or shortly after surgery (6).

There are several important questions for which answers are needed before surgery can be recommended with confidence. These include the following:

1) Will the incidence of myocardial infarction or sudden death be reduced in patients that have bypass procedures?
2) Will the rate of development of coronary atherosclerosis in the native vascular bed be altered?
3) Is there significant functional improvement in the majority of patients, or does the function of the heart deteriorate as a result of surgery?
4) What are the long-term effects of operation-related myocardial infarctions?

Until the answers to these questions are known, our group will follow a conservative course.

At this time we consider the following to be the major indications for saphenous vein coronary bypass surgery:

1) angina pectoris not responding to good medical management and interfering with the patient's life style and
2) in conjunction with aortic valve replacement if significant coronary artery obstruction is present.

Other indications for surgery on the coronary arteries, such as pre-infarction angina, young patients, and patients with recent myocardial infarctions, are less certain, and further data are needed before they become major considerations.

Since the above major indications for surgery necessarily require visualization of the coronary arteries, they are therefore the major indications for coronary arteriography. The number of patients who fit these indications is not large. Further consideration must be given to those patients who might have the so-called lethal lesions; that is, stenosis of the main left or proximal left anterior descending coronary arteries. Also, the physician cannot help but be concerned about the possible existence of severe stenosis of the right coronary artery or more peripheral lesions of the left side in patients who are still at the moment relatively asymptomatic.

TREADMILL TESTING

It is our current belief that "lethal lesions" and significant stenosis at other sites can be ruled out in most patients by means of symptom-limited treadmill stress testing. The protocol followed in our clinic is a modification of that recommended by Bruce, utilizing a treadmill with variable speed and variable height; we record nine ECG leads rather than the one lead recommended by Bruce. We have correlated the results of the test with coronary arteriography in a group of

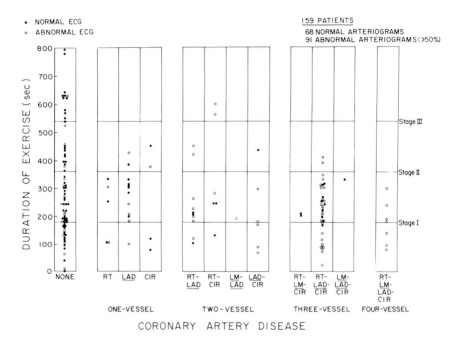

Fig. 1. Relationship between the duration of exercise and the location of significant obstructive lesions in the coronary arteries. The exercise was continued until the patient developed chest pain, fatigue, or electrocardiographic abnormalities such as frequent premature ventricular beats and more than two millimeters of ST segment depression.

75 patients who had normal resting electrocardiograms, were not taking any digitalis preparation, and were normotensive. Utilizing the criteria of one millimeter of horizontal ST depression in any lead as indicative of ischemia, and 50% occlusion of a major coronary artery as significant, the sensitivity was 96%. There were approximately 10% false positive treadmill tests which occurred primarily in women. We are confident that in patients without prior evidence of heart disease on their electrocardiogram, we can determine the presence or absence of significant coronary artery disease (i.e., stenosis of 50% or more).

Can the severity of coronary artery disease be determined without resorting to coronary arteriography? The duration of exercise in 159 patients was correlated with the severity of coronary artery disease with particular attention to the vessels involved (Fig. 1). Two patients with normal electrocardiograms (no myocardial infarctions or left bundle branch block) and lesions of the left anterior descending coronary artery were able to exercise longer than stage II. In one patient the lesion was only 50% occlusive and in the other the lesion was in the mid portion of the left anterior descending artery. No patients with left main coronary artery disease (> 50% occlusion) were able to complete stage II.

The information derived from the stress testing has been of considerable help in the formulation of the management of patients with or suspected of having angina pectoris (Fig. 2). If the patient has a normal resting electrocardiogram and a negative treadmill test (heart rate response adequate), the patient's workup is directed toward other causes of chest pain. If the test is positive and exercise

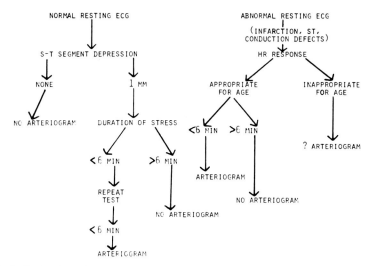

Fig. 2. Evaluation of classical angina pectoris by treadmill stress test (no valvular disease, hypertension, or digitalis).

tolerance is greater than stage II, the patient is placed on medical therapy. If he remains symptomatic after an adequate trial of medical therapy, he is studied by the technique of coronary arteriography and surgery is considered. If the patient becomes essentially asymptomatic on a good medical regimen, he is not considered for surgery and thus is not subjected to coronary arteriography. When a patient is repeatedly unable to complete six minutes of exercise because of the appearance of ischemic changes on the electrocardiogram, angina pectoris, or fatigue, an arteriogram and hence surgery are contemplated. In a patient with an abnormal resting electrocardiogram to begin with, the considerations are the same. If he completes stage II exercises, then decisions regarding further investigation depend on other clinical information. Several of our patients with previous myocardial infarctions and proximal lesions of the left anterior descending coronary artery have been able to exercise into stage III, but these patients have already exhibited the nature of their disease. Furthermore, we have been concerned about patients in whom the heart rate response has been inappropriate for their age. If we do not reach at least 90% of the predicted maximal heart rate in this group, decision making again is based on the other available information, such as the type of stress the patient is likely to encounter in day-to-day living.

REFERENCES CITED

1. Ross, R. S., and Gorlin, R. 1968. Coronary arteriography. Circulation 38 Suppl. III-67.
2. Selzer, A., Anderson, W. L., and March, H. W. 1971. Indications for coronary arteriography: Risks vs. benefits. California Med. 115:1–6.
3. Abrams, H. L. Personal communication.
4. Abrams, H. L., Adelstein, S. J., Elliott, L. P., Ellis, K., Greenspan, R. H., Judkins, M. P., and Viamonte, M. 1971. Optimal radiologic facilities for examination of the chest and the cardiovascular system. Circulation 43:A–135.
5. Morris, G. C., Reul, G. J., Howell, J. F., Crawford, E. S., Chapman, D. W., Beazley, H. L., Winters, W. L., Peterson, P. K., and Lewis, J. M. 1972. Follow-up results of distal coronary artery bypass for ischemic heart disease. Amer. J. Cardiol. 29:180–185.
6. Brewer, D., Bilbro, R., and Bartel, A. 1972. Myocardial infarction as a complication of coronary artery bypass surgery. Circulation 45 Suppl. II-69.
7. Bruce, R. A., and Hornsten, T. R. 1969. Exercise stress testing in evaluation of patients with ischemic heart disease. Prog. Cardiov. Dis. 11:371–390.

DETERMINANTS AND FUNCTIONAL SIGNIFICANCE OF THE CORONARY COLLATERAL CIRCULATION IN ISCHEMIC HEART DISEASE

RICHARD R. MILLER, EZRA A. AMSTERDAM, ROBERT ZELIS, RASHID A. MASSUMI, and DEAN T. MASON

The clinical role of the coronary collateral circulation has been a subject of great interest and controversy for many years. Despite extensive investigations in experimental animals (1–7) and pathologic studies in patients (8–12), the fundamental significance and determinants of the development of the collateral circulation of the myocardium in clinical coronary artery disease remain unclarified (13–19). It is now generally agreed that these auxiliary vessels are congenitally derived channels and that their function is promoted by coronary stenosis and myocardial ischemia. Although the anatomic presence of these collateral vessels implies a protective effect, and experimental studies have shown substantial blood flow conveyed by them, the precise importance of the coronary collateral circulation in patients with coronary artery disease has not been determined.

COLLATERALS IN VARIABLE NUMBER OF OBSTRUCTED CORONARY ARTERIES

In order to evaluate objectively the role of coronary collaterals in patients with coronary artery disease, we recently have studied the relationships among these collateral vessels, as observed by selective coronary arteriography, and certain clinical features and cardiac performance variables. In the first study of this series of investigations, patients with obstruction (greater than 75% stenosis) of one or more of the three major coronary arteries were assessed to determine the relationship between specific clinical factors and myocardial collateralization (20–22).

Patient age and sex were found not to be determinants of collateral formation. Further, a relationship between these auxiliary vessels and coronary risk factors was not observed. However, there was a direct relationship between the extent of coronary artery disease and the presence of collateral channels (Fig. 1).

Supported in part by Research Program Project Grant HL-14780 from the National Institutes of Health, Bethesda, Maryland. The authors gratefully acknowledge the secretarial assistance of Barbara Giles and Margaret Phister.

R. R. Miller *et al.*

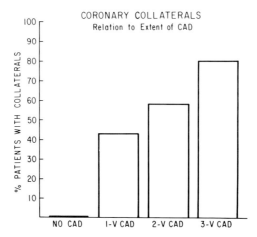

Fig. 1. Relation between extent of coronary artery disease (*CAD*) and presence of coronary collaterals. *V* = vessel (major coronary artery) with significant obstruction (greater than 75% stenosis).

Collaterals were not observed in individuals with normal coronary arteries or in patients with coronary artery disease without major vessel obstruction. However, the percentage of patients with collaterals was related directly to the number of coronary arteries obstructed: there was progressive increase in the number of patients with collaterals in the groups with one-, two-, and three-vessel coronary artery stenosis, respectively (20–22).

The presence of collaterals per number of coronary vessels obstructed was related to electrocardiographic features (20–22). Normal ECG occurred more often in those patients without collaterals, while pathologic Q waves indicating previous myocardial infarction were more frequent in individuals with these auxiliary vessels. Thus, the existence of collaterals does not appear to offer a protective effect in terms of electrocardiographic analyses of ventricular ischemia and infarction.

Concerning cardiac performance in coronary artery disease, left ventricular end-diastolic pressure and cardiac index did not differ significantly between patients with and without collaterals, as demonstrated in Figure 2 (20–22). Indeed, hemodynamics tended to be more disturbed in the patients with collateral vessels. Moreover, in coronary artery disease, patients with collaterals had a greater frequency of dyssynergy than those without collateral channels (20–22). Therefore, no protective effect of collateralization was observed on left ventricular function in coronary artery disease in terms of end-diastolic filling pressure, cardiac output, and segmental contraction.

In addition, characteristics of coronary heart disease were related to the number of major coronary arteries receiving collaterals (20–22). The duration of

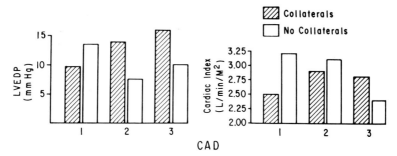

Fig. 2. Relation of the presence or absence of coronary collaterals to left ventricular end-diastolic pressure (*LVEDP*) and to cardiac index in patients with coronary atherosclerosis (*CAD*) with significant obstruction (greater than 75% stenosis) of one, two, and three of the major coronary arteries, as determined by selective coronary cineangiography.

angina pectoris correlated positively with the number of collateral vessels. Thus, in coronary patients with angina pectoris for longer than five years, there were significantly more individuals with collaterals to all three coronary arteries than those without collaterals or with auxiliary vessels to one or two obstructed major arteries. Therefore, when angina pectoris is taken as an index of myocardial ischemia, the collateralization response appears to be related in part to the duration of ischemia. Further, the coronary patients with collaterals demonstrated greater frequency of pathologic Q waves on ECG than did coronary patients without collaterals. With respect to left ventricular function in coronary artery disease, the frequency of dyssynergy was greater in patients with collaterals, and there were no significant differences in cardiac index and end-diastolic pressure related to the presence or number of collateral channels. Patients with collaterals had significantly greater frequency of three major vessel obstructive coronary disease than did coronary patients without collaterals, and the occurrence of obstruction in all three coronary arteries tended to correlate with the extent of collateralization. From these observations, it appears that the degree of coronary collateral circulation is related directly to the extent and duration of coronary artery disease itself and to the severity of cardiac disturbances resulting from coronary obstruction.

COLLATERALS IN THREE-VESSEL CORONARY DISEASE

The observation that stenosis involving all three major coronary arteries is associated closely with collateral formation indicates that assessment of effects of collaterals on clinical features and ventricular performance should be carried out in patients who have the common denominator of equal extent of coronary artery disease. Since the study described above included patients with one, two, or three coronary vessel obstructions, a second study was performed which was comprised only of patients with greater than 75% stenosis of all three major coronary vessels, in order that the functional significance of collaterals in clinical coronary disease might be evaluated more critically (23).

In patients with three-vessel coronary obstruction, the frequency of previous myocardial infarction defined by pathologic Q waves did not differ between patients with and without collaterals (23). Further, the percentage of three-vessel disease patients with positive postexercise ECG treadmill tests was the same in patients with and without collateral channels (23). Thus, in these coronary patients matched by obstruction in all three coronary arteries, collaterals did not appear to confer special protective benefit against the presence of active myocardial ischemia and development of myocardial infarction, if these collateral vessels were present prior to infarction.

Patients with three-vessel disease exhibited no difference in cardiac performance dependent on presence or absence of collaterals or on the number of obstructed vessels receiving collaterals (23). Thus, the left ventricular end-diastolic pressure was elevated equally, and the cardiac output was at the lower limits of normal in each of these groups of patients.

The relation of collaterals to the pattern of left ventricular segmental contraction was assessed in these patients with three-vessel coronary obstruction (23). Dyssynergy was present with greater frequency in patients with collaterals than in those without collateral formation. Thus, in this relatively homogeneous group of patients with obstructive artery disease in all three major coronary vessels, the presence of one or multiple collaterals was not associated with favorable differences in ischemic ECG response, previous myocardial infarction, or left ventricular dynamics, in comparison to three-vessel disease patients without collaterals. In fact, in general, left ventricular abnormalities caused by coronary obstruction tended to be more frequent in patients with multiple collaterals than in those with a single auxiliary channel with equal extent of coronary obstruction.

COLLATERALS IN LEFT ANTERIOR DESCENDING CORONARY DISEASE

Having first studied clinical coronary artery disease as a whole, and second having studied patients with coronary disease with three-vessel obstruction, we undertook a third, more precisely controlled analysis of the collateral circulation in patients equally matched for both extent and location of coronary obstruction (24, 25). Under evaluation in this study was the functional significance of collaterals to the left anterior descending coronary artery, the coronary vessel supplying the largest portion of the left ventricular myocardium; obstruction of this coronary artery appears to be the most important of the three major coronaries relative to sudden death and myocardial infarction shock (26, 27). Each patient had complete or greater than 75% obstruction of the proximal left anterior descending coronary artery and equal extent of coronary artery disease in the right and circumflex coronary arteries. These patients were divided into two groups, those with and those without collaterals to the left anterior descending coronary artery below the obstruction. Thus, the presence or absence of collaterals to the distal patent left anterior descending coronary artery was the only apparent variable.

Collateral vessels were evaluated relative to ECG evidence of previous anterior myocardial infarction and to positive exercise ECG treadmill tests (24, 25). Again, as in our first two studies, the presence of collaterals to the left anterior descending coronary artery did not appear to influence the existence of previous infarction or current active ischemia.

In the same group of patients with matched coronary artery disease and left anterior descending occlusion differing only by whether or not the distal portion of this artery received collaterals, left ventricular function was evaluated by examination of end-diastolic pressure, cardiac output, and the pattern of contraction (24, 25), as seen in Figure 3. No significant difference was observed in ventricular filling pressure or cardiac output based on the presence or absence of collaterals, and there was greater frequency of left ventricular dyssynergy in those patients with collaterals supplying the distal left anterior descending coronary artery.

In addition, the possible importance of the nature of collaterals to the left anterior descending coronary artery in these patients with matched three-vessel coronary artery disease was examined (25). Patients with intercoronary collaterals (right coronary artery to the left anterior descending coronary artery) were

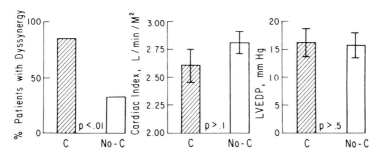

Fig. 3. The relation of the presence of coronary collateral vessels to regional ventricular contraction pattern, cardiac output, and left ventricular filling pressure in patients with severe obstruction of the left anterior descending coronary artery and equivalent disease of the remaining major coronary vessels. In one group of patients, collateral vessels to the diseased left anterior descending coronary artery were present (*hatched bars, C*) in contrast to their absence (*white bars, no-C*) in the other patients.

compared to patients with intracoronary (bridge) collaterals (proximal left anterior descending coronary artery to the distal left anterior descending coronary artery). There was no significant difference in the apparent benefit provided by collaterals between inter- and intracoronary collaterals analyzed by variables of cardiac performance: left ventricular end-diastolic pressure, cardiac index, and ventricular synergy. Thus, again, the fundamental determinant of abnormalities of cardiac function appeared to be the presence of left anterior descending disease itself, with no significant influence by collateral vessels.

CONCLUSIONS

The foregoing observations on the role of the coronary collateral circulation suggest that these vessels do not appear to provide a major degree of selective protection in coronary artery disease in terms of left ventricular function, abnormal regional ventricular contraction, occurrence of myocardial infarction, and symptoms and objective evidence of ventricular ischemia. These findings concerning the limited value of collaterals in clinical coronary artery disease are derived even when the extent of coronary artery disease among patients is matched as equally as possible by selective coronary angiography.

More recently, we have extended these observations to the electrical activity of the heart. Thus, the frequency of ventricular extrasystoles and the occurrence of their more serious forms (multiple, multifocal, and premature beats on T waves) are not influenced by the presence of coronary collateral vessels (28).

Consistent with this view of the lack of significance of collateral vessels in coronary disease is current clinical information which suggests that clinical improvement derived from exercise training programs by angina patients is not associated with coronary collateralization (29–32). Rather, the beneficial effect of exercise training is derived from extracardiac mechanisms affecting the peripheral circulation and function of skeletal muscles, allowing greater physical activity with less myocardial mechanical effort.

On the other hand, it is important to point out that these observations suggesting a limited role of the myocardial collateral circulation are not conclusive. Thus, the patients reported here were preselected for coronary arteriography necessary for clinical management. Further, selective angiography may not allow complete definition of collaterals, and the extent of coronary artery disease itself is difficult to quantitate precisely by this technique. Also, no information regarding blood flow in these collateral channels is provided. Nevertheless, it is noteworthy that no demonstrable benefit from collateral vessels could be shown by these clinical analyses.

The possibility should be recognized that these collateral channels may be promoted by means other than the factors evaluated in the present study, such as the opening of collaterals on the mechanical basis of increasing aortic diastolic blood pressure by counterpulsation techniques (33). In addition, some studies in experimental and clinical occlusive disease have indicated nitroglycerin-induced dilation of coronary collaterals with improved flow to ischemic areas conveyed by these auxiliary channels (34–37). Also, the rapidity of coronary obstruction appears to be important in determining the degree of collateral function; infarctions are infrequent and small with gradual occlusion over several days, whereas sudden ligation leads to large areas of necrosis and high mortality in dogs (38).

It is of interest that other workers have made similar observations concerning the limited benefit of coronary collaterals in patients with coronary artery disease (39–46). Thus, the presence or number of collaterals did not favorably influence left ventricular function, level of physical activity, duration of angina pectoris, and frequency of previous myocardial infarction (39–42). Also, metered coronary blood flow intraoperatively was diminished equally in obstructed coronary arteries with or without collaterals (46). Although collaterals did not protect against active ischemia as assessed by the Master two-step (39) and treadmill stress tests (42), death was perhaps less frequent with coronary episodes of myocardial ischemia and infarction (42). Also, improved survival has been reported in patients with collaterals to their obstructed left anterior descending coronary artery (47).

Present clinical information suggests that coronary collaterals provide a relatively limited protective role in coronary artery disease. These auxiliary vessels appear to be inherently involved in the response to stenosis in the native coronary arterial circulation itself. Further, these channels are most related to the severity of coronary obstruction, and they serve as markers of coronary artery disease. The coronary collateral vessels appear to supply only marginal blood flow in coronary disease, and they likely are incapable of increasing coronary flow adequately to ischemic areas with acute demand of the heart for oxygen. Collateral formation does not appear to represent a major compensatory mechanism within the framework of the natural history of coronary artery disease, thus providing additional benefit by allowing superior cardiac function in comparison to that in patients without collateral vessels. Finally, the coronary collateral circulation may play a small but perhaps critical role in improving survival with acute coronary events.

REFERENCES CITED

1. Tennant, R., and Wiggers, C. J. 1935. Effect of coronary occlusion on myocardial contraction. Amer. J. Physiol. 112:351.
2. Kattus, A. A., and Gregg, D. E. 1959. Some determinants of coronary collateral blood flow in the open-chest dog. Circ. Res. 7:628.
3. Kong, Y., Chen, J. T., Zeft, H. J., Whalen, R. E., and McIntosh, H. D. 1969. Natural history

of experimental coronary occlusion in pigs: A serial cineangiographic study. Amer. Heart J. 77:45.

4. Elliot, E. C., Bloor, C. M., Jones, E. L., Mitchell, W. J., and Gregg, D. E. 1971. Effect of controlled coronary occlusion on collateral circulation in conscious dogs. Amer. J. Physiol. 220:857.

5. Schaper, W., De Brabander, M., and Lewi, P. 1971. DNA synthesis and mitoses in coronary collateral vessels of the dog. Circ. Res. 28:671.

6. Gregg, D. E. 1971. The role and functional significance of collateral vessels. Page 44 *in* R. R. Ross and F. Hoffman, eds. Myocardial ischemia. Excerpta Medica, New York.

7. Schaper, J., Borgers, M., and Schaper, W. 1972. Ultrastructure of ischemia-induced changes in the precapillary anastomotic network of the heart. Amer. J. Cardiol. 29:851.

8. Schlesinger, M. J. 1938. Injection plus dissection study of coronary artery occlusions and anastomoses. Amer. Heart J. 15:528.

9. Blumgart, J. L., Schlesinger, M. J., and Davis, D. L. 1940. Studies on the relation of the clinical manifestations of angina pectoris, coronary thrombosis and myocardial infarction to the pathologic findings. Amer. Heart J. 19:1.

10. Snow, P. J. D., Jones, A. M., and Daber, K. S. 1955. Coronary disease: A pathological study. Brit. Heart J. 17:305.

11. Spain, D. M., Bradess, V. A., Iral, P., and Cruz, A. 1963. Intercoronary anastomotic channels and sudden unexpected death from advanced coronary atherosclerosis. Circulation 27:12.

12. Baroldi, G. 1973. Coronary heart disease: Significance of the morphologic lesions. Amer. Heart J. 85:1.

13. Gensini, G. G., and Da Costa, B. C. 1969. The coronary collateral circulation in living man. Amer. J. Cardiol. 24:393.

14. Rees, J. R. 1969. The myocardial collateral circulation. Brit. Heart J. 31:1.

15. Sheldon, W. C. 1969. On the significance of coronary collaterals. Amer. J. Cardiol. 24:303.

16. James, T. N. 1970. The delivery and distribution of coronary collateral circulation. Chest 58:183.

17. Mason, D. T., Amsterdam, E. Z., Miller, R. R., Hughes, J. L., Bonanno, J. A., Iben, A. B., Hurley, E. J., Massumi, R. A., and Zelis, R. 1971. Consideration of the therapeutic roles of pharmacologic agents, collateral circulation and saphenous vein bypass in coronary artery disease. Amer. J. Cardiol. 28:608.

18. Schaper, W. 1971. The collateral circulation of the heart. American Elsevier, New York.

19. Wells, R. 1972. Microcirculation and coronary blood flow. Amer. J. Cardiol. 29:847.

20. Miller, R., Mason, D. T., Zelis, R., Bonanno, J. A., and Amsterdam, E. A. 1971. Determinants of the coronary collateral circulation in man: Development principally related to severity of regional atherosclerosis. Clin. Res. 19:117.

21. Miller, R. R., Mason, D. T., Zelis, R., Bonanno, J., and Amsterdam, E. A. 1971. The coronary collateral circulation in man: Relation to regional atherosclerosis and evaluation of protective role on clinical course and cardiac function. Clin. Res. 19:328.

22. Miller, R., Mason, D. T., Bonanno, J. A., Zelis, R., and Amsterdam, E. A. 1971. Clinical significance of the coronary collateral circulation: Correlation solely with severity of regional atherosclerosis, abnormal segmental contraction and ventricular dysfunction. Chest 60:299.

23. Miller, R., Salel, A., Bonanno, J., Massumi, R., Zelis, R., Mason, D. T., and Amsterdam, E. A. 1972. The functional significance of the coronary collateral circulation in man. Clin. Res. 20:208.

24. Miller, R., Zelis, R., Mason, D. T., and Amsterdam, E. A. 1971. Relation of coronary collateral vessels to ventricular function in patients with equal extent of coronary artery disease. Circulation 44:202.

25. Miller, R., Mason, D. T., Salel, A., Zelis, R., Massumi, R. A., and Amsterdam, E. A. 1972. Determinants and functional significance of the coronary collateral circulation in patients with coronary artery disease. Amer. J. Cardiol. 29:281.

26. Amsterdam, E. A., Most, A. S., Wolfson, S., Kemp, H. G., and Gorlin, R. 1970. Relation

of degree of angiographically documented coronary artery disease to mortality. Ann. Internal Med. 72:780.

27. Friesinger, G. C., Page, E. E., and Ross, R. S. 1970. Prognostic significance of coronary angiography. Trans. Assoc. Amer. Physicians 83:78.

28. Amsterdam, E. A., Vismara, L., Massumi, R. A., Zelis, R., and Mason, D. T. 1973. Relationship of ventricular ectopic rhythms to angiographically defined coronary artery disease. Conference of Council on Epidemiology, American Heart Association, New Orleans, March 12.

29. Hellerstein, H. K. 1968. Exercise therapy in coronary disease. Bull. N.Y. Acad. Med. 44:1028.

30. Clausen, J. P., Larsen, O. A., and Trap-Jensen, J. 1969. Physical training in the management of coronary artery disease. Circulation 40:143.

31. Kattus, A. A., and Grollman, J. 1972. Patterns of coronary collateral circulation in angina pectoris: Relation to exercise training. Page 352 in H. Russek and B. Zohman, eds. Changing concepts of cardiovascular disease. Williams and Wilkins Co., Baltimore.

32. Kennedy, C. C., Spiekerman, R. E., Lindsay, M. I., Frye, R. L., Mankin, H. T., Cantwell, J. D., and Harbold, N. B. 1973. Evaluation of a one-year graduated exercise program for men with angina pectoris by physiologic studies and coronary arteriography. Amer. J. Cardiol. 31:141.

33. Banas, J. S., Brilla, A., Soroff, H. S., and Levine, J. J. 1972. Evaluation of external counterpulsation for the treatment of severe angina pectoris. Circulation 46(Suppl. 2):74.

34. Fam, W. M., and McGregor, M. 1964. Effect of coronary vasodilator drugs on retrograde flow in areas of chronic myocardial ischemia. Circ. Res. 15:355.

35. Horwitz, L. D., Gorlin, R., Taylor, W. J., and Kemp, H. G. 1971. Effects of nitoglycerin on regional myocardial blood flow in coronary artery disease. J. Clin. Invest. 50:1578.

36. Cohen, M. V., Downey, J. M., Urschel, C. W., Sonnenblick, E. H., and Kirk, E. S. 1973. Enhancement of myocardial contractility by dilation of coronary collaterals. Amer. J. Cardiol. 31:126.

37. Goldstein, R. E., Stinson, E. B., and Epstein, S. E. 1973. Effects of nitroglycerin on coronary collateral function in patients with coronary occlusive disease. Amer. J. Cardiol. 31:135.

38. Schaper, W. 1971. Pathophysiology of coronary circulation. Prog. Cardiov. Dis. 14:275.

39. Most, A. S., Kemp, H. G., and Gorlin, R. 1969. Postexercise electrocardiography in patients with arteriographically documented coronary artery disease. Ann. Internal Med. 71:1043.

40. Helfant, R. H., Kemp, H. G., and Gorlin, R. 1970. Coronary atherosclerosis, coronary collaterals, and their relation to cardiac function. Ann. Internal Med. 73:189.

41. Tuna, N., and Amplatz, K. 1970. The significance of coronary collateral circulation. Coronary arteriographic and electrovectorcardiographic correlations. Amer. J. Cardiol. 26:663.

42. Helfant, R. H., Vokonas, P. S., and Gorlin, R. 1971. Functional importance of the human coronary collateral circulation. New Engl. J. Med. 284:1277.

43. Goldschlager, N., Cake, D., and Cohn, K. 1972. Significance of exercise-induced ventricular arrhythmias. Circulation 46(Suppl. 2):73.

44. Harris, C. N., Kaplan, M. A., Parker, D. P., Aronow, W. S., and Ellestad, M. H. 1972. Anatomic and functional correlates of intercoronary collateral vessels. Amer. J. Cardiol. 30:611.

45. Knoebel, S. B., McHenry, P. L., Phillips, J. F., and Pauletto, F. J. 1972. Coronary collateral circulation and myocardial blood flow reserve. Circulation 46:84.

46. Smith, S. C., Gorlin, R., Herman, M. V., Taylor, W. J., and Collins, J. J. 1972. Myocardial blood flow in man: Effects of coronary collateral circulation and coronary artery bypass surgery. J. Clin. Invest. 51:2556.

47. Moberg, C. H., Webster, J. S., and Sones, F. M. 1972. Natural history of severe proximal coronary disease as defined by cineangiography (200 patients, 7 year followup). Amer. J. Cardiol. 29:282.

Clinical Decisions in Therapy

WHAT CONSTITUTES ADEQUATE MEDICAL THERAPY FOR THE PATIENT WITH ANGINA PECTORIS?

HENRY I. RUSSEK

Ideally, any rational approach to treatment of ischemic heart disease should be directed toward three major objectives: 1) alleviation of the symptoms of disability, 2) prevention of myocardial ischemia, and 3) control of the underlying atherosclerotic process. Despite the existing potential for achieving these goals in angina pectoris, therapy for this syndrome is frequently no better today than it was a century ago when physicians attempted to deal with this problem. This anachronism is a consequence of a lack of knowledge or of faith in currently available methods of treatment. Moreover, the unfortunate consequences of "casual" rather than "optimal" medical management no longer can be estimated solely from the inadequacy of the medical regimen. These consequences have been compounded further in recent years by the morbidity and mortality of revascularization procedures needlessly undertaken in patients for whom proper trial of intensive medical therapy may have proved more effective and less hazardous (1–3). Thus, it is in the hope of avoiding such pitfalls and of establishing proper criteria for patient selection for surgical intervention that the physician carefully must examine the question: "What constitutes adequate medical therapy for the patient with angina pectoris?"

RELIEF OF SYMPTOMS

Removal of Precipitating and Contributing Factors

Most patients with classical angina pectoris improve or become asymptomatic simply as the result of reassurance, the establishment of a good doctor-patient relationship, and the use of nitroglycerin when indicated. In some, the elimination of contributing factors and the application of measures designed to reduce the work of the heart also may be essential for adequate control. Thus, effective prophylaxis often is established by reduction in the speed of walking, allowance of more time for dressing in the morning, a change in the manner of transportation, avoidance of overloading the stomach and of walking after meals or in cold weather, and by elimination of emotional outbursts, prolonged conversation, straining at stool, or watching competitive sports. Similarly, reduction in weight, correction of hypertension, abstinence from tobacco and stimulants, the resolution of emotional conflicts, and a program of physical reconditioning all may prove to be effective measures for the relief of symptoms.

Effective Use of Antianginal Drugs

When a change in habits is not feasible or when avoidance of precipitating and contributory factors has not brought satisfactory improvement despite the appropriate use of nitroglycerin, the syndrome must not be classified prematurely as "intractable." In such cases, earnest effort to reduce the frequency and severity of anginal episodes by means of other potent therapeutic agents, notably the long-acting nitrates and propranolol, may prove singularly successful. Failure to prescribe these drugs, particularly in combination (3–7), or their administration in an ineffectual manner frequently has been responsible for the abandonment of medical therapy in favor of surgical intervention. It is not yet recognized widely that even when propranolol and sublingual isosorbide dinitrate, respectively, produce insignificant results, the response to their combined administration may be strikingly beneficial (3–7), as shown in Figure 1. Thus, the trial of either agent without success or of both improperly administered cannot be accepted as evidence of the failure of optimal medical therapy. The

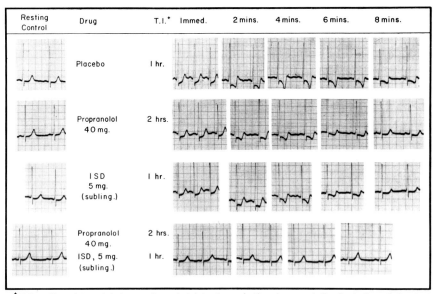

[+] T.I. - *Time interval between the administration of the drug and the beginning of the test.*

Fig. 1. Comparative EKG responses (lead V_s) to standard exercise (26 trips) following propranolol and/or isosorbide dinitrate (*ISD*) (R.D., 65-year-old male). It can be seen that although propranolol and isosorbide dinitrate were ineffective when used alone, striking response was obtained from combined administration.

unique synergistic phenomenon observed when propranolol is administered in combination with sublingual isosorbide dinitrate is the net result of the summation of favorable effects accompanied by cancellation of negating actions attending the use of the respective drugs (3–7). For this synergism to be obtained, propranolol must be administered in sufficient dosage three or four times a day to achieve a resting heart rate of 55–60 beats/min in each case. The effective dose may vary from as little as 10 mg to 160 mg three or four times daily and can be determined only by careful titration in the individual patient. The prescription of a fixed dose for treatment of all subjects (8) obviously indicates a lack of understanding of the rationale of therapy. The use of a *sublingual* long-acting nitrate is preferred because *oral* nitrates *in standard dosage* are relatively ineffectual as a result of rapid degradation in the liver. Much larger doses of oral preparations than those now commonly used are necessary to escape hepatic degradation and to produce a significant therapeutic response (Fig. 2). The most useful of the sublingual long-acting nitrates is isosorbide dinitrate administered in the range of 2.5–10 mg according to tolerance and response; however, erythrityl tetranitrate, which is associated with a higher incidence of headache, also may be effective.

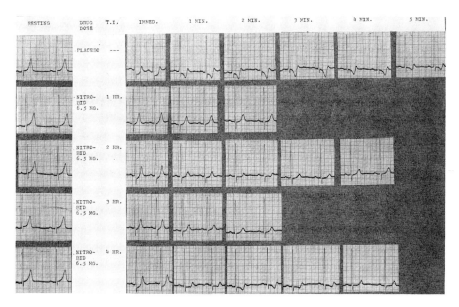

Fig. 2. Comparative electrocardiographic responses (lead V_s) to standard exercise following placebo or a sustained action preparation of nitroglycerin (Nitro-BID). Despite failure of response to 2.5-mg doses of Nitro-BID, note favorable response to 6.5-mg dosage of the preparation. Such findings indicate the ability of nitrates in large doses to escape degradation in the liver.

Propranolol-Nitrate Synergism:
Coordination of Therapy with Chronology of Symptoms

Consideration of the time of onset and duration of action of propranolol and sublingual isosorbide dinitrate (ISDN), respectively, helps to provide an optimal formula for their administration in a combined treatment program. The following facts must be kept in mind in establishing a schedule for therapy:

1. The patient's most vulnerable period is following the ingestion of food.

2. Propranolol requires 30–60 minutes for therapeutic effect, while ISDN is active within 5 minutes.

3. Propranolol in a single dose has a duration of action of 4–5 hours, while ISDN sublingually exerts its influence for only 1.5–2 hours.

In order to provide the longest period of maximal prophylaxis during physical stress, the following routine is recommended:

1. The patient is instructed to rest for at least half an hour after each meal whenever possible.

2. The dose of propranolol is administered before each meal, so that the drug is fully active on the resumption of activity following the postprandial rest period.

3. Isosorbide dinitrate is taken sublingually 5 minutes before the termination of the rest period following each meal.

Given in this manner, both drugs become active at about the time that physical exertion is resumed, and no portion of the prophylactic effect is wasted during the sedentary dining period. Since ISDN tapers in its effect after 1.5–2 hours, it should be taken again between meals by those engaged in continuous activity or before any contemplated exertion by those who have no established routine of work or play. If this practice is not followed, it is evident that only the limited benefits from propranolol may be available to the patient during certain periods of activity when maximal protection may be indicated.

Avoidance of Side-Effects of Beta-Blockade

Side-effects from therapy are rarely serious. Some patients complain of tiredness in the legs, light-headedness, or diarrhea and, rarely, syncope. Marked bradycardia or postural hypotension occasionally may be associated with dizziness, weakness, or faintness. All of these manifestations frequently respond to adjustment in dosage. Shortness of breath or overt evidence of congestive heart failure occur occasionally, but after digitalization and the use of diuretics, propranolol-nitrate therapy generally may be resumed with safety. Careful attention to body weight may provide a subtle clue to impending congestive heart failure. Because of the hazard of bronchospasm, therapy generally is avoided in patients with bronchial asthma.

Intractability Caused by Improper Choice of Drugs

As has been indicated, one of the principal causes of intractability in angina pectoris unfortunately often resides with the attending physician himself. The common reliance on so-called sustained action oral formulations, which are relatively ineffectual in recommended dosage, rather than on potent, sublingual, long-acting nitrates is a common cause of failure. Moreover, even when potent antianginal drugs are employed, it is fundamental that their action be permitted to coincide in time with the known pattern of occurrence of the anginal episodes in the individual patient.

**Removal of Physiologic,
Emotional, and Other Noncoronary Causes**

Angina pectoris also may become refractory to treatment primarily as a result of physiologic or emotional disturbance, some additional cardiovascular problem, or complicating noncoronary disease. Marked intensification of myocardial ischemia may result when any one of these factors augments the coronary-myocardial imbalance already imposed by coronary atherosclerosis. Thus, resistance to usual treatment may ensue from recurrent paroxysmal tachycardia or bradycardia, from hypoxia associated with congestive heart failure, and from progressive hypertension or valvular heart disease, notably aortic stenosis. A relatively mild angina also may be transformed into an intractable problem by prolonged emotional distress, anger, or conflict, and by anemia, infection, hyperthyroidism, or obstructive prostatic hypertrophy. On the other hand, substantial improvement may follow corrective measures such as antiarrhythmic therapy, digitalis, antihypertensive drugs, the resolution of emotional conflicts, replacement of blood loss, antibiotics, or surgery. Consequently, for optimal therapy in any given case of intractable angina pectoris, the physician must consider not only the probable status of organic changes in the coronary system, but also the possible role of complicating cardiac, noncardiac, and environmental factors.

Hospitalization

When the severity of symptoms has incapacitated the patient to a major degree despite the prudent use of potent antianginal agents, it has been accepted practice to institute a broad therapeutic regimen of coordinated measures designed primarily to correct the noncoronary factors contributing to the intractability of angina. In brief, this consists of a period of bed rest in hospital to ensure a reduction in physical activity and isolation from stressful environment; a bland, low-calorie, low-fat diet; abstinence from tobacco, coffee, and alcohol; and the use of sedatives, nitrates such as nitroglycerin and isosorbide dinitrate, and digitalis, if indicated. If propranolol in combination with nitrate therapy has not yet been prescribed, hospitalization affords an opportunity to titrate carefully the optimal doses of the respective drugs. With the resolution of conflicts, adjustments in interpersonal relationships, or psychotherapy, improvement often develops, and dramatic relief sometimes may ensue.

Intensive Therapy for Accelerated
Angina and Impending Myocardial Infarction

Similar management is usually remarkably effective when a sudden reduction in coronary reserve produces a characteristic alteration in the usual pattern of the anginal syndrome. In these cases, symptoms become refractory to usual treatment as the result of a recent anatomic change characterized by partial or complete occlusion of a coronary artery without infarction or evident subendocardial necrosis. The episode of discomfort frequently becomes more prolonged and more severe, occurring at rest and even without obvious cause. It may occur especially upon recumbency, with some degree of relief on sitting or standing. It may occur more frequently and with less and less provocation, so that rest or nitroglycerin or both may produce little or no relief. In these cases, viability of heart muscle may be maintained by collateral circulation, despite the critical level of coronary reserve. Physical and emotional rest, reduction in myocardial oxygen consumption, and improvement in regional coronary blood flow are crucial factors in management. The combined administration of propranolol and sublingual ISDN in the manner outlined frequently provides the key to success when all other measures have failed. In a series of 34 consecutive cases, such therapy not only has proved strikingly effective in the control of symptoms but has been followed by sustained improvement without a single hospital mortality (unpublished observations). Moreover, on repeated occasions, patients with impending infarction for whom immediate bypass surgery was already under consideration have become asymptomatic following the first dose of propranolol in combination with ISDN and have maintained such progress on continued treatment (unpublished observations). It seems clear, therefore, that surgery for accelerated angina and impending infarction cannot be justified without initial trial of intensive medical therapy which includes the prudent use of beta-blockade in combination with nitrate therapy.

PREVENTION OF MYOCARDIAL ISCHEMIA

With the amelioration of symptoms under medical management, it commonly is assumed by the practicing physician that recurrent myocardial ischemia has been checked and its dangers averted. The fallacy in this presumption should be evident from the frequency with which classical ischemic electrocardiographic patterns are observed in the absence of pain in anginal patients monitored during exercise stress. Such evidence of ischemia may be observed not only in anginal patients who are asymptomatic during therapy or during spontaneous periods of remission and in patients who have been without complaint following myocardial infarction, but also in asymptomatic subjects without clinical disease. In these cases, it is clear that pathophysiologic abnormalities are accompanying the activities of daily living in the absence of overt manifestations. Such subclinical myocardial alterations would be less disturbing if they were not known to possess the potential for triggering electrophysiologic disturbances predisposing to serious arrhythmias and sudden death. Since the majority of sudden coronary death patients have had a previously known history of cardiac disease and often were free of symptoms for a period preceding their demise, the need for prophylactic control of even subclinical ischemic episodes is strongly suggested. Consequently, while the relief of symptoms still remains a major objective of therapy, the persistence of ischemic patterns in standard exercise-electrocardiographic tests, despite amelioration or disappearance of angina during treatment, would appear to dictate the need for a more comprehensive approach with appropriate drugs and other measures. Thus, the adequacy of therapy and the index of benefit can best be determined when the relief of pain is viewed against the background of the ischemia which has caused it.

From these considerations, it would seem that exercise-electrocardiographic tests are indicated in all patients with angina pectoris when feasible, in order to determine whether or not optimal therapy has been achieved. With such an approach, limited benefits from nitroglycerin or long-acting nitrates may be converted to striking response when these agents are employed in combination with propranolol for their synergistic interaction. Similarly, these tests may underscore the need for more diligent attention to aggravating but reversible factors such as obesity, hypertension, diabetes, tobacco consumption, and other noncoronary influences.

CONTROL OF ATHEROSCLEROSIS

The chief risk factors in coronary heart disease generally are considered to be a positive heredity, high-fat diet, hypercholesterolemia, high blood pressure, emotional stress, diabetes, cigaret smoking, obesity, and lack of exercise. In Western society, atherosclerosis begins as a pediatric disorder, so that by the time the disease becomes clinically manifest, treatment is in large measure focused on the end result of a disease process rather than on its prophylaxis. Nevertheless, there appears to be justification for efforts directed at the retardation of the inexorable progression of the disease, at least in the young and mature adult and even in the patient of middle age. When angina pectoris occurs in these age groups, the elimination of all risk factors in the individual case would appear to be a worthwhile goal. Thus, a regimen designed to achieve optimal weight and to correct hyperlipidemia, hypertension, and diabetes should be seriously pursued. The resolution of stressful life patterns without compromising the zest for living, graduated exercise, and abstinence from tobacco and stimulants are also measures worthy of application. Whether useful or not in slowing the progression of atherosclerosis, such approaches are of undisputed value in reducing myocardial oxygen consumption and anginal symptoms and therefore warrant intelligent application, particularly in refractory cases.

On the other hand, it seems equally apparent that while aggressive medical management in the treatment of angina pectoris is a desirable objective in most cases, for some patients such an approach may be self-defeating. The physician with keen insight and sound judgment has no difficulty in recognizing, for example, that little can be expected from therapy which deprives the elderly of the already dwindling pleasures which they possess in the contracted life space of old age. Yet it is not uncommon to encounter patients in their middle or late seventies who have been conditioned by their physicians to be fearful of ingesting an occasional egg or a scoop of ice cream. Obviously compromises should be made even in the young when the "cure" is viewed as worse than the disease.

DISCUSSION

Recent advances have made it evident that the therapy of angina pectoris no longer can be considered to begin and end with the use of nitroglycerin. Nevertheless, scores of patients currently undergoing revascularization surgery have been found to have had little or no prior medical management, except perhaps for the use of nitroglycerin and the advice to "take it easy." A recent survey of patients admitted to hospital for bypass surgery actually has shown that more than 50% had previously received no other antianginal agent but nitroglycerin and that even this drug frequently had been prescribed only to abort an attack rather than to prevent it (unpublished observations). In many instances, little effort had been expended by patient or physician to eliminate either precipitating factors for angina pectoris or risk factors for atherosclerosis. Such "casual" treatment of angina pectoris frequently fails not only to provide relief of symptoms but also to correct underlying myocardial ischemia and its associated hemodynamic, metabolic, and electrophysiologic abnormalities. Indeed, even when angina has been controlled in this manner, the appearance of ischemic patterns in standard exercise-electrocardiographic tests provides strong indication for more intensive and effectual therapy. Since electrophysiologic disturbances evoked in this way eventually may trigger serious arrhythmias and sudden death, the physician no longer can remain secure with the relief of symptoms as his sole objective of therapy.

In recent years, the introduction of propranolol and its use in conjunction with isosorbide dinitrate sublingually has provided antianginal and anti-ischemic prophylaxis never imagined possible. While propranolol *alone* is helpful in many patients with angina pectoris, the improvement in exercise tolerance resulting from its use is often only modest, and in a large segment of patients is negligible. Consequently, unless the drug is used synergistically with a long-acting nitrate such as isosorbide dinitrate sublingually, only very limited benefits may be available. Unfortunately, this fact either is being ignored by a large proportion of physicians or remains unknown to them. Paracelsus (9) in the 16th century pointed out that the same drug can be inert, poisonous, or therapeutic, depending on how it is used and the dosage in which it is given. This characterization of therapeutic agents is certainly most applicable to the administration of propranolol. The remarkable synergism between beta-adrenergic blocking agents and the nitrates is a consequence of the summation of favorable responses coupled with the fortuitous cancelling out of negating actions of the respective drugs. Thus, even when each agent evokes poor response when used separately in patients with severe angina pectoris, combined administration may be surprisingly effective (Fig. 1). Such medicinal therapy in conjunction with a comprehensive program of medical management actually has been shown to have improved markedly the quality of life in more than 90% of a series of 133 patients with severe and refractory forms of angina pectoris studied prospectively over a period of five years (3). Moreover, the annual fatality rate in those of the series manifesting good left ventricular function was only 1.2%, a mortality figure not unlike that for the same age group in the general population.

This experience makes it clear that excellent medical therapy now exists for the treatment of angina pectoris even in its severest forms. To achieve optimal results, the physician must act aggressively with enthusiasm and a high degree of intensity of purpose not unlike that displayed by his surgical colleagues. "Casual" therapy of angina pectoris, like "casual" therapy of hypertension, represents in most instances a disservice to the patient. A full range of treatment should be instituted that is aimed not only at the relief of symptoms, but also at the prevention of myocardial ischemia and the control of the underlying atherosclerotic process. Too often, striking clinical improvement has followed the application of such therapy after unsuccessful surgical revascularization. The same effort prior to surgery obviously might have eliminated the need for this heroic step. Success in treatment depends on an intimate knowledge of the nature and life style of the individual patient, of the diseases which afflict him, and of the prudent use of drugs and other measures. It is only when treatment has been carried out intensively in this manner that a valid decision can be reached in the individual case as to the possible merit of surgical revascularization.

REFERENCES CITED

1. Russek, H. I. 1969. Medical versus surgical therapy for angina pectoris. Dis. Chest 55:269.
2. Russek, H. I. 1970. Medical versus surgical therapy in angina pectoris. Geriatrics 25:93.
3. Russek, H. I. 1972. Prognosis in severe angina pectoris: Medical versus surgical therapy. Amer. Heart. J. 83:6.
4. Russek, H. I. 1967. Propranolol and isosorbide dinitrate synergism in angina pectoris. Amer. J. Med. Sci. 254:406.
5. Russek, H. I. 1968. Propranolol and isosorbide dinitrate synergism in angina pectoris. Amer. J. Cardiol. 21:44.
6. Russek, H. I. 1969. New dimension in angina pectoris therapy. Geriatrics 24:81.
7. Russek, H. I. 1970. Intractable angina pectoris. Med. Clin. N. Amer. 53:2.
8. Aronow, W. S., and Kaplan, M. A. 1969. Propranolol combined with isosorbide dinitrate versus placebo in angina pectoris. New Engl. J. Med. 280:847.
9. Paracelsus paraphrased by Erik Jorpes. 1965. *In* I. M. Vigran, ed. Clinical anticoagulant therapy. Lea & Febiger, Philadelphia.

Acute Myocardial Infarction

Changing Patterns
in Acute Coronary Care

BRADYCARDIA, ATROPINE, AND NITROGLYCERINE IN ACUTE MYOCARDIAL INFARCTION

STEPHEN E. EPSTEIN, DAVID R. REDWOOD, KENNETH M. KENT,
ELDON R. SMITH, and ROBERT E. GOLDSTEIN

Approximately 50% of all deaths from acute myocardial infarction (AMI) occur during the first two hours after onset of symptoms as diagrammed in Figure 1 (1, 2). As a result, approximately two-thirds of patients with AMI die prior to receiving medical attention (2–5). On the basis of data gathered by the mobile coronary care unit, it appears that most of these deaths result from ventricular fibrillation (6). Clearly, then, any intervention that can successfully modify or eliminate those factors that predispose to ventricular fibrillation during the prehospital phase of acute myocardial infarction will have a profound influence on the natural history of coronary artery disease.

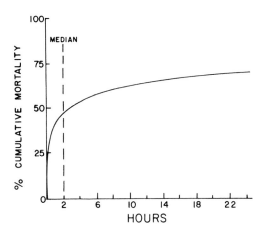

Fig. 1. Cumulative percentage mortality in the first 24 hours after the onset of symptoms of myocardial infarction [modified from Fulton et al. (2)].

BRADYCARDIA AS A RISK FACTOR

In this section we will assess bradycardia as a risk factor in the prehospital phase of acute myocardial infarction.

One of the important observations evolving from the early mobile coronary care unit experience is that bradycardia occurs quite commonly during AMI

101

within the first few hours of the onset of the attack. The incidence averages about 25% for patients seen within the first hour of symptoms (7, 8), but is even higher in patients seen within the first 30 minutes (7) (see Fig. 2). The relatively frequent occurrence of bradycardia at a time when patients are at greatest risk from ventricular fibrillation (VF) raises the question whether bradycardia predisposes to VF during the prehospital phase of acute myocardial infarction. This possibility was reinforced by several clinical and experimental observations. For example, it has been shown experimentally that a wider range of ventricular refractory periods is present in contiguous areas of myocardium during bradycardia than during faster heart rates (9), a finding believed to be associated with a greater propensity for the development of reentrant arrhythmias. Moreover, the vulnerability of the ventricle to fibrillate has been reported to increase with bradycardia (9). Studies on the occurrence of arrhythmias during AMI also have been reported that are apparently compatible with these electrophysiologic studies. Thus the incidence of ventricular ectopic beats occurring during acute myocardial ischemia in the open-chest anesthetized dog was inversely related to the ventricular rate (10); the incidence of ventricular tachycardia in hospitalized patients was found to be higher in patients with bradycardia (11); ventricular ectopic activity present during bradycardia may be abolished following atropine-induced tachycardia (11, 12). In addition, several other observations implicate bradycardia as a cause of the high mortality in the early phases of AMI: an optimum cardiac output and arterial pressure response

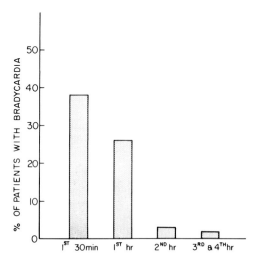

Fig. 2. Prevalence of sinus bradycardia at initial examination related to time after onset of symptoms [plotted from data of Adgey et al. (18)].

in patients with acute myocardial infarction and complete heart block occur at a paced rate of 100 beats/min (13); and, finally, bradycardia is not infrequently associated with a lowered arterial pressure (8, 14), a finding that has been shown experimentally to increase the ischemic insult during acute coronary occlusion in the dog (15, 16).

Thus, bradycardia is a commonly occurring, apparently unstable rhythm that might predispose to arrhythmic death in the prehospital phase of AMI. On the basis of this evidence, it has been suggested that atropine should be administered to every patient with an acute myocardial infarction who has bradycardia, whether he is within the confines of the hospital (17) or prior to hospitalization (18).

As indicated above, the case favoring the use of atropine in the patient with bradycardia and AMI appears to be supported by a sizeable number of independent observations. When critically examined, however, the evidence is found to lack convincing documentation. For example, what is the evidence that patients with acute myocardial infarction and associated bradycardia have an increased mortality? As we reported elsewhere (19), a review of the literature and tabulation of all of the available series does not bear out this impression. Thus, pooled data indicate that 346 individuals with untreated sinus bradycardia (mortality rate 13%) fared at least as well as the remaining 2,012 individuals without sinus bradycardia (mortality rate 28%). In four of these studies where more detailed information was offered (20–23), the pooled data again indicated that mortality rate in patients in sinus rhythm with heart rates of 60 or less was not higher (and even tended to be slightly lower) than that in patients in sinus rhythm with rates between 61 and 99. Moreover, in a recently published, well-documented study of 735 patients, 152 patients with sinus bradycardia (76% of whom did not receive atropine*) had only a 6% mortality (24). This figure was significantly lower than the 15% mortality observed in patients with heart rates between 60 and 100 (Fig. 3). There obviously may be selection factors influencing these data; thus, it is possible that the most seriously ill patients with bradycardia died before being admitted to the hospital. It is also possible that the patients with bradycardia had smaller, less serious infarcts, and if they all were treated with atropine, their mortality might have been even lower. Nevertheless, the point to be made is that there is no convincing evidence to suggest that bradycardia in the hospitalized patient predisposes to a higher mortality; if anything, the data suggest a diminished risk.

Although studies using the experimental animal have obvious drawbacks when attempts are made to apply the results to disease in man, there are many situations in which it is extremely difficult or impossible to derive the essential

---

* R. M. Norris, personal communication

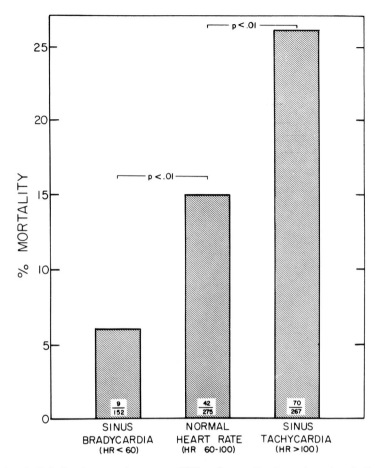

Fig. 3. Relation between heart rate (*HR*) and mortality in patients hospitalized with acute myocardial infarction [plotted from data of Norris et al. (24)]. Numerator of the fraction at the bottom of each bar is the number of deaths in each group; the denominator is the total number of patients in each group.

information from clinical experiences. Certainly, many important practical problems confront the investigator attempting to study the early phase of acute myocardial infarction in man. As a result, several attempts have been made to evaluate the role of bradycardia during AMI in the experimental animal. Thus, Han and co-workers (10) originally showed that slower heart rates during experimental acute myocardial ischemia are associated with an increased incidence of premature ventricular contractions (PVC's). This study served as an important impetus to the hypothesis that bradycardia is deleterious during acute myocardial infarction. However, the significance of these findings is severely restricted

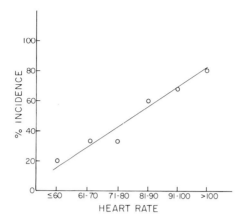

Fig. 4. Total incidence of occlusion arrhythmias in control animals as a function of heart rate measured after 10 minutes of coronary occlusion. Each open circle represents the arrhythmia incidence of the corresponding 10 beats/min subgroups shown on the horizontal axis. Reproduced by permission of Circulation (26).

by the conditions of study: observations were made mainly within the first one to three minutes of onset of acute coronary occlusion in an open-chest, anesthetized dog (with the attendant increase in circulating catecholamines, faster control heart rates, etc.).

A somewhat different picture emerges from the experimental observations of Scherlag and co-workers (25). These investigators, following their animals (open-chest anesthetized dogs) over a slightly longer time period, demonstrated that ventricular slowing produced by vagal stimulation caused *disappearance* of ventricular ectopic beats. These same investigators also reported that when hearts were paced rapidly (200 beats/min), the incidence of ventricular arrhythmias during coronary occlusion increased. Interpretation of these findings obviously is complicated by the possibility that the very fast paced heart rate was particularly deleterious. Moreover, their study was not specifically designed to answer the question of whether slow heart rates during acute coronary occlusion predispose to serious ventricular arrhythmias and death.

In an attempt to employ an experimental model more closely related to acute myocardial infarction as it occurs in man, we produced acute coronary occlusion in the closed-chest sedated dog (26). Coronary occlusion was effected by injecting saline solution into an exteriorized Silastic tube connected to a balloon cuff that had been placed around the left anterior descending coronary artery (LAD) 10–14 days prior to the study. This model was chosen so that the arrhythmic tendencies of a more physiologic range of heart rate could be evaluated in the absence of the reflex and humoral changes that unavoidably are present in the open-chest dog. Using this closed-chest model, we found that the

incidence of ventricular arrhythmias observed during 3–4 hours of acute coronary occlusion was *directly* related to the spontaneous heart rate measured 10
minutes after onset of coronary artery occlusion (Fig. 4). Thus, slower heart
rates were associated with a considerably lower incidence of arrhythmias than
were faster rates.

In the above analysis, as well as in most other previous studies, the arrhyth-
mogenic tendencies of any given condition (i.e., bradycardia) or the antiarrhythmic effects of an intervention (i.e., atropine) generally have been determined by
assessing the frequency of all types of ventricular arrhythmias. While this
approach may be valid, there is increasing evidence that not all types of
ventricular ectopic rhythms predispose to a fatal outcome. Therefore, we might
ask what is the evidence that the type of PVC's or ventricular tachycardia that
occurs during bradycardia is associated with a high incidence of VF and death?
For example, it is not at all uncommon (27–29) to observe a patient with an
idioventricular rhythm ("slow ventricular tachycardia") occurring during an AMI
(Fig. 5). However, this rhythm rarely leads to a fatal outcome, a finding
suggesting to some observers that this type of ventricular arrhythmia need not be
treated (27–29). In this regard, we recently analyzed the type of arrhythmias
that occurred prior to the onset of VF when acute coronary artery occlusion was
produced in the closed-chest unanesthetized dog (26, 30). Of 127 dogs studied,
34 developed VF. Prior to fibrillation, all 34 dogs had ectopic ventricular beats
that followed a preceding beat by less than 0.43 sec (equivalent to a heart rate of
140 beats/min); VF never appeared in the 21 dogs that had only those PVC's or
ventricular tachycardia with longer R-R intervals. Attesting to the malignancy of
the closely coupled arrhythmias was the finding that of dogs developing this
type of ectopic activity, 43% (34/81) eventually developed VF.

Using the above data, we classified ventricular arrhythmias into benign
(coupling intervals $\geqslant 0.43$ sec) and malignant (coupling intervals < 0.43 sec). We

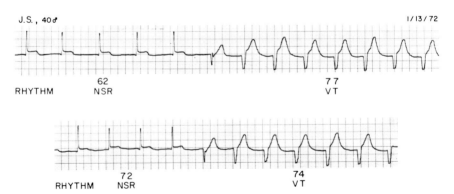

Fig. 5. Idioventricular rhythm appearing in a patient with acute myocardial infarction.

then explored the interaction of heart rate and ventricular arrhythmias by analyzing both the frequency and type of ventricular arrhythmias observed during acute coronary artery occlusion (26). Twelve animals exhibited brady-cardia (heart rate below 60) at some time during coronary artery occlusion, while 15 other dogs had heart rates remaining between 60 and 110. Of the bradycardia group, only 16% had benign arrhythmias, and the remaining 84% had no ventricular arrhythmias at all. In marked contrast, 73% of dogs without bradycardia had either malignant PVC's, malignant ventricular tachycardia, or VF. Thus, these results, in addition to those previously cited, suggest that slower heart rates do *not* favor the development of serious ventricular arrhythmias in our canine model. On the contrary, slow heart rates seem to exert a protective action.

To examine the effects of more pronounced and consistent bradycardia, we electrically stimulated the vagus nerves of 24 dogs to maintain ventricular rate between 40 and 60 during a one-hour period of LAD occlusion (26). The results in this group were compared to those in a similarly treated control group in

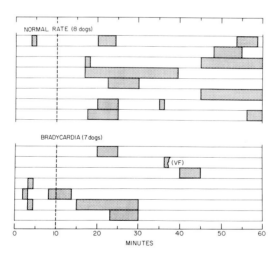

Fig. 6. Time course of serious arrhythmia (in this context, PVC's and VT with coupling interval < 0.43 sec) in those eight dogs of the normal heart group (*upper panel*) and those seven dogs of the bradycardia group which showed serious arrhythmia at any time during coronary occlusion. Shaded portions of each horizontal bar depict times when serious arrhythmias were present in each individual dog. The vertical dashed line indicates the 10 minute point when heart rate control was initiated. One animal died (*VF*) after 36 minutes of occlusion. Of the six dogs in the bradycardia group alive between 45 and 60 minutes, none had serious arrhythmias, in contrast to 5 of 8 of the control group. Moreover, one animal in the bradycardia group (*lower panel, fourth from top*) had serious arrhythmia before but not after vagal bradycardia. In a second animal (*lower panel, fifth from top*), serious arrhythmia disappeared soon after initiating vagal bradycardia. Reproduced by permission of Circulation (26).

which heart rate was maintained between 80 and 100. Once again, the results indicated that bradycardia per se did not predispose to serious ventricular arrhythmias. In fact, serious arrhythmias tended to disappear in the dogs with bradycardia during the last 15 minutes of occlusion, while arrhythmias in the dogs with normal heart rates tended to persist (Fig. 6). Thus, while there were no statistically significant differences in the incidence of arrhythmias shortly after the onset of occlusion, after 45 minutes of occlusion the proportion of dogs with serious ventricular arrhythmias in the bradycardia group was significantly lower than in the group with normal heart rates.

EFFECTS OF ATROPINE ON ARRHYTHMIAS

In this section we will consider the effects of atropine on arrhythmias occurring during acute coronary occlusion.

If bradycardia does not predispose to serious ventricular arrhythmias, what is the evidence that speeding the heart rate with atropine is effective in abolishing those arrhythmias which, if untreated, might lead to VF or death?

The available evidence is based mainly on the clinical and experimental demonstration that atropine can effectively abolish ventricular ectopic activity as heart rate is increased (11, 12). However, no analysis has ever been performed on the relative efficacy of atropine in abolishing the more malignant, close-coupled PVC's. To evaluate this question, two experiments were conducted in the closed-chest model of acute coronary occlusion described above. In the first

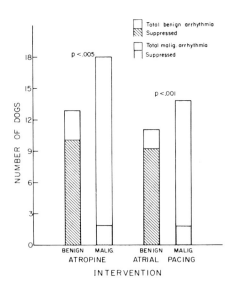

Fig. 7. Suppression of benign and malignant (*malig.*) arrhythmias.

(30), treatment was begun after arrhythmias appeared: they were treated either with atropine (in progressively increasing doses until the arrhythmias disappeared or a heart rate of 120 beats/min was reached) or with atrial pacing at a rate of 120 beats/min. Surprisingly, we found that while increasing heart rate with either atropine or pacing was extremely effective in abolishing what we have termed benign arrhythmias, it was considerably less effective in eliminating the close-coupled arrhythmias frequently associated with the eventual development of VF (Fig. 7). Although atropine or pacing successfully suppressed 19 of 24 benign ventricular arrhythmias, these interventions suppressed a total of only 4 out of 32 arrhythmias characterized as malignant.

In the second experiment, we tested the efficacy of *prophylactically* administered atropine by increasing heart rate during coronary occlusion *before* the onset of arrhythmias (26). Animals with previously implanted LAD balloon

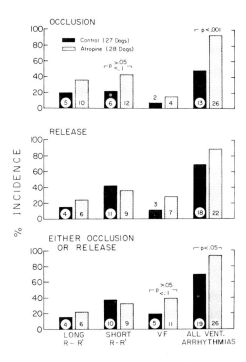

Fig. 8. Incidence of each type of ventricular (*vent.*) arrhythmia occurring during acute coronary occlusion (*upper panel*), following release of occlusion (*middle panel*), and occurring during either occlusion or release periods (*lower panel*). Long R-R′ = minimum coupling interval of PVC's or VT $\geq$ 0.43 sec. Short R-R′ = minimum coupling interval < 0.43 sec. VF = ventricular fibrillation; *HR* = heart rate. Each dog is categorized according to the most serious arrhythmia manifested (Long R-R′ < Short R-R′ < VF). P values are shown for all differences attaining or approaching significance. Number of animals in each category appears at bottom of corresponding bar. Reproduced by permission of Circulation (26).

cuffs were given either atropine (in doses sufficient to raise heart rate by an average of 21 beats/min) or placebo. Atropine administration was begun 10 minutes after cuff inflation and was repeated as often as needed to sustain the rise in heart rate throughout the two-hour observation period. The results are shown in Figure 8. In each of the arrhythmia categories during coronary occlusion (*upper panel*), the 28 atropine-treated animals tended to have more arrhythmias than did the 27 control animals. The overall incidence of arrhythmias during the occlusion period and after release of occlusion (*lower panel*) was significantly greater in the atropine-treated dogs. Furthermore, although the numbers in the VF category were too small to achieve statistical significance, the incidence of VF in the atropine-treated group was twice that of the control group. Thus, there was no evidence that prophylactically administered atropine was protective in our infarction model. Indeed, it appeared to augment the frequency of serious arrhythmias and death.

In summary, when acute anterior myocardial infarction is produced in the normotensive closed-chest dog, sustained bradycardia, even when moderately severe, does not appear to increase the frequency of serious ventricular arrhythmias. Conversely, heart rates above 80 beats/min, either occurring spontaneously or resulting from atropine administration, may be associated with an *augmented* risk of serious ventricular arrhythmia. Direct application of these findings to the clinical setting requires considerable caution because of the many differences between the experimental model and the patient with coronary artery disease. Nonetheless, several examples of serious ventricular arrhythmias, including VF, have been reported to occur very soon after the administration of atropine to patients with myocardial infarction and bradycardia (14, 32–34).

EFFECTS OF ALTERING HEART RATE

In this section we will assess the effects of altering heart rate during coronary occlusion on the degree of ischemic injury and electrical stability of the myocardium.

Since vagally induced bradycardia does not augment serious ventricular arrhythmias in dogs with acute myocardial ischemia, it becomes particularly important to scrutinize the evidence relating to the conclusion that bradycardia exerts deleterious electrophysiologic effects during AMI. It had been demonstrated that both bradycardia (studied in the nonischemic heart) and ischemia independently increase the disparity of the duration of ventricular refractory periods (thereby favoring the development of reentrant arrhythmias) and decrease VF threshold (9, 35). These data have been interpreted as supporting the hypothesis that increasing the heart rate of a patient with AMI and bradycardia will diminish the risk of arrhythmic death (17, 36, 37). Although this might have been true, we questioned the validity of extrapolating data relating to the electrophysiologic effects of bradycardia (obtained in the absence of ischemia) to the ischemic situation. Our skepticism originated from the finding that increasing heart rate, even from rates as slow as 30–40/min, increased the degree of ischemic injury in the closed-chest, conscious dog (38). These latter studies were carried out in the same closed-chest conscious dog model previously described. The degree of myocardial ischemia was estimated by measuring S-T segment elevation recorded from leads attached to 12 myocardial electrodes previously implanted into the area supplied by the LAD. The degree of myocardial ischemia was expressed as the sum of the S-T segment elevations of all 12 myocardial leads in mv (Σ S-T). Heart rate was either increased from control (by atrial pacing or atropine) or decreased by electrical stimulation of the right cervical vagus nerve exposed under local anesthesia. As can be seen in Figure 9, ischemic injury was directly related to heart rate over the entire range of heart rates studied (from 30 to 215 beats/min). Thus, in a normotensive model of acute myocardial infarction, lowering heart rate reduces the degree of myocar-

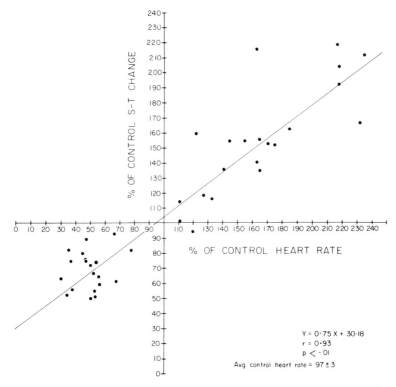

Fig. 9. Effect of alterations in heart rate at normal arterial pressures on the degree of S-T segment elevation at 5 minutes of occlusion. Reproduced by permission of Circulation (16).

dial ischemia. Conversely, increasing heart rate, even in the presence of very slow rates, intensifies ischemic injury.

If the propensity for arrhythmias to develop after coronary occlusion is directly related to the degree of associated myocardial ischemia, then slowing heart rate during acute coronary occlusion might have just the opposite electro-physiologic effects than those observed under nonischemic conditions. To deter-mine whether this hypothesis was valid, we defined the relation of heart rate to disparity of refractory periods and to VF threshold in dogs with and without acute LAD occlusion (39).

Mongrel dogs were anesthetized with sodium pentobarbital. The chest was opened and an adjustable ligature was placed around the LAD approximately 2 cm from its origin. The disparity of refractory periods was determined by measuring the relative refractory periods of eight closely spaced electrodes positioned in the area of distribution of the LAD before and during ischemia. The disparity of refractory periods was defined as the maximum difference of the eight refractory periods measured in each animal during a given intervention. Ventricular fibrillation threshold was defined as the current (in milliamps) required to produce fibrillation by delivering a 200-msec train of 3-msec pulses to the left ventricle during the vulnerable period.

Our results demonstrated that in the nonischemic heart, the maximum difference of refractory periods decreased an average of 30% as heart rate was increased from 60 to 120 beats/min, and decreased a total of 46% as heart rate was increased to 180 (Fig. 10, *left*). However, *opposite* results were obtained in *ischemic* myocardium (Fig. 10, *right*). Thus, as heart rate was increased from 60 to 180 beats/min, the disparity of refractory periods increased 88% ($p < 0.02$).

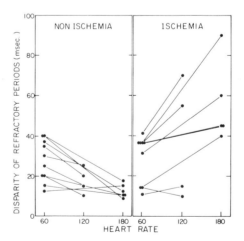

Fig. 10. Influence of heart rate on the disparity of refractory periods in the absence of ischemia (*left*) and during ischemia (*right*). Reproduced by permission of Circulation (39).

To determine the effects of smaller increments in heart rate, another group of animals was studied at heart rates of 50–60, 90, 120, and 180 beats/min. As heart rate was increased from 50–60 to 90 beats/min, disparity of refractory periods increased in three of the six dogs tested; at 120 beats/min, it increased in four of six animals; and at 180 beats/min, large increases occurred in each of the dogs studied.

Similar results were observed when the effects of altering heart rate on VF threshold were determined in the presence and absence of ischemia. In the absence of ischemia, the current required to produce VF showed no consistent relation to heart rate; in the ischemic myocardium, however, VF threshold was inversely related to heart rate (Fig. 11).

From additional studies, we suspected that vagal stimulation, independent of any induced changes in heart rate, might also have an effect on VF threshold. We carried out a series of experiments to test this hypothesis, and Figure 12 demonstrates that when heart rate was held constant at 180 beats/min by ventricular pacing, vagal stimulation increased VF threshold by an average of 180%. Moreover, while the decrease in VF threshold was not consistent when heart rate was increased *by ventricular pacing* from 50 to 90 beats/min, VF threshold consistently decreased in all animals tested (average 37%, $p < 0.05$) when the same increase in heart rate was achieved by reducing the intensity of stimulation of the vagus nerve (Fig. 13).

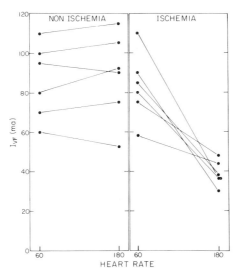

Fig. 11. Influence of heart rate on ventricular fibrillation threshold (I_{VF}) in the absence of ischemia (*left*) and during ischemia (*right*) in six animals. Reproduced by permission of Circulation (39).

114   S. E. Epstein *et al.*

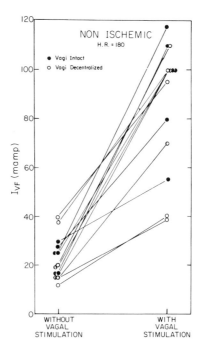

Fig. 12. Effect of vagal stimulation on ventricular fibrillation threshold (I_{VF}). Bilateral vagal stimulation at an intensity to slow the atrial rate to 50–60 beats per min was used. The vagi were either intact or decentralized and the peripheral vagi were stimulated.

Thus, our results demonstrate that in experimental acute myocardial ischemia: (1) increasing heart rate increases the nonhomogeneity of refractory periods in contiguous areas of myocardium and increases the vulnerability of the ventricle to fibrillation; and (2) reducing vagal tone, independent of changes in heart rate, leads to diminished electrical stability of the heart. Both of these effects were demonstrated to occur at a physiologic heart rate range, and both effects would be potentially deleterious consequences of increasing heart rate with atropine during AMI. That these experimental findings may be relevant to AMI in man is suggested by several recent reports of serious ventricular arrhythmias, including VF, that occurred after administration of atropine to patients with AMI (14, 32–34).

Definitive evidence relating to the mechanism by which vagal stimulation directly decreases vulnerability of the ventricle to fibrillate is lacking. Although vagal stimulation per se (i.e., in the absence of associated heart rate reduction) does reduce vulnerability to fibrillation, we also noted that it does not influence disparity of refractory periods in contiguous areas of myocardium. This contrasts with the effects of altering heart rate, which has a profound influence on both of these electrophysiologic parameters. On the other hand, Bailey et al.

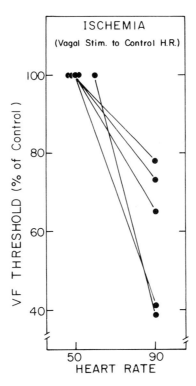

Fig. 13. Ventricular fibrillation threshold as a function of heart rate (*H.R.*) in five animals during ischemia. Heart rate was controlled by altering vagal stimulation (*STIM.*). Reproduced by permission of Circulation (39).

(40) have shown that acetylcholine depresses the slope of diastolic depolarization and increases the rise time, amplitude, and conduction velocity of action potentials recorded in the proximal portion of the His-Purkinje system of the canine ventricle. It is not known whether these actions of acetylcholine reflect a physiologic function of the vagus on propagation of the ventricular action potential. If they do, then vagal stimulation might minimize any tendency for decremental conduction to occur and thereby create a less favorable electro-physiologic environment for reentrant arrhythmias, whereas inhibition of vagal stimulation would produce the opposite effects.

EFFECTS OF NITROGLYCERIN

In this section we will consider the effects of nitroglycerin on the degree of ischemic injury and electrical stability of the myocardium during experimental acute coronary occlusion.

Nitroglycerin has been used for more than a century in the treatment of angina pectoris. However, this agent generally is not employed in the treatment of pain caused by acute myocardial infarction, on the grounds that the nitroglycerin-induced decrease in arterial pressure and reflex increase in heart rate might extend the ischemic process. The fear of hypotension is amply justified and originates, in large part, from the poor outcome of patients who develop cardiogenic shock. Under these circumstances, hypotension is a result of pump failure caused by massive myocardial damage, but the diminished arterial pressure itself undoubtedly plays a causal role in the usually lethal cycle characterized by diminished coronary perfusion pressure, greater ischemic injury, more severe hypotension, etc. Indeed, we and others have shown that hypotension induced either by hemorrhage (15, 16) or by stimulation of the carotid baroreceptors (41) tends to increase ischemic injury occurring during experimental acute coronary occlusion. These considerations understandably have focused the physician's attention on the prompt treatment of hypotension and the avoidance of any drugs that may reduce blood pressure in patients with AMI.

However, nitroglycerin has complex actions on the cardiovascular system, with the potential to alter preload, afterload, and myocardial blood flow (42–45). Since the relative importance of each of these factors on the extent of ischemic injury is unknown, an *a priori* judgment cannot be made as to whether nitroglycerin would be beneficial or deleterious when given to the patient with acute infarction. We therefore studied the net effect of nitroglycerin on the degree of ischemia (46) and on the vulnerability of the myocardium to fibrillation (47) in the canine model.

To study the effect of nitroglycerin on the degree of ischemic injury, the closed-chest sedated dog model, as described previously, was employed. The effects of 15-minute periods of LAD occlusion in control animals were compared to studies in which an intravenous bolus of 400 μg of nitroglycerin followed by a continuous infusion of the drug (200–400 μg/min) were administered just prior to and during coronary occlusion.

Despite an average decrease of 14 mm Hg in mean arterial pressure and an increase of 20 beats/min in heart rate, occlusions during nitroglycerin infusion caused significantly less S-T segment elevation than that present during control conditions (Fig. 14). The beneficial effects of nitroglycerin on S-T segment elevation contrast with the deleterious effects that occurred when identical pressure and heart rate changes were induced by venous hemorrhage (Fig. 15). It should be noted that when the nitroglycerin-induced pressure and heart rate changes were reversed by the simultaneous administration of an alpha-adrenergic agonist (methoxamine or phenylephrine), the degree of ischemia was even less than when nitroglycerin was administered alone (Fig. 16). This salutary effect on ischemic injury was still evident when the drugs were administered as long as two hours after the onset of total occlusion of the coronary artery.

The beneficial effects of nitroglycerin and methoxamine during experimental

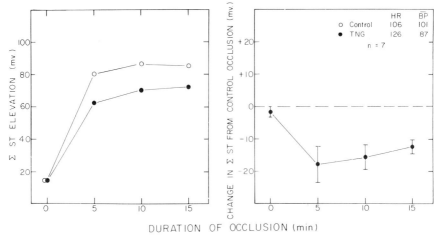

Fig. 14. Effect of nitroglycerin (*TNG*) on total S-T segment elevation during 15 minute coronary artery occlusions. *Left,* abscissa, duration of occlusion in minutes; ordinate, total S-T segment elevation (Σ S-T) in millivolts. The data points represent the mean of the results in seven dogs. *Right,* the results are replotted to depict better the spread of the data. Abscissa, duration of occlusion; ordinate, the difference in total S-T segment elevation (mv) between occlusions during nitroglycerin and control occlusions (dashed line). The vertical bars represent two S.E. Despite an increase in heart rate (*HR*) and decrease in mean arterial pressure ($\overline{BP}$), occlusions during administration of nitroglycerin resulted in significantly less Σ S-T than occurred during control occlusions. Reproduced by permission of Circulation (46).

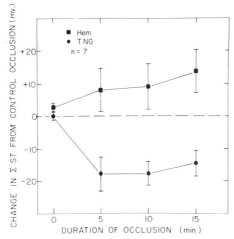

Fig. 15. Comparison of the effects of hemorrhage (*Hem*) and nitroglycerin (*TNG*) on S-T segment elevation during 15 minutes of coronary occlusion. Identical changes in mean arterial pressure and heart rate were produced by both interventions. Abscissa, duration of occlusion; ordinate, the difference in S-T segment elevation between control occlusions (dashed line), occlusions after hemorrhage (solid squares), and occlusions after nitroglycerin administration (solid circles). The mean difference in S-T segment elevation between the two interventions was statistically significant ($p < 0.02$). Reproduced by permission of Circulation (46).

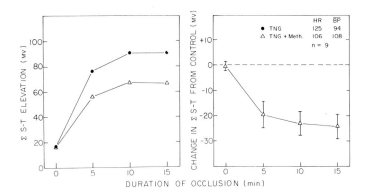

Fig. 16. Effects of nitroglycerin (*TNG*) alone and nitroglycerin plus methoxamine (*Meth.*) on Σ S-T. *Left,* absolute Σ S-T values; *right,* differences in Σ S-T between nitroglycerin alone (dashed line) and nitroglycerin plus methoxamine (*Meth.*). Nitroglycerin plus methoxamine resulted in significantly less Σ S-T than nitroglycerin alone. Reproduced by permission of Circulation (46).

coronary occlusion have recently been confirmed and extended. Thus, we have demonstrated that the extent of myocardial infarction (quantitated by measuring the depression of myocardial creatine phosphokinase activity) produced by five hours of LAD occlusion is considerably less in dogs treated by an infusion of nitroglycerin and methoxamine than in a control group (48).

Thus, our experimental data indicate that nitroglycerin reduces the degree of myocardial ischemia during acute coronary occlusion in the dog; this action is potentiated when the nitrate-induced arterial pressure and heart rate changes are prevented by the simultaneous administration of an alpha-receptor agonist. It therefore appears that the reduction of ischemia produced by nitroglycerin does not depend upon a diminution of systemic arterial pressure. Indeed, our data suggest that nitroglycerin-induced hypotension actually augments the degree of ischemia during acute coronary occlusion; potentially deleterious effects of reduced blood pressure, however, seem to be overridden by other actions that lead to a net reduction in ischemic injury. Whether the net benefit results from actions of nitroglycerin that decrease myocardial wall tension, and thereby, $M\dot{V}O_2$ (by causing venous pooling and decreased ventricular volume), or from the capacity of nitroglycerin to increase blood flow to ischemic areas (by effects on coronary arterial or collateral flow), is unknown. With regard to the latter point, recent studies performed in collaboration with Dr. Edward Stinson (45) have demonstrated that nitroglycerin does have the capacity to decrease resistance to collateral flow in patients undergoing coronary bypass surgery. Nonetheless, it remains to be determined whether results obtained during coronary bypass operations are applicable to the clinical situation. It also is unknown whether nitroglycerin will lead to a net reduction in ischemic injury in the patient with multivessel disease who is experiencing acute myocardial ischemia since, in the presence of widespread occlusive disease, vasodilators (including nitroglycerin) could theoretically act detrimentally by diverting collateral blood flow from ischemic to nonischemic areas (49).

Although it is as yet unknown whether the beneficial effects of nitroglycerin on ischemic injury caused by acute coronary occlusion in the dog are clinically applicable, recent studies in man have demonstrated that vasodilators improve the pumping performance of the heart in some patients with acute myocardial infarction. Thus, Gold and his colleagues (50) administered nitroglycerin sublingually to a group of patients with acute myocardial infarction. In those patients with persistent refractory left ventricular failure, nitroglycerin resulted in a fall in pulmonary capillary wedge pressure and an increase in output. Similar results were obtained by Franciosa and co-workers (51), who infused the vasodilator, sodium nitroprusside, in patients with acute myocardial infarction. The improvement in hemodynamics observed in some patients after treatment with vasodilators does not necessarily imply that ischemic injury is reduced. For

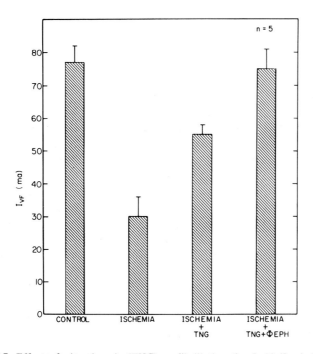

Fig. 17. Effect of nitroglycerin (*TNG*) on fibrillation threshold (I_{VF}). The bars represent the average value for five dogs with two S.E. Nitroglycerin produced a significant increase in I_{VF}. When phenlyephrine (*ΦEPH*) was administered in a dose sufficient to reverse the nitrate-induced decrease in arterial pressure, a further increase in I_{VF} occurred.

example, the enhanced performance could be caused by favorable alterations in preload and afterload which improve the pumping capacity of the nonischemic myocardium. These results, however, in conjunction with our experimental data, support the hypothesis that nitroglycerin might be uniquely valuable in the ischemic heart, and they certainly indicate that more extensive trials are warranted.

Once we found that nitroglycerin decreases the degree of experimental myocardial ischemia, we next studied the effect of this agent on the electrical stability of the myocardium (47). In the open-chest dog, complete heart block was induced by formalin injection of the atrioventricular nodal region, and the ventricles were paced at a rate of 120 beats/min. Myocardial ischemia was produced by occlusion of the LAD. As before, ischemia diminished VF threshold markedly. Nitroglycerin, infused intravenously at a rate sufficient to decrease mean arterial pressure an average of 19 mm Hg, caused a significant increase in fibrillation threshold. Moreover, when the same dose of nitroglycerin was administered but the decrease in arterial pressure was prevented by the simultaneous administration of phenylephrine, VF threshold increased still further (Fig. 17).

CONCLUSIONS

The results presented above do not provide definitive answers regarding the approach to a patient with bradycardia who has an AMI or to the use of vasodilators in the treatment of AMI. The results do point out, however, that the pharmacologic approach to therapy of AMI is undergoing evolution; old concepts are being questioned, and new ones are being explored. It is possible that increasing heart rate by means of atropine might exert beneficial effects in the patient with bradycardia and acute infarction. However, in experimental myocardial infarction, the administration of atropine (1) increases the degree of ischemic injury; (2) decreases electrical stability of the ventricle; and (3) increases the incidence of serious ventricular arrhythmias. Thus, considerably more information must be accumulated before a public health program advocating self-administration of atropine during the prehospital phase of acute myocardial infarction by all patients with bradycardia can be justified.

Once the patient is under the care of a physician, candidates for atropine therapy can be selected more critically. For example, when severe hypotension complicates the course of the patient with bradycardia, correction of the hypotension is mandatory. In these circumstances, hypotension generally responds to atropine administration. However, considering the potential complications of atropine, it might be asked whether any other therapeutic options are available besides the administration of this drug. The bradycardia-hypotension complex that occurs following myocardial infarction simulates quite closely the reflex syndrome of vasovagal syncope. During vasovagal syncope reflex, loss of arteriolar tone plays a significant role in reducing blood pressure (52–56). An extremely effective method for raising pressure under these circumstances is to have the patient lie supine with legs elevated (Fig. 18). It is therefore possible that this maneuver might be as effective as atropine in treating the bradycardia-hypotension syndrome seen following acute myocardial infarction. Moreover, the usual course of events following this postural maneuver in patients with vasovagal syncope is for pressure to increase without an immediate significant increase in heart rate. In contrast to the situation following atropine administration, coronary perfusion pressure would therefore increase without complications that might accompany a concomitant rise in heart rate. If this postural maneuver is not completely successful in raising arterial pressure, another alternative approach would be to administer phenylephrine. This drug also would raise arterial pressure without raising heart rate; experimentally, we have found that when phenylephrine or methoxamine is used to raise arterial pressure either from previously depressed level or from normal control levels, the extent of ischemic injury occurring during coronary occlusion is significantly reduced (38).

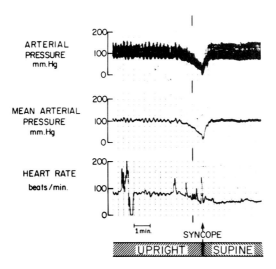

Fig. 18. Vasovagal syncope occurring during 80° head-up tilt. After several minutes in the 80° head-up tilt position, a rapid decrease in arterial pressure occurs, accompanied by a fall in heart rate. After resumption of the supine position with legs elevated, arterial pressure reverts to normal within 30 seconds. Heart rate, however, remains slow, averaging about 50 beats/min.

The above remarks were directed to the relatively unusual situation in which extreme bradycardia is accompanied by severe hypotension. However, let us consider the patient who has only moderate degrees of bradycardia and hypotension. Lown and co-workers (11) have indicated that moderate hypotension unassociated with impaired mentation, clinical evidence of vasoconstriction, or reduced regional perfusion does not significantly increase mortality in hospitalized patients with AMI. Thus, while administration of atropine in this situation would raise heart rate and blood pressure, the beneficial effects of these changes would be questionable, and the patient would be exposed to the potentially deleterious effects of a faster heart rate.

Another potentially serious consequence of the administration of atropine in these circumstances was reported recently by the Belfast mobile coronary care unit group (14). These investigators found that despite careful titration of the atropine dosage, 35% of the patients who were given atropine by the attending physician for bradycardia and hypotension "developed an inappropriately rapid heart rate." Most of these patients developed heart rates that were in excess of 100 beats/min, and some developed ventricular tachycardia or ventricular fibrillation.

In summary, we cannot as yet define the precise role of atropine in the treatment of AMI, either when treatment is considered as a public health approach to the prehospital phase of acute myocardial infarction, or when the physician is in attendance and has to administer to the individual patient. We now recognize, however, that atropine is *not* a benign drug which is invariably harmless in the context of AMI. Unquestionably, there are individual situations in which atropine should be administered promptly. In particular, the patient with marked bradycardia and severe hypotension would be in this category (although, as discussed, there may be alternative modes of therapy even for this patient). However, our studies in the experimental animal, and several published clinical examples of atropine-induced ventricular tachycardia or fibrillation, indicate that a cautious approach is warranted whenever use of this drug is contemplated.

With respect to the use of vasodilators in myocardial infarction, definitive answers are once again not available. Our results suggest, however, that the effects of hypotension on myocardial ischemic injury cannot be predicted without also taking into consideration the specific conditions in which the hypotension occurs: different hemodynamic changes evolve when hypotension is produced by vasodilators than when it is the result of hemorrhage or massive myocardial necrosis.

Although the relation between nitroglycerin-induced hypotension and ischemic injury is complex, it is clear that the long-standing clinical caveat not to administer nitroglycerin or other hypotensive agents to patients with AMI needs reevaluation. Moreover, it is possible that nitroglycerin (taken by the patient while lying supine with legs elevated to avoid the risks of excessive hypotension) may be useful in the prehospital phase of acute myocardial infarction. In the hospital environment, it is possible that nitroglycerin or other vasodilators (administered, if necessary, in conjunction with an alpha-adrenergic agonist or perhaps balloon counterpulsation to obviate any hypotensive effects) might reduce infarct size and decrease the risk of serious arrhythmias.

Regardless of the final answers that emerge, we hope that a greater understanding of the complex actions of various pharmacologic interventions during AMI will lead to new methods of therapy capable of ameliorating ischemic injury and of reducing the morbidity and mortality of acute myocardial infarction.

REFERENCES CITED

1. Armstrong, A., Duncan, B. Oliver, M. F., Julian, D. G., Donald, K. W., Fulton, M., Lutz, W., and Morrison, S. L. 1972. Natural history of acute coronary heart attacks. A community study. Brit. Heart J. 34:67.
2. Fulton, M., Julian, D. G., and Oliver, M. F. 1969. Sudden death and myocardial infarction. Circulation 40(Suppl. 4):182.
3. Kuller, L., Lilienfeld, A., and Fisher, R. 1966. Epidemiological study of sudden and unexpected deaths due to arteriosclerotic heart disease. Circulation 34:1056.
4. Weinblatt, E., Shapiro, S., Frank, C. W., and Sager, R. V. 1968. Prognosis of men after first myocardial infarction: Mortality and first recurrence in relation to selected parameters. Amer. J. Publ. Health 58:1329.
5. McNeilly, R. H., and Pemberton, J. 1968. Duration of last attack of 998 fatal cases of coronary disease and its relation to possible cardiac resuscitation. Brit. Med. J. 3:139.
6. Adgey, A. A. J., Nelson, P. G., Scott, M. E., Geddes, J. S., Allen, J. D., Zaidi, S. A., and Pantridge, J. F. 1969. Management of ventricular fibrillation outside hospital. Lancet 1:1169.
7. Adgey, A. A. J., Allen, J. D., Geddes, J. S., James, R. G. G., Webb, S. W., Zaidi, S. A., and Pantridge, J. F. 1972. Acute phase of myocardial ischemia. Circulation 46:323.
8. Grauer, L. E., Gershen, B. J., Orlando, M. M., and Epstein, S. E. Bradycardia and its complications in the prehospital phase of acute myocardial infarction. Amer J. Cardiol. (In press).
9. Han, J., Millet, D., Chizzonitti, B., and Moe, G. K. 1966. Temporal dispersion of recovery of excitability in atrium and ventricle as a function of heart rate. Amer. Heart J. 71:481.
10. Han, J., De Traglia, J., Millet, D., and Moe, G. K. 1966. Incidence of ectopic beats as a function of basic rate in the ventricle. Amer. Heart J. 72:632.
11. Lown, B., Vassaux, C., Hood, W. B., Jr., Fakhro, A. M., Kaplinsky, E., and Roberge, G. 1967. Unresolved problems in coronary care. Amer. J. Cardiol. 20:494.
12. Adgey, A. A. J., Geddes, J. S., Mulholland, H. C., Keegan, D. A. J., and Pantridge, J. F. 1968. Incidence, significance, and management of early bradyarrhythmia complicating acute myocardial infarction. Lancet 2:1097.
13. Lassers, B. W., Anderton, J. L., George, M., Muir, A. L., and Julian, D. G. 1968. Hemodynamic effects of artificial pacing in complete heart block complicating acute myocardial infarction. Circulation 38:308.
14. Webb, S. W., Adgey, A. A. J., and Pantridge, J. F. 1972. Autonomic disturbance at onset of acute myocardial infarction. Brit. Med. J. 3:89.
15. Maroko, P. R., Kjekshus, J. K., Sobel, B. E., Watanabe, T., Covell, J. W., Ross, J., Jr., and Braunwald, E. 1971. Factors influencing infarct size following experimental coronary artery occlusion. Circulation 43:67.

16. Redwood, D. R., Smith, E. R., and Epstein, S. E. 1972. Coronary artery occlusion in the conscious dog. Effects of alterations in heart rate and arterial pressure on the degree of myocardial ischemia. Circulation 46:323.
17. Lown, B., and Wolfe, M. 1971. Approaches to sudden death from coronary heart disease. Circulation 44:130.
18. Adgey, A. A. J., Allen, J. D., Geddes, J. S., James, R. G. G., Webb, S. W., Zaida, S. A., and Pantridge, J. F. 1971. Acute phase of myocardial infarction. Lancet 2:501.
19. Epstein, S. E., Redwood, D. R., and Smith, E. R. 1972. Atropine and acute myocardial infarction. Circulation 45:1273.
20. Imperial, E. S., Carballo, R., and Zimmerman, H. A. 1960. Disturbances of rate, rhythm and conduction in acute myocardial infarction: A statistical study of 153 cases. Amer. J. Cardiol. 5:24.
21. Hurwitz, M., and Eliot, R. S. Arrhythmias in acute myocardial infarction. Dis. Chest 45:616.
22. Lawrie, D. M., Greenwood, T. W., Goddard, M., Harvey, A. C., Donald, K. W., Julian, D. G., and Oliver, M. F. 1967. A coronary-care unit in the routine management of acute myocardial infarction. Lancet 2:109.
23. Master, A. M., Dack, S., and Jaffe, H. L. 1937. Disturbances of rate and rhythm in acute coronary artery thrombosis. Ann. Internal Med. 11:735.
24. Norris, R. M., Mercer, C. J., and Yeates, S. E. 1972. Sinus rate in acute myocardial infarction. Brit. Heart J. 34:901.
25. Scherlag, B. J., Helfant, R. H., Haft, J. I., and Damato, A. N. Electrophysiology underlying ventricular arrhythmias due to coronary ligation. Amer. J. Physiol. 219: 1665.
26. Goldstein, R. E., Karsh, R. B., Smith, E. R., Orlando, M., Norman, D., Farnham, G., Redwood, D. R., and Epstein, S. E. 1973. The influence of atropine and of vagally mediated bradycardia on the occurrence of ventricular arrhythmias following acute coronary occlusion in closed-chest dogs. Circulation 47:1180.
27. Rothfeld, E. L., Zucker, I. R., Parsonnet, V., and Alinsonorin, C. A. 1968. Idioventricular rhythm in acute myocardial infarction. Circulation 37:203.
28. Logic, J. R., Morrow, D. H., and Gatz, R. N. 1969. Idioventricular tachycardia complicating experimental myocardial infarction. Dis. Chest 56:477.
29. Schamroth, L. 1969. Idioventricular tachycardia. Dis. Chest 56:466.
30. Epstein, S. E., Beiser, G. D., Rosing, D. R., Talano, J. V., and Karsh, R. B. 1973. Experimental acute myocardial infarction. Characterization and treatment of the malignant premature ventricular contraction. Circulation 47:446.
31. Norris, R. M., Mercer, C. J., and Yeates, S. E. 1972. Sinus rate in acute myocardial infarction. Brit. Heart J. 34:901.
32. Massumi, R. A., Mason, D. T., Amsterdam, E. A., Demaria, A., Miller, R. R., Scheinman, M. M., and Zelis, R. 1972. Ventricular fibrillation and tachycardia after intravenous atropine for treatment of bradycardias. New Engl. J. Med. 287:336.
33. Zipes, D. P., and Knoebel, S. B. 1972. Rapid rate-dependent ventricular ectopy; adverse responses to atropine-induced rate increase. Chest 62:255.
34. Morgensen, L., and Orinius, E. 1971. Arrhythmic complications after parasympatholytic treatment of bradyarrhythmia in a coronary care unit. Acta Med. Scand. 190:495.
35. Han, J. 1969. Ventricular vulnerability during acute coronary occlusion. Amer. J. Cardiol. 24:857.
36. Zipes, D. P. 1969. The clinical significance of bradycardic rhythms in acute myocardial infarction. Amer. J. Cardiol. 24:814.
37. Han, J. 1971. The concepts of reentrant activity responsible for ectopic rhythms. Amer. J. Cardiol. 28:253.
38. Redwood, D. R., Smith, E. R., and Epstein, S. E. 1972. Coronary artery occlusion in the conscious dog. Effects of alterations in heart rate and arterial pressure on the degree of myocardial ischemia. Circulation 46:323.

39. Kent, K. M., Smith, E. R., Redwood, D. R., and Epstein, S. E. 1973. Electrical stability of acutely ischemic myocardium: Influences of heart rate and vagal stimulation. Circulation 47:291.

40. Bailey, J. C., Greenspan, K., Elizari, M. C., Anderson, G. J., and Fisch, C. 1972. Effects of acetylcholine on automaticity and conduction in the proximal portion of the His-Purkinje specialized conduction system of the dog. Circ. Res. 30:211.

41. Thibault, G. E., Farnham, G. S., Myers, R. W., Goldstein, R. E., and Epstein, S. E. Increased myocardial ischemia caused by reflexly induced hypotension during coronary occlusion in the conscious dog. (Submitted for publication.)

42. Williams, J. F., Jr., Glick, G., and Braunwald, E. 1965. Studies on cardiac dimensions in the intact unanesthetized man. V. Effects of nitroglycerin. Circulation 32:767.

43. Bernstein, L., Friesinger, G. C., Lichtlen, P. R., and Ross, R. S. 1966. The effect of nitroglycerin on the systemic and coronary circulation in man and dogs. Circulation 38:107.

44. Horowitz, L. D., Gorlin, R., Taylor, W. J., and Kemp, H. G. 1971. Effects of nitroglycerin on regional myocardial blood flow in coronary artery disease. J. Clin. Invest. 50:1578.

45. Goldstein, R. E., Stinson, E. B., and Epstein, S. E. 1973. Effects of nitroglycerin on coronary collateral function in patients with coronary occlusive disease [abstract]. Amer. J. Cardiol. 31:135.

46. Smith, E. R., Redwood, D. R., McCarron, W. E., and Epstein, S. E. 1973. Coronary occlusion in the conscious dog: Effects of alterations in arterial pressure produced by nitroglycerin, hemorrhage and alpha-adrenergic agonists on the degree of myocardial ischemia. Circulation 47:51.

47. Kent, K. M., Smith, E. R., Redwood, D. R., and Epstein, S. E. Beneficial electrophysiologic effects of nitroglycerin during acute myocardial infarction. (Submitted for publication.)

48. Hirshfeld, J. W., Jr., Borer, J. S., Goldstein, R. E., and Epstein, S. E. 1973. Reduction in extent of myocardial infarction when nitroglycerin and methoxamine are administered during coronary occlusion [abstract]. Circ. Res. 31:426.

49. Forman, R., Kirk, E. S., Downey, J. M., and Sonnenblick, E. H. 1972. Reduced subendocardial blood flow and ventricular contractile force caused by nitroglycerin [abstract]. Amer. J. Cardiol. 29:262.

50. Gold, H. K., Leinbach, R. C., and Sanders, C. A. 1972. Use of sublingual nitroglycerin in congestive failure following acute myocardial infarction. Circulation 46:839.

51. Franciosa, J. A., Guiha, N. H., Limas, C. J., Rodriguera, E., and Cohn, J. N. 1972. Improved left ventricular function during nitroprusside infusion in acute myocardial infarction. Lancet 1:650.

52. Lewis, T. 1932. Vasovagal syncope and the carotid sinus mechanism. Brit. Med. J. 1:873.

53. Barcroft, H., Edholm, O. G., McMichael, J., and Sharpey-Schafer, E. P. 1944. Posthemorrhagic fainting: Study by cardiac output and forearm flow. Lancet 1:489.

54. Barcroft, H., and Edholm, O. G. 1945. On the vasodilation in human skeletal muscle during posthaemorrhagic fainting. J. Physiol. 104:161.

55. Greene, M. A., Boltax, A. J., and Ulberg, R. J. 1961. Cardiovascular dynamics of vasovagal reactions in man. Circ. Res. 9:12.

56. Epstein, S. E., Stampfer, M., and Beiser, G. D. 1968. Role of the capacitance and resistance vessels in vasovagal syncope. Circulation 37:524.

FREQUENCY OF ARRHYTHMIA PRECIPITATED BY PSYCHOGENIC FACTORS IN A CORONARY CARE UNIT

STEWART WOLF

Probably the most worrisome problem in a coronary care unit is the ever present hazard of serious arrhythmia. To many observers in the early days of such units, the obvious drama and the imposing instrumentation appeared to predispose to psychologically induced arrhythmias. This fear was not substantiated. The instrumentation turned out to be more reassuring than frightening. Nevertheless, it appeared that some arrhythmias in the coronary care unit were triggered by psychosocial stimuli. Thus a concentration of interest on the physical arrangements of the coronary care units followed. Should the patients be isolated from the sight and sound of each other, or should the beds all be in one room with only curtain separations? The findings were conflicting.

Leigh and associates (1) compared the "open" with a "closed" unit and found no difference in measures of anxiety or in the incidence of arrhythmia or death. The disturbances and disruptions of the open unit were apparently balanced by the reassuring quality of human interaction. In the closed unit, although the patient was protected against excitement, he was susceptible to feeling isolated, lonely, and unloved—almost abandoned. Which arrangements were anxiety producing depended on the person. People are different. Leigh's group was able to identify those with high risk of cardiac arrhythmias on the basis of psychological criteria including test scores indicating high separation anxiety and high hostility directed inward, but low overt hostility (Fig. 1).

It has gradually become clear that far more crucial than imposing instrumentation or the geographical arrangements of the coronary care unit are the people in attendance, the degree to which their attitudes and behavior affect susceptible patients, and the general psychological atmosphere of the place.

Dr. Burch emphasized the physiological importance of a reassuring attitude on the part of the doctor and nurse—the importance to the patient of the feeling that things are well in hand. It has now been thoroughly documented by measurements of serum fatty acids and cortisol, and by urinary catecholamine measurements as they correlate with bouts of arrhythmia, that disruptions on the ward, the behavior of staff, and the presence of emotionally significant visitors, are highly important to the smooth regulation of cardiac rate and rhythm (2,3).

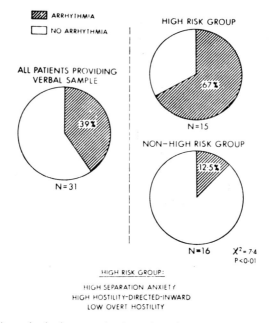

Fig. 1. Cardiac arrhythmias occurring in patients in coronary care units, either "open" or "closed," who completed a Gottschalk verbal sample test. Reprinted from Leigh, H., M. A. Hofer, J. Cooper, and M. F. Reiser. 1972. J. Psychosom. Res. 16:453.

In animal experiments in which the heart is completely denervated, ligation of a coronary artery is much less likely to induce a fatal arrhythmia than when the nerve supply is intact. Cardiologists may have been slow to recognize the importance of the brain in the control of the heart because of the heart's remarkable intrinsic regulatory capability, even when separated from the body. In the intact individual, however, the central nervous system exerts a continuous regulatory tone and can make powerful adjustments (4).

The importance of central nervous system connections in the matter of sudden death after myocardial infarction was pointed out nearly 40 years ago by Leriche and co-workers (5). Their demonstration that survival is enhanced by cardiac denervation has been confirmed repeatedly and most recently by the careful studies of Ebert et al. (6).

Subsequent to cardiac transplantation in animals or man there may be pump failure, but arrhythmias have not been a problem until sufficient time has elapsed for regeneration of the nerve supply. Thus, it would appear that cardiac arrhythmias following myocardial infarction are mainly reflex, and that the disturbance may be enhanced by emotionally charged situations, perhaps because of deficient modulation by connections from a supratentorial network of inhibitory neurons that normally regulate autonomic responses (7,8).

In human subjects who have sustained massive central nervous system damage, especially to the brain stem, and when an automatic respirator is required, the cardiac rhythm is usually remarkably regular. Conversely, in the presence of lesser degrees of central nervous system involvement (9) and with an irritable myocardium, as after an infarct, there is a loss of normal damping of autonomic effects on the heart. Lynch and associates (10) compared the automatically monitored EKG in patients in a coronary care unit when alone and undisturbed, with the pattern observed during very minor disturbances such as a nurse taking the pulse. During such events, bursts of ectopic beats and conduction changes were observed including, for example, the Wenkebach phenomenon. Dr. Burch has told us that in a suspected myocardial infarction his first order is "cancel all hospital routines."

In a previous chapter I mentioned that both the emotional state of the patient and his cognitive state are important to the regulation of the heart beat—not just the former. Somehow during intense concentration or mental absorption, modulating forces seem to come into play that tend to regularize the heart beat. The opposite was observed during periods of distraction and confusion (11).

The problem of controlling the experimental situation makes it very difficult to evaluate in a critical way studies of the effects of psychosocial forces on the cardiac mechanism.

Bruhn et al. (12) studied the patients on a coronary care unit continuously over a three-month period and found not only increased heart rate variability and ectopic beats, but very marked changes in blood pressure during disruptions on the ward, especially upon the death of another patient. One patient experienced ventricular tachycardia while the nurses were attempting to revive an arrested patient in the next bed.

Because the neural control of the heart beat and of other cardiovascular parameters is altered during various stages of sleep and because, as Master (13) showed several years ago, one out of five coronary deaths occur during sleep, we undertook to study a series of healthy subjects and compare them to asymptomatic individuals who had suffered a myocardial infarction a year or more in the past and to patients hospitalized for a recent myocardial infarction. We recorded EEG, eye movements, respiration, EKG, and cardiotachogram and counted ectopic beats, principally ventricular premature contractions, during various stages of sleep throughout the night. Ectopic beats occurred in all stages of sleep and wakefulness and especially in association with wide swings in heart rate. These occurred most typically during REM (rapid eye movements) or dreaming sleep or in transitions from one stage to another. When the subjects were sleeping in the laboratory, we noted marked variation in the number of ectopic beats in the same subject from night to night. The variability was clearly correlated with day-to-day life experiences. Days marked by emotional conflicts were followed by frequent ventricular premature contractions during sleep at night.

Dr. Burch has stated that a coronary care unit can produce a myocardial infarction. We found that it can certainly produce ventricular premature contractions. Four asymptomatic postcoronary patients who had been monitored during sleep repeatedly in the laboratory were admitted to vacant beds in the coronary care unit. In every case more ventricular premature contractions were counted during sleep in the coronary care unit than in the laboratory.

The study of arrhythmias in sleep in patients confined to the coronary care unit because of recent myocardial infarction was particularly revealing. The likelihood of nighttime arrhythmias was greatest following a day that included an emotionally disturbing visitor, a conflict with a member of the staff, or a catastrophe on the ward.

Finally, in the laboratory at night, we studied effects of barbiturates and alcohol on sleep patterns and on the frequency of ectopic beats in three patients who had suffered a well-documented myocardial infarction a year or more in the past. Generally, there were fewer ectopic beats when the patient was under the influence of either barbiturates (0.2 gm sodium pentobarbital) or 8 ounces of 86 proof whiskey. In two of the subjects, however, an emotionally stressful day was followed by more ectopic beats on a sedated than on a nonsedated night, in one subject after taking alcohol and in the other after taking barbiturates.

It appears that the lesson from all this is the complexity and extensive ramifications of neural mechanisms that control the heart beat. It is of paramount importance to understand the patient as a person and to be alert to his attitudes and vulnerabilities as they may affect the circuitry that controls the rate and rhythm of the heart.

REFERENCES CITED

1. Leigh, H., Hofer, M. A., Cooper, J., and Reiser, M. F. 1972. A psychological comparison of patients in "open" and "closed" coronary care units. J. Psychosom. Res. 16:449–457.
2. Green, W. A., Moss, A. J., Goldstein, S., Levy, A. L., and Klein, R. F. 1972. Psychosocial, hormonal, and arrhythmia precursors of the early pre-hospital phase of myocardial infarction. Presented at the American Psychosomatic Society Annual Meeting, April 1972, Boston, Massachusetts.
3. Wallace, A. G. 1968. Catecholamine metabolism in patients with acute myocardial infarction. In D. G. Julian and M. F. Oliver, eds. Acute myocardial infarction, p. 237. Livingstone, Edinburgh.
4. Randall, W. C. ed. 1965. Nervous control of the heart. Williams and Wilkins, Baltimore.
5. Leriche, R. L., Herrmann, L., and Fontaine, R. 1931. Ligature de la coronaire gauche et fonction chez l'animal intact. C.R. Soc. Biol. 107:545.
6. Ebert, P. A., Allgood, R. J., and Sabiston, D. C. 1967. Effect of cardiac denervation on arrhythmia following coronary artery occlusion. Surg. Forum 18:114.
7. Clemente, C. D. 1968. Forebrain mechanisms related to internal inhibition and sleep. Cond. Reflex 3:145–174.

8. Wolf, S. 1970. Evidence on inhibitory control of autonomic function. Int. J. Psychobiol. 1:27–33.
9. McGraw, C. P., Tindall, G. T., Iwata, K., and Parent, A. D. 1972. Response of comatose head injured patients to stimulation. Presented at the Twelfth Annual Meeting of the Society for Psychophysiological Research, November, 1972. Boston, Mass.
10. Lynch, J. J., Thomas, S. A., Mills, M. E., and Malinow, K. 1973. Heart rate reactions of patients in a coronary care unit to social interactions. New Engl. J. Med. (in press).
11. Long, J., Bynum, T. E., and Wolf, S. Unpublished data.
12. Bruhn, J. G., Thurman, A. E., Jr., Chandler, B. C., and Bruce, T. A. 1970. Patients' reactions to death in a coronary care unit. J. Psychosom. Res. 14:65–70.
13. Master, A. M., Dack, S., and Jaffe, H. L. 1940. The relation of effort and trauma to acute coronary occlusion. Industrial Med. 9:359–364.

HEMODYNAMIC MEASUREMENTS IN THE CHOICE
AND EVALUATION OF THERAPEUTIC INTERVENTIONS

H. J. C. SWAN, KANU CHATTERJEE, and
WILLIAM GANZ

It is now recognized that the usual early hospital course of acute myocardial infarction is a metabolically dynamic event. The initial pathologic process consists of an area of extreme ischemia in which myocardial cells have undergone or are undergoing necrosis. Intermingled with these areas of dead or dying cells are areas of tissue which are functionally inactive, yet which have not progressed to that metabolic state in which death has occurred or is inevitable. These areas of ischemia can potentially recover and function may be restored. Under unfavorable metabolic states, they progress to a nonreversible state of infarction.

These pathologic and metabolic processes are accompanied by changes in the hemodynamic state of the circulation, according to alterations in the quantity of contractile myocardium, the functional state of the ischemic but not yet infarcted myocardium, cardiovascular compensatory mechanisms, and the presence of associated mechanical defects. Disturbances of heart rate and rhythm also contribute adversely to the depression of cardiovascular function. A wide spectrum of initial hemodynamic presentation is therefore possible, from the situation in which only a small and geographically unimportant area of myocardium is affected to that pertaining when a left main coronary artery or a primary branch thereof is occluded totally so that a large segment of contractile myocardium is acutely deprived of its blood flow. The prognosis and consequences of these two strikingly different subsets of the same "disease" are as different as those pertaining to rubella or smallpox.

Although clinical signs have proved helpful in identifying those patients in whom greater or lesser degrees of depression of cardiovascular function exists, they permit gross appraisal only, and do not always precisely identify the hemodynamic state. Further, significant changes in hemodynamic state may occur without accompanying changes in clinical signs. Hence, the reliability of current clinical examination using currently accepted methods is less than adequate to allow rapid decision-making concerning immediate prognosis and

Supported in part by Contract No. PH-43-NHLI-68-1333-M under Myocardial Infarction Program, National Heart and Lung Institute, NIH Department, HEW.

rational therapy. New noninvasive methods are desirable to allow for this precise definition, but until then invasive techniques appear necessary for the initial evaluation, determination of prognosis, selection of appropriate therapy, and the identification of favorable or unfavorable responses to the therapy.

At the present time heart rate may be measured reliably and systemic arterial blood pressure recorded adequately by the indirect or Korotkoff method in the majority of patients. However, when severe depression of cardiovascular function associated with vasoconstriction exists, then the recording of arterial pressure by the indirect method is likely to indicate erroneously low values (1). Hence, in patients thought to be close to or in the shock state, the direct recording of intra-arterial pressure is a necessity for adequate evaluation.

BALLOON FLOTATION CATHETER

Introduction of the balloon-guided flotation catheter has now allowed additional important performance parameters to be obtained safely and regularly in the acutely ill patient (2). By means of this device pressure in the pulmonary artery may be recorded. Unlike conventional cardiac catheterization, this procedure is accomplished at the bedside without fluoroscopy. A small balloon at the tip of an extruded polyvinyl-chloride catheter is inflated with 0.8 ml of air when its tip is judged to lie in the great intrathoracic veins or in the right atrium. The inflated balloon guides the tip of the catheter into the right ventricle, pulmonary artery, and distal into a pulmonary arterial branch where an "occluded" or (wedged) pulmonary arterial pressure is obtained (3). This pressure is closely related in amplitude and phase to the pressure in the left atrium and pulmonary vein. The mean pulmonary arterial occluded pressure is also closely correlated with the mean left ventricular diastolic pressure (4). At high levels of left ventricular end-diastolic pressure and/or when the ventricular compliance is severely reduced, end-diastolic left ventricular pressure is substantially greater than mean occluded pulmonary artery pressure. Pulmonary artery diastolic pressure relates closely to the mean "occluded pulmonary artery" pressure in most instances, but is greater in patients with obstructive lung disease or pulmonary embolus. Under such circumstances, the pulmonary arterial diastolic pressure is higher than the left ventricular filling pressure or left atrial pressure. It has now been demonstrated beyond a doubt that in clinical practice central venous or right atrial pressure relates poorly to left atrial pressure in acute myocardial infarction and use of this value in prognostic and therapeutic decision-making may lead to erroneous therapy (5).

The addition of a thermistor to a larger model of the balloon flotation device, with the provision of a second lumen for injection of cold ($0-5°C$) solution into the right atrium, allows for the measurement of cardiac output by the thermo-

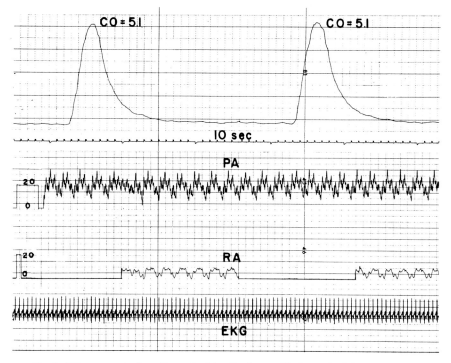

Fig. 1. Measurement of cardiac output by the thermodilution principle.

dilution principle (6) by detection of the resultant change of pulmonary arterial blood temperature (Fig. 1).

Application of Data

From data on the filling pressure on the left side of the circulation it is possible to make prognostic and therapeutic decisions relative to pulmonary vascular congestion. By measurement of "occluded" pulmonary artery pressure a relatively precise numerical identification of the level of pulmonary venous congestion can be obtained. X-rays of the lung fields and auscultation of the chest reveal abnormalities in most instances in which the pulmonary "occluded" and pulmonary pressure exceeds 20 mm Hg. However, changes in pulmonary vascular dynamics will precede x-ray changes and physical signs. The lag between changes in pressure and recognizable changes revealed by clinical method may vary from hours to days.

The practical ability to calculate the output of the heart at the bedside provides the physician with one of the most important cardiac performance indicators. To reason that a knowledge of the absolute value for cardiac output and the changes in this value is without practical importance is to ignore the fundamental principles of science in general and of applied cardiovascular physiology in particular. Figure 2 demonstrates by means of such hemodynamic data the wide spectrum of hemodynamic alterations that occurs in a hetero-geneous group of patients under a single diagnostic term—acute myocardial infarction. While the patients who are represented in the upper segment of this display have an excellent prognosis, those in the right lower section have markedly depressed cardiac performance, may or may not demonstrate the clinical shock syndrome, and their outlook with conventional therapy is omi-nous, indeed. These two subsets of what is generally considered to be the same illness, acute myocardial infarction, are an indictment of the precision of our taxonomy from a pragmatic standpoint both in regard to concept, prognosis, and therapy.

PROGNOSTIC INDEX

The development of precise, consistently reliable indices which are rapidly obtainable is of fundamental importance in decision-making in the management of acute myocardial infarction. In those patients deemed to have a good prognosis in terms of natural history the advisability of any form of pharmaco-

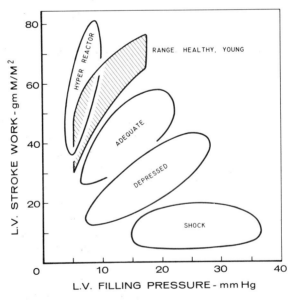

Fig. 2. Wide spectrum of hemodynamic alterations in a heterogeneous group of patients with acute myocardial infarcts.

logic therapy can be questioned; in those patients with a poor prognosis, vigorous measures must be undertaken with the least possible delay. The developed ability to categorize precisely large numbers of patients on a hemodynamic subclassification should markedly improve the prognostic decision-making precision and hence allow the more rational selection of appropriate therapy.

Figure 2 indicates four arbitrary categories or subsets of patients with acute myocardial infarction. Clearly these overlap to some degree but they are useful in considering the heterogeneous needs of such patients (Table 1). Patients with normal or hypernormal function whose cardiac performance may be elevated for the sedated situation, having a stroke work index in excess of 60 gm-m per m^2 per beat and a mean left ventricular filling pressure of 10 mm Hg or less, have an excellent prognosis. Under ordinary circumstances there is no significant hemodynamic deficiency in such patients and unless a dysrhythmia supervenes or the infarcted area extends in magnitude, the hospital mortality should be negligible. In contrast, patients characterized by a stroke work index of less than 20 gm-m per m^2 per beat with a mean left ventricular filling pressure in excess of 20 mm Hg will have an unfavorable outcome in approximately 90% of instances under conventional therapeutic regimens.

Those patients having adequate cardiac function will not infrequently experience a period of pulmonary congestion of short duration, possibly caused by changes in ventricular compliance. The overall risk rate in this group should not amount to more than 5%. Patients who have depressed cardiovascular function (a stroke work index of 20–40 gm-m per m^2 per beat at a filling pressure of 15 mm Hg or greater would appear to experience a mortality rate which ranges

Table 1. Hemodynamic Subsets and Clinical Implications

Functional state	C.I.[a]	L.V.F.P.[b]	S.W.I.[c]	Possible therapy
Hypertensive	N[d]	N or ↑	↑	Reduce blood pressure
Hyperdynamic	↑	N	↑	Propranolol
Normal	N	N	N	None
Pulmonary congestion	N	↑	N	Diuretics
Moderate depression	↓	↑	↑	Diuretics, time, digitalis (?)
Severe depression	↓↓	↑	↓↓	Impedance reduction, early surgery

[a]C.I. - cardiac index
[b]L.V.F.P. = left ventricular filling pressure
[c]S.W.I. = stroke work index
[d]N = normal

from 15 to 25%. While clinical examination may serve to categorize such patients in general, it is at present impossible to promptly assign a given patient to an individual subset on discrete and clearly defined clinical criteria alone. Nevertheless, definition of such patients as within certain of these categories may have important and fundamental therapeutic implications (Table 1).

SELECTION OF THERAPY

Certain patients, particularly those with posterior or inferior infarction, have normal cardiac function and in some instances a cardiac output and/or level of blood pressure and heart rate which is above the normal. This may be caused by circulating catecholamines or reflexes initiated by the acute infarction process causing sympathetic augmentation. Such patients occasionally maintain high heart rates and continued chest discomfort, although they are sedated and under adequate hospital care. Some have responded to small doses of propranolol (Inderal) by a reduction of circulatory performance parameters to the normal range with, it is to be hoped, preservation of "at risk" myocardium. Patients within the category of adequate cardiac function in the absence of evidence of autonomic hyperactivity seldom need specific treatment. Exceptions include those patients with normal performance parameters who also experience a high left ventricular filling pressure with associated dyspnea, chest rales, and even pulmonary edema (Group 2, Fig. 2). Hemodynamic evaluation will demonstrate that these patients lie in the upper right part of the cardiovascular profile. Stroke work indices in excess of 50 gm-m per m^2 per beat or stroke volume indices of 50 ml per m^2 per beat are frequently seen. It is possible that changes so defined are reflections of transient phases of decreased left ventricular compliance—increased stiffness—which makes an increase in left-sided filling pressure mandatory for the maintenance of forward flow. These changes will usually revert to normal in two to three days but with a maintenance of adequate cardiac performance. Specifically, there is no positive relationship between cardiac performance and increased levels of ventricular filling pressure above 15 mm Hg. Conversely, a reduction in left ventricular filling pressure to approximately this level will not cause any diminution in cardiac performance. The reduction in left ventricular filling pressure which is usually spontaneous is accompanied by a resolution of the physical findings of pulmonary congestion and left ventricular diastolic hypertension—increased S_4 and the presence of S_3. If the patient is uncomfortable, the physician may utilize diuretics to diminish mean left ventricular filling pressure to approximately 15 mm Hg. Under such circumstances all patients in this category should have an uneventful convalescence and experience minimal mortality.

Patients with more severe depression of cardiac function have both an increase in pressure and reduction in cardiac performance. The initial choice of drugs is the diuretic group. As indicated above, filling pressure must be maintained at approximately 15 mm Hg because a marked reduction in cardiac performance will occur if left ventricular filling pressure is caused to decline below this value. This is of particular significance in patients with moderate to severe depression of cardiac function. This hemodynamic state is believed to be caused by the involvement of a significant proportion of the contractile elements comprising 15–30% of normal myocardium, with an increased stiffness of viable but ischemic myocardium. The development of hypotension in these patients may suggest the temporary use of inotropic agents such as norepinephrine in small doses, or newer approaches may be called for. However, it has been found that whereas moderate responses in terms of cardiovascular performance parameters may be observed in patients with acute myocardial infarction and adequate cardiac function, those patients with more severe depression of cardiac function and hence the need for therapeutic interventions respond less well or not at all. If such changes in function are observed within a few hours of the onset of symptoms and there are reasons to believe that the process remains largely ischemic, then the possible benefit of immediate coronary angiography and immediate bypass surgery should be considered.

Extreme depression of cardiac performance is seen in patients with stroke work indices of less than 20 gm-m per m^2 per beat and a filling pressure in excess of 20 mm Hg. Some of these patients exhibit the shock syndrome on admission. In the others if the hemodynamic status cannot be improved promptly the shock state will supervene in hours or in a very few days. Frequently patients will present with stroke work indices and stroke volume values of less than 10 gm-m per m^2 per beat and 10 ml per m^2 per beat, respectively. In these patients a mortality of 100% may be expected with conventional treatment. Control of heart rate and rhythm and a prompt reduction of pulmonary venous pressure to values of approximately 15 mm Hg is desirable to reduce the work of breathing and to improve arterial hypoxia. However, unless the patient's circulatory performance is rapidly improved, the likelihood of survival remains extremely small.

Several new interventions may be currently considered since the patient's response to them may be evaluated within a few minutes by the hemodynamic measurements outlined previously. These interventions include evaluation of the effects of newer pharmacologic agents such as dopamine, glucagon, glucose-insulin-potassium solutions, etc., aortic impedance reduction by regitine or sodium nitroprusside infusions, and the use of mechanical circulatory assist by either the invasive (balloon) or the noninvasive (cardiassist) methods.

Sudden depression of left ventricular function of an extreme degree in a previously healthy patient suggests an extensive process involving the anterior wall of the left ventricle caused by a high grade obstructive lesion in the left main coronary artery or in the proximal portion of the left anterior descending coronary artery. If the patient is young, without a previous history of heart disease or of myocardial infarction, if the heart is small, and a short period of time has intervened since the onset of symptoms, prompt revascularization under skilled hands is indicated (7). Delays in decision-making as to such interventions can be avoided if specific and precise hemodynamic measurements are promptly available to indicate the disastrous situation which pertains in actuality and to assist the physician in the avoidance of optimistic procrastina- tion. Logistically it is possible to perform coronary arteriography and coronary vein bypass surgery in a time span sufficiently short to prevent massive myo- cardial necrosis. In patients operated on at times in excess of ten hours following the development of symptoms and the shock syndrome, the results have been less satisfactory. However, in reports now being made on a small group of patients from across the country, early surgery has resulted in the most favorable mortality figures for cardiogenic shock.

CONCLUSION

The disease entity known as acute myocardial infarction is a dynamic phenome- non in which myocardial tissue is dominantly ischemic at the beginning of the illness and probably dominantly necrotic as the illness progresses. The functional derangement so produced is highly variable and cannot always be adequately assessed from clinical examination. Measurement of a cardiac performance parameter—cardiac output, stroke volume index, or left ventricular stroke work index—allows a decision to be made as to whether the performance level is above normal (greater than 60 gm-m per m^2 per beat), within the normal range (40–60 gm-m per m^2 per beat), depressed (20–40 gm-m per m^2 per beat), or probably not compatible with prolonged survival (less than 20 gm-m per m^2 per beat). The level of congestion of the pulmonary vascular bed may be defined by measure- ment of "occluded" pulmonary arterial pressures. Values in excess of 18 mm Hg are progressively associated with increasing degrees of pulmonary congestion and pulmonary edema. No change in cardiac performance parameters is seen as mean left ventricular filling pressure is reduced from pulmonary edema values to 15 mm Hg. The latter value is the optimal level at which filling pressure should be maintained in the presence of depression of cardiac function.

The data for the establishment of the major subsets of acute myocardial infarction can be obtained at the bedside without fluoroscopy by means of the more advanced versions of the balloon-tipped flotation catheter technique. This is an acceptable and safe procedure and provides the data which are reliable and relevant to important clinical decision-making. A judgment on the specific therapy and the urgency of its implementation as well as the positive or negative circulatory responses thereto can materially assist the practicing physician in the treatment of acute myocardial infarction.

REFERENCES CITED

1. Cohn, J. N., and Luria, M. H. 1964. Studies in clinical shock and hypotension. The value of bedside hemodynamic observations. J.A.M.A. 190:113.
2. Swan, H. J. C., Ganz, W., Forrester, J., Marcus, H., Diamond, G., and Chonette, D. 1970. Catheterization of the heart in man with use of a flow-directed balloon-tipped catheter. New Engl. J. Med. 283:447.
3. Fitzpatrick, G. F., Hampson, L. G., and Burgess, J. H. 1972. Bedside determination of left atrial pressure. Can. Med. Assoc. J. 106:1293.
4. Rahimtoola, S. H., Loeb, H. S., Ehsani, A., Sinno, M. Z., Chuguimia, R., Lal, R., Rosen, K., and Gunnar, R. M. 1972. Relationship of pulmonary artery to left ventricular diastolic pressures in myocardial infarction. Circulation 46:283.
5. Forrester, J. S., Diamond, G., McHugh, T., and Swan, H. J. C. 1971. Filling pressures in the right and left side of the heart in acute myocardial infarction. New Engl. J. Med. 285:190.
6. Forrester, J. S., Ganz, W., McHugh, T., Chonette, D. W., and Swan, H. J. C. 1972. Thermodilution cardiac output determination with a single flow-directed catheter. Amer. Heart J. 83:306.
7. Matloff, J. M., Sustaita, H., Fields, J., Marcus, H. S., Chatterjee, K., and Swan, H. J. C. 1973. The rationale for surgery in preinfarction angina. Ann. Thoracic Surg. (in press).

RECENT ADVANCES IN PATHOPHYSIOLOGY AND THERAPY OF MYOCARDIAL INFARCTION SHOCK

DEAN T. MASON, EZRA A. AMSTERDAM, RICHARD R. MILLER,
RASHID A. MASSUMI, and ROBERT ZELIS

With the advent of the coronary care unit in the past decade, effective management of cardiac arrhythmias has reduced the death rate in acute myocardial infarction from 30 to 15% in many medical centers (1, 2). However, efforts to overcome myocardial infarction shock have been unsatisfactory and the remaining hospital mortality is largely caused by this complication. Approximately 15% of patients with transmural myocardial infarction develop cardiogenic shock which is fatal in more than 90% of instances (1, 2). Cardiogenic shock now constitutes the major cause of mortality in patients reaching the hospital with infarction and accounts for about 100,000 deaths yearly in the United States.

CARDIAC DYSFUNCTION

Shock following myocardial infarction is fundamentally characterized by profound depression of cardiac performance which leads to lowered cardiac output, diminished arterial blood pressure, and inadequate organ perfusion. The basic physiologic defect in this condition is severe decrease of ventricular contractility, principally caused by loss of myocardial contractile units. The degree of impairment of cardiac function and contractile state is governed by the extent of the infarction itself, and shock occurs when more than 40% of the left ventricular muscle mass is destroyed (1–3).

Ventricular function is diminished in nearly all patients with acute transmural myocardial infarction, including those without complications (4–6). Thus there is a spectrum of depression of ventricular performance in transmural infarction: most extreme in cardiogenic shock, intermediate in congestive heart failure without hypotension, and least in uncomplicated infarction (Fig. 1). In addition to loss of contractile units, cardiac dysfunction results from diminished inotropic state in ischemic areas and from regional ventricular dyssynergy. Further, in some patients, there may be mitral insufficiency caused by papillary muscle incompetence and rupture of the interventricular septum. Viewed in terms of the Frank-Starling principle which relates cardiac performance to ventricular filling pressure (Fig. 2), the ventricular function curve is most depressed and flattened in cardiogenic shock. Thus, despite operation of the heart at the apex

ACUTE MYOCARDIAL INFARCTION

	UNCOMPLICATED	CHF	SHOCK
BP:	N	N	↓
CO:	N	N/↓	↓/↓↓
LVEDP:	N/↑	↑/↑↑	↑↑/↑↑↑
PVR:	N	N/↑	↑
CVP:	N	N/↑	↑

Fig. 1. Hemodynamics in acute myocardial infarction (MI): uncomplicated transmural MI, MI with congestive heart failure (*CHF*), and MI with cardiogenic shock. *BP* = systemic arterial blood pressure; *CO* = cardiac index; *LVEDP* = left ventricular end-diastolic pressure; *PVR* = peripheral vascular resistance; *CVP* = central venous pressure; *N* = normal value.

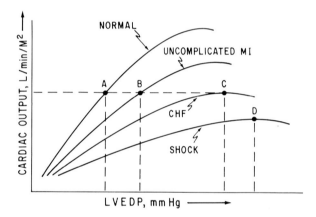

Fig. 2. Ventricular function curves in normal subject, acute uncomplicated transmural myocardial infarction (MI), acute MI with congestive heart failure (*CHF*), and acute MI with cardiogenic shock, Points *A, B,* and *C* all represent the same cardiac output, but each is at a different level of left ventricular end-diastolic pressure (*LVEDP*) shown by the vertical broken lines. In shock, despite operation of ventricle at apex of function curve (point *D*) with marked elevation of LVEDP, an adequate cardiac output cannot be delivered and hypotension results. (Reproduced with permission: Mason, D. T. et al. 1972. Page 137 *in* R. Eliot, ed. The acute cardiac emergency. Futura, Mt. Kisco, N.Y.)

of this abnormal curve in cardiogenic shock, cardiac output is reduced to such a marked degree that organ perfusion is too low to maintain life.

Severe pump failure occurs more commonly with extensive acute anterior myocardial infarction than it does with inferior wall infarction (7, 8). Experimental evidence suggests that the size of the infarction is related to myocardial oxygen requirements at the time of coronary occlusion (9). Although ventricular compliance may be transiently increased in the first day following infarction

(10), compliance is usually diminished throughout the initial five days of the acute episode (10–12). This increased stiffness of the chamber actually tends to improve the lowered stroke volume from the dysfunctioning ventricle by raising left ventricular end-diastolic pressure and preload and by diminishing ventricular distensibility during ejection (12). The persistency of an abnormal pattern of segmental contraction following infarction correlates temporally with the presence of pathologic Q waves and the nature and extent of chronic dyssynergy is related to ST-T wave changes (13).

A poor prognosis in myocardial infarction is portended by persistently low cardiac indices and marked elevation of left ventricular end-diastolic pressure, failure to augment stroke volume in response to plasma volume expansion, marked reduction of stroke work index, sustained systemic arterial desaturation, and low urine output (1, 2, 14, 15). Since right ventricular function is often normal in myocardial infarction, systemic venous pressure may be normal. However, right ventricular performance may be directly impaired in patients with right coronary occlusion and diaphragmatic infarction (16). Pulmonary blood volume is usually increased, while total blood volume is normal or even reduced following treatment with sympathomimetic drugs. Systemic arterial hypoxemia is attributable to impaired alveolar-capillary diffusion and venous admixture caused by pulmonary edema. Metabolic acidosis in cardiogenic shock is consequent to marked reduction of cardiac output.

In at least 50% of patients with cardiogenic shock, shock occurs early within a few hours of the infarction (17). These patients are usually relatively young, in their fourth and fifth decades of life, with acute anterior myocardial infarction resulting from thrombotic occlusion of the left anterior descending coronary artery. Further, they often have accelerated coronary disease and atherosclerosis risk factors. Cardiomegaly may be absent and usually is no more than moderate. Left ventriculography has demonstrated extensive dyskinesis of the anterior free wall and apex, usually greater than 50% of the ventricular silhouette, with increased extent and velocity of shortening of the posterior base of the chamber (18), as demonstrated in Figure 3. Selective coronary arteriography has shown complete obstruction of the proximal left anterior descending coronary artery (18) and pathologic examination has revealed that there is often distal patency of this vessel (17), although the patency may not be evident on angiography (18).

In approximately 16% of patients in cardiogenic shock, severe mechanical abnormalities are also present, such as mitral incompetence, ventricular septal defect (Fig. 4) or cardiac tamponade (17). In our experience it is unusual for a patient with diaphragmatic infarction to develop cardiogenic shock based solely on loss of left ventricular muscle; when shock occurs with this location of infarction it is usually caused by the added insult to cardiac function of a mechanical disturbance for which a careful search should be carried out (Fig. 5).

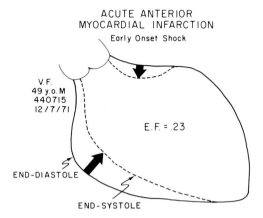

Fig. 3. Diagram of left ventricular cineangiogram (right anterior oblique view) in a 49-year-old man with immediate onset of severe pump failure which was present on admission to the hospital coronary care unit following acute anterior myocardial infarction. Extensive akinetic anterior-apical wall is shown with increased compensatory extent and velocity of basal segmental shortening. *EF* = ejection fraction.

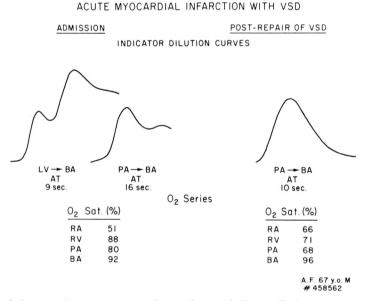

Fig. 4. Preoperative and postoperative cardiogreen indicator-dilation curves and right heart oxygen series in a 67-year-old man with acute anterioseptal myocardial infarction and acquired ventricular septal defect (*VSD*) with a pulmonary-to-systemic flow ratio of 3.4 to 1 and cardiogenic shock. Successful immediate VSD repair was accomplished in first day of infarction and septal rupture. Following surgery, cardiac pump failure was reversed and chronic survival achieved. *AT* = appearance time; O_2 *sat* = oxygen saturation; *LV* = left ventricle; *PA* = pulmonary artery; *RA* = right atrium; *RV* = right ventricle; *BA* = brachial artery.

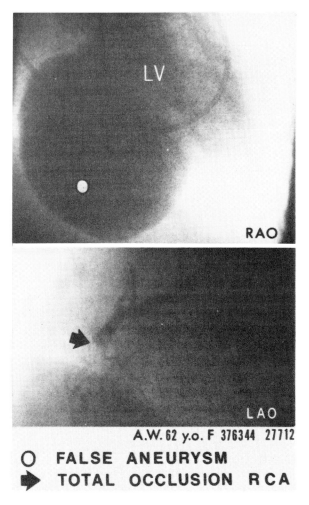

O **FALSE ANEURYSM**
➡ **TOTAL OCCLUSION R CA**

Fig. 5. 62-year-old woman with acute diaphragmatic myocardial infarction and rupture of posterior wall with cardiogenic shock. *Top:* Left ventricular cineangiogram showing false aneurysm at site of ventricular rupture. *RAO* = right anterior oblique view. *Bottom:* Selective right coronary artery (*RCA*) angiogram demonstrating complete proximal RCA occlusion. *LAO* = left anterior oblique view.

In the remaining 33% of patients with myocardial infarction shock, this syndrome develops more slowly within several days of severe intractable conges- tive heart failure following acute infarction (17). These patients usually have moderate to marked cardiomegaly (Fig. 6) and chronic symptomatology of ventricular pump dysfunction with previous episodes of myocardial ischemia and infarction. In addition, they usually are older, more than 60 years of age, and

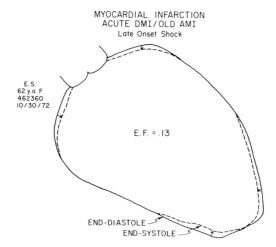

Fig. 6. Diagram of left ventricular cineangiogram (RAO view) in a 62-year-old woman with late onset of refractory cardiogenic shock gradually developing on fifth day following acute diaphragmatic myocardial infarction (*DMI*). She had a chronic history of cardiac dysfunction subsequent to an old anterior myocardial infarction (*AMI*). Generalized hypokinesis and akinesis of the entire ventricle are demonstrated. LVEDP = 40 mm Hg.

have diffuse multivessel coronary disease. Pump dysfunction in these individuals can often be considered terminal heart failure resulting from generalized left ventricular disease. On occasion, however, congestive heart failure and gradual development of shock occur with localized coronary stenosis in younger individuals in whom the extent of anterior infarction is somewhat less than that which produces acute onset of cardiogenic shock.

ROLE OF THE PERIPHERAL CIRCULATION

Although failure of cardiac pumping action with consequent decline of cardiac output is the major determinant in the initiation and persistence of myocardial infarction shock, abnormal integrity of circulatory response appears to play a secondary role in this condition. Thus, in many patients with shock following myocardial infarction, there is incomplete rise of systemic vascular resistance when cardiac output falls; this is postulated to result from competitive reflex vasodilation, initiated by stretch and chemoreceptors in the left ventricular wall, opposing carotid and aortic baroreceptor vasoconstrictor activity (19). Thereby the increase of peripheral vascular resistance is insufficient to maintain blood pressure at a normal level in the presence of low cardiac output.

Supporting this hypothesis of incomplete vascular constriction in myocardial infarction shock are studies carried out in experimental animals (19, 20) and in

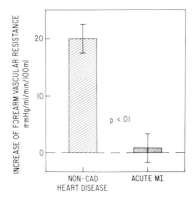

Fig. 7. Reflex forearm vascular resistance responses to head-upright tilting in acute myocardial infarction (*MI*) compared to hospitalized cardiac patients without coronary artery disease (*non-CAD*).

patients (21, 22). In this regard, utilizing plethysmographic techniques, we have shown arteriolar dilation in the forearm, consequent to selective coronary angiography in patients (21). Further, we have observed (22) impairment of reflex vasoconstriction in the forearm and in total systemic resistance with head-up tilting and the Valsalva maneuver in patients with acute myocardial infarction (Fig. 7).

MEDICAL THERAPY

At the beginning of consideration of treatment, the physiologic importance of maintaining normal blood pressure in this particular type of cardiogenic shock should be recognized (23). Thus, in myocardial infarction shock with low coronary arterial perfusion pressure, autoregulation of myocardial blood flow is impaired in the diseased coronary bed and the coronary vessels become dependent on adequate levels of systemic arterial diastolic pressure to maintain coronary blood flow. With very low levels of arterial blood pressure, the critical closing pressure of the coronary vasculature may be reached. Therefore, prolonged hypotension produces death of ischemic but potentially viable myocardium surrounding the infarcted area and results in greater depression of left ventricular function. Thus there is further decline of cardiac output and more profound lowering of arterial pressure, which leads to additional reduction of coronary blood flow, continued deterioration of cardiac function, and ultimately a fatal outcome. Consequently, in myocardial infarction shock, primary therapeutic consideration should be given to maintenance of coronary perfusion pressure to supply adequate flow through the stenotic atherosclerotic vessels, thus improving the contractile state of the ischemic myocardium.

In the treatment of myocardial infarction shock, adverse factors other than loss of myocardial contractile units should be considered and corrected. Thus, arrhythmias producing either excessively rapid or slow heart rate may reduce cardiac output in themselves. Hypoxia resulting from disturbances of respiratory function and pulmonary venous admixture can contribute to impairment of cardiac function. Excessive pain may be an additive influence in the production of shock. Detrimental iatrogenic factors should be considered, such as impairment of cardiorespiratory function provoked by large doses of morphine. When all such contributory factors to cardiogenic shock are eliminated and the severely depressed hemodynamic state persists, therapy with volume expansion and vasoactive agents is indicated.

It has become evident, however, that the most judicious employment of pharmacologic therapy in acute myocardial infarction shock allows successful outcome in no more than 10% of these patients. In our experience, survival is most likely to be achieved in the small proportion of patients who respond quickly with an increase in systemic blood pressure and a fall in the elevated left ventricular end-diastolic pressure. We emphasize that the very severely depressed ventricular function curve characteristic of myocardial infarction shock is inadequate to sustain life for more than a few hours in the presence of hypotension, or for more than a few days in the presence of severe intractable congestive failure without hypotension.

In the medical management of cardiogenic shock, volume expansion is used first when the left ventricular end-diastolic pressure is below 15 mm Hg to elevate ventricular preload, cardiac output and arterial blood pressure without inducing pulmonary congestion (24). However, the usefulness of this approach is limited since the flatness of the disturbed ventricular function curve does not

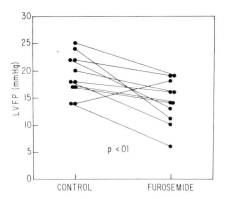

Fig. 8. Effect of intravenous furosemide on left ventricular end-diastolic pressure in patients with acute myocardial infarction and congestive heart failure without shock. *LVFP* = left ventricular filling pressure measured as mean pulmonary capillary wedge pressure using the Swan-Ganz PA catheter.

provide much rise in output with increasing end-diastolic pressure. Further, the end-diastolic pressure is often too high, above 15 mm Hg, to allow trial of volume expansion.

In the case of severe hypotension (systolic arterial pressure below 75 mm Hg), blood pressure is increased by administration of the vasoconstrictor-positive inotropic agent norepinephrine (25). When hypotension is not marked, a positive inotropic drug which also causes relatively mild generalized vasodilation, such as dopamine, is given (25) and, if hypotension is not corrected, pharmacologic therapy is switched to norepinephrine.

In the presence of congestive heart failure without shock, marked elevations of left ventricular end-diastolic pressure above 18 mm Hg are reduced to below 15 mm Hg by the administration of furosemide (26), as indicated in Figure 8. Digitalis is usually ineffective in cardiogenic shock but produces salutary changes in approximately 50% of patients in congestive failure without hypotension (26, 27) as shown in Figure 9. Pertinent to the mechanism of the attenuated hemodynamic improvement with digitalis in some patients with acute myocardial infarction is the experimentally documented diminution of positive inotropic action of the glycoside in the hypoxic myocardium (Fig. 10).

At the present time, new approaches to pharmacologic therapy have not improved survival in myocardial infarction shock, although certain of them have not been thoroughly tested. These agents include glucagon (28), steroids (29), alpha-adrenergic blockade (30), mannitol (31), glucose and insulin (32), hyaluronidase (33), and allopurinol (34). Since the fundamental pathologic defect in cardiogenic shock is the extent of loss of ventricular muscle, it is difficult to anticipate that new drugs per se will offer major advances in the future in the management of cardiogenic shock. Still a different mechanism of treatment to be evaluated in myocardial infarction is antithrombosis with urokinase and streptokinase.

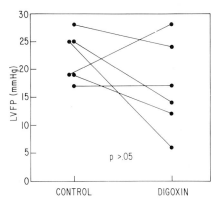

Fig. 9. Effect of intravenous digoxin on left ventricular end-diastolic pressure in patients with acute myocardial infarction and congestive heart failure without shock.

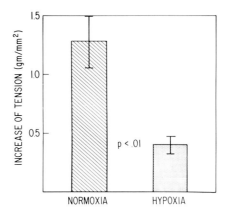

Fig. 10. Comparison of the effect of ouabain on peak isometric tension between normally oxygenated (*normoxia*) and hypoxic right ventricular cat papillary muscles.

MECHANICAL ASSISTANCE

Several mechanical devices have been developed for the temporary support of the damaged left ventricle after infarction. These devices are designed on the physiologic principle of reducing myocardial oxygen demands and improving coronary blood flow, while providing support of the systemic circulation. With the short-term application of circulatory assistance, time is allowed for the possible recovery of cardiac muscle with the hope that improved ventricular function can be maintained when artificial support is discontinued.

The most practical and beneficial technique is that of counterpulsation in which phasic alterations of aortic pressure are applied synchronously with the cardiac cycle. In this approach, an intraaortic balloon catheter is inserted into the descending thoracic aorta through the femoral artery (35). Diastolic augmentation of coronary blood flow is achieved by raising ascending aortic diastolic pressure by rapid inflation of the balloon during ventricular relaxation. During subsequent deflation of the balloon during systole, the resistance to left ventricular ejection is reduced and thereby myocardial oxygen requirements are diminished. The counterpulsation method has been extended to noninvasive devices which utilize intermittent external body compression synchronized with the cardiac cycle (36). Such an apparatus is the lower extremity suit which hydraulically provides phasic positive and negative ambient pressures in diastole and systole respectively (37).

Although hemodynamic improvement attends counterpulsation, this salutary effect is usually temporary and deterioration of pump function often follows discontinuation of assistance. Thus only a relatively small fraction of patients with myocardial infarction shock unresponsive to pharmacologic management have recovered as a result of application of counterpulsation. Perhaps a more beneficial application of counterpulsation in the future may be in patients with a high risk of developing cardiogenic shock, such as those with acute anterior myocardial infarction even without hypotension or congestive failure, in an effort to save as much ventricular myocardium as possible.

CARDIAC SURGERY

In certain patients with refractory cardiogenic shock and severe intractable heart failure, emergency left ventricular angiography and coronary arteriography can be performed with reasonable safety to determine whether acute revascularization by saphenous vein bypass, infarctectomy, mitral valve replacement or repair of a ruptured interventricular septum is likely to be efficacious (38–41). The extremely high mortality rate of myocardial infarction shock, despite careful pharmacologic management, argues for an aggressive approach in this grave situation, particularly in middle-aged and younger patients without a history of heart failure before the acute infarction. Our current policy is to carry out

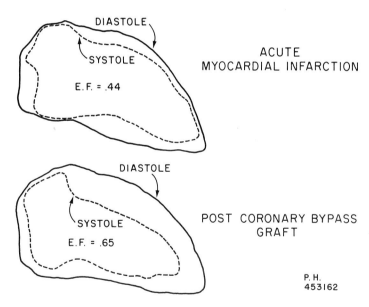

Fig. 11. Diagrams of left ventricular cineangiograms (RAO view) in a patient with acute myocardial infarction, pump dysfunction, and sustained myocardial ischemic pain. Segmental hypokinesis and reduced ejection fraction (*top*) were markedly improved (*bottom*) and chest pain was relieved by double aortocoronary saphenous vein bypass graft carried out in the early period following myocardial infarction.

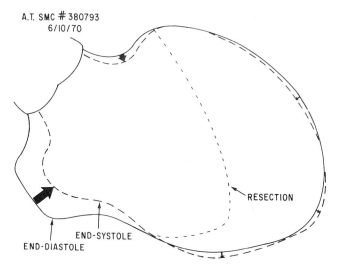

A.T. SMC # 380793
6/10/70

RESECTION

END-SYSTOLE
END-DIASTOLE

Fig. 12. Diagram of preoperative left ventricular angiogram (RAO view) in a 54-year-old man with profound intractable shock in the immediate period following acute anterior myocardial infarction. Dyssynergy of the anterior-apical wall is shown with normal contraction pattern of the basal segment. The *short dashes* represent the area of surgical excision carried out at successful emergency infarctectomy. Postoperatively cardiogenic shock disappeared and chronic survival was achieved. (Reproduced with permission: Mason, D. T. et al., reference 41.)

ventriculography and coronary arteriography as soon as it is established that the patient is unresponsive to medical treatment, within an hour or two with cardiogenic shock and between one to three days in the case of marked, refractory congestive failure without hypotension. From the information thereby obtained, surgical intervention with saphenous bypass is recommended as the procedure of choice when satisfactory patency is demonstrated of the distal portion of the proximally obstructed left anterior descending coronary artery (Fig. 11). For revascularization to restore myocardial function, success appears to be substantially enhanced when the bypass is carried out within 2−6 hours following infarction and shock.

When the obstructed left anterior descending vessel is not suitable for bypass, acute segmental ventricular resection may be successful as the primary procedure if the segment with abnormal motion, most often the anterior apical portion of the left ventricle, is well defined and there is normal or increased extent and velocity of shortening of the remaining myocardium (Fig. 12), usually the posterior-diaphragmatic area (41). Appropriate candidates for this operative intervention may have areas of dyssynergy of greater than 60% of the chamber, and extensive resections up to 50% in patients with ventricular dilation have been accomplished with survival.

CONCLUSIONS

The basic physiologic defect in acute myocardial infarction shock is marked depression of ventricular performance which is principally related to the extent of loss of contractile units. Thus, hypotension is primarily the result of reduced cardiac output. In addition, an inadequate rise in systemic vascular resistance contributes secondarily to the diminished blood pressure. This incomplete constriction in the systemic arteriolar beds is postulated to be the result of competitive reflex vasodilation, initiated by stretch and chemoreceptors within the left ventricular wall, which opposes carotid and aortic arch baroreceptor reflex vasoconstrictor activity.

Specific drug therapy is applied in cardiogenic shock after establishing that adequate plasma volume has not reversed the hemodynamic derangement. However, an ideal agent for this purpose is lacking and is unlikely to become available. Judicious medical therapy is successful in about 10% of patients with myocardial infarction shock and the use of mechanical assist devices allows survival in perhaps an additional 10%. Emergency coronary and ventricular angiography with coronary bypass revascularization or infarctectomy might prove to be life-saving in possibly 20% more of the patients. However, the mortality in this shock syndrome remains distressingly high, the outcome proving fatal in most patients. The major inroads in the management of myocardial infarction shock must await the development of a permanently implantable artificial heart.

REFERENCES CITED

1. Scheidt, S., Ascheim, R., and Killip, T. 1970. Shock after acute myocardial infarction. Amer. J. Cardiol. 26:556.
2. Swan, H. J. C., Forrester, J. S., Danzig, R., and Allen, H. N. 1970. Power failure in acute myocardial infarction. Prog. Cardiov. Dis. 12:568.
3. Page, D. L., Caulfield, J. B., Kaster, J. A., DeSanctis, R. W., and Saunders, C. A. 1971. Myocardial changes associated with cardiogenic shock. New Engl. J. Med. 285:133.
4. Shillingford, J., and Thomas, M. 1967. Hemodynamic effects of acute myocardial infarction in man. Prog. Cardiov. Dis. 9:571.
5. Ratshin, R. A., Rackley, C. A., and Russell, R. O., Jr. 1970. Hemodynamic evaluation of left ventricular failure in cardiogenic shock complicating acute myocardial infarction. Amer. J. Cardiol. 26:655.
6. Hamosh, P., and Cohn, J. N. 1971. Left ventricular function in acute myocardial infarction. J. Clin. Invest. 50:523.
7. Russell, R. O., Jr., Hunt, D., and Rackley, C. E. 1970. Left ventricular hemodynamics in anterior and inferior myocardial infarction. Amer. J. Cardiol. 26:658.
8. Hughes, J. L., Salel, A. F., Massumi, R. A., Zelis, R., Amsterdam, E. A., and Mason, D. T. 1971. The electrocardiogram as a predictor of ventricular function and cardiogenic shock in acute myocardial infarction. Circulation 44 (Suppl. 2):179.
9. Maroko, P. R., Kjekshus, J. K., Sobel, B. E., Watanabe, T., Covell, J. W., Ross, J., Jr., and Braunwald, E. 1971. Factors influencing infarct size following experimental coronary artery occlusions. Circulation 43:67.

10. Forrester, J. S., Diamond, G., Parmley, W. W., and Suran, J. J. C. 1972. Early increase in left ventricular compliance following acute myocardial infarction. J. Clin. Invest. 51:598.
11. Hood, W. B., Jr., Bianco, J. A., Kumar, R., and Whiting, R. B. 1970. Experimental myocardial infarction: IV. Reduction of left ventricular compliance in the healing phase. J. Clin. Invest. 49:1316.
12. Swan, H. J. C., Forrester, J. S., Diamond, G., Chatterjee, K., and Parmley, W. W. 1972. Hemodynamic spectrum of myocardial infarction and cardiogenic shock: A conceptual model. Circulation 45:1097.
13. Miller, R. R., Mason, D. T., Massumi, R. A., Zelis, R., and Amsterdam, E. A. 1972. ECG determination of nature, location and extent of abnormal ventricular segmental contraction in coronary artery disease. Circulation 46(Suppl. 2):9.
14. Russell, R. O., Jr., Rackley, C. E., Pombo, J., Hunt, D., Potanin, C., and Doge, H. T. 1970. Effects of increasing left ventricular filling pressure in patients with acute myocardial infarction. J. Clin. Invest. 49:1539.
15. Ramo, B. W., Myers, N., Wallace, A. G., Starmer, F., Clark, D. O., and Whalen, R. E. 1970. Hemodynamic findings in 123 patients with acute myocardial infarction on admission. Circulation 42:567.
16. Vismara, L., Mason, D. T., Amsterdam, E. A., and Zelis, R. 1972. Right ventricular muscle mechanics in myocardial infarction: Implications concerning indices of left ventricular filling. Circulation 46(Suppl. 2): 232.
17. Swan, H. J. C. 1972. Cardiogenic Shock, Abstracts of Papers: Fifth Asian-Pacific Congress of Cardiology, Oct. 8–13, 1972, Singapore, p. 21.
18. Amsterdam, E. A., Choquet, Y., Bonanno, J. A., Massumi, R. A., Zelis, R., and Mason, D. T. 1973. Correlative hemodynamics and angiography in acute coronary syndromes. Clin. Res. 21:232.
19. Constantin, L. 1963. Extracardiac factors contributing to hypotension during coronary occlusion. Amer. J. Cardiol. 11:205.
20. Toubes, D. B., and Brody, M. D. 1970. Inhibition of reflex vasoconstriction of experimental coronary embolization in the dog. Circ. Res. 26:211.
21. Zelis, R., Mason, D. T., Spann, J. F., Jr., and Amsterdam, E. A. 1970. Stimulation of myocardial chemoreceptors in man: Forearm arteriolar dilation induced by contrast media during coronary arteriography. Circulation 46(Suppl. 3):42.
22. Miller, R., Mason, D. T., Zelis, R., Hughes, J. L., Massumi, R. A., and Amsterdam, E. A. 1972. Attenuation of peripheral reflex vasoconstriction in patients with acute and chronic ischemic heart disease. Clin. Res. 20:388.
23. Braunwald, E. 1968. Acute myocardial infarction with shock: Physiological, pharmacological and clinical consideration. *In* H. L. Blumgart, ed. Symposium on Coronary Heart Disease. American Heart Association Monograph No. 2, p. 110.
24. Amsterdam, E. A., Massumi, R. A., Zelis, R., and Mason, D. T. 1972. Evaluation and management of cardiogenic shock. Part I. Approach to the patient. Heart and Lung. 1,3:402.
25. Amsterdam, E. A., Massumi, R. A., Zelis, R., and Mason, D. T. 1972. Evaluation and management of cardiogenic shock. II: Drug Therapy. Heart and Lung 1:663.
26. Amsterdam, E. A., Huffaker, H. K., DeMaria, A., Vismara, L. A., Choquet, Y., Massumi, R. A., Zelis, R., and Mason, D. T. 1972. Hemodynamic effects of digitalis in acute myocardial infarction and comparison with furosemide. Circulation 46(Suppl. 2):113.
27. Rahimtoola, S. H., Sinno, M. Z., Chuquimia, R., Loeb, H. S., Rosen, K. M., and Gunnar, R. M. 1972. Effects of ouabain on the left ventricle in acute myocardial infarction. New Engl. J. Med. 287:527.
28. Amsterdam, E. A., Zelis, R., Spann, J. F., Jr., Hurley, E. J., and Mason, D. T. 1970. Comparison of glucagon and catecholamines in congestive heart failure and coronary shock. Circulation 42(Suppl. 3):82.
29. Libby, P., Maroko, P. R., Sobel, B. E., Bloor, C. M., Covell, J. W., and Braunwald, E. 1972. Reduction in infarct size following experimental coronary occlusion by hydrocortisone treatment. Clin. Res. 20:207.

30. Corday, E., Vyden, J. K., Lang, T. W., Boxzormenyi, E., Carvalho, M., Gold, H., Goldman, A., and Rosselot, E. 1969. Reevaluation of the treatment of shock secondary to cardiac infarction. Chest 56:200.
31. Amsterdam, E. A., Foley, D., Massumi, R. A., Zelis, R., and Mason, D. T. 1972. Influence of increased glucose availability and mannitol on performance of hypoxic myocardium. J. Clin. Invest. 51:4a.
32. Amsterdam, E. A., Foley, D., Massumi, R., Zelis, R., and Mason, D. T. 1972. Effects of glucose loading and insulin on myocardial function during experimental hypoxia. Fifth International Congress on Pharmacology, San Francisco, p. 6.
33. Maroko, P. R., Libby, P., Bloor, C. M., Sobel, B. E., and Braunwald, E. 1972. Reduction by hyaluronidase of myocardial necrosis following coronary artery occlusion. Circulation 46:430.
34. Miller, R. R., Choquet, Y., Zelis, R., Massumi, R. A., Mason, D. T., and Amsterdam, E. A. 1973. Positive inotropic effect of allopurinol and enhancement of cardiac contractile function during hypoxia. Amer. J. Cardiol. 31:147.
35. Kantrowitz, A., Krakauer, J. S., and Butner, A. M. 1969. Phase-shift balloon pumping in cardiogenic shock. Prog. Cardiov. Dis. 12:293.
36. Cohen, L. S., Mitchell, J. H., Mullins, C. B., and Porterfield, D. 1969. Cardiovascular effects of sequenced external counterpulsation. Circulation 40(Suppl. 3):59.
37. Soroff, H. S., Cloutier, C. T., Birtwell, W. C., Banas, J. S., Brilla, A. H., Begley, L. A., and Messer, J. V. 1972. Clinical evaluation of external counterpulsation in cardiogenic shock. Circulation 45(Suppl. 2):75.
38. Heimbecker, R. O., Lemire, G., and Chen, C. 1968. Surgery for massive myocardial infarction: An experimental study of emergency infarctectomy with a preliminary report on the clinical application. Circulation 38(Suppl. 2):3.
39. Daggett, W. M., Burwell, L. R., Lawson, D. W., and Austen, W. G. 1970. Resection of acute ventricular aneurysm and ruptured interventricular septum after myocardial infarction. New Engl. J. Med. 283:1507.
40. Mundth, E. D., Yurchak, P. M., Buckley, M. J., Leinbach, R. C., Kantrowitz, A., and Austen, W. G. 1970. Temporary mechanical circulatory assistance and emergency direct coronary artery surgery for the treatment of cardiogenic shock complicating acute myocardial infarction. New Engl. J. Med. 283:1382.
41. Mason, D. T., Amsterdam, E. A., Miller, R. R., Hughes, J. L., Bonanno, J. A., Iben, A. B., Hurley, E. J., Massumi, R. A., and Zelis, R. 1971. Consideration of the therapeutic roles of pharmacologic agents, collateral circulation and saphenous vein bypass in coronary artery disease. Amer. J. Cardiol. 28:608.

ACHIEVEMENTS AND POTENTIAL OF COUNTERPULSATION IN CORONARY ARTERY DISEASE

DWIGHT EMARY HARKEN

Presentations and publications on assisted circulation have been met with a notable lack of active clinical implementation. Could it be that those clinicians in a position to make this modality useful are put off by the mass of solid scientific laboratory and clinical supporting evidence? Could it be that another type of sound must be made to reach the right ears? After all, presentations are only as reliable as the person making them. Such a set of circumstances prompts a narrative presentation here. Hopefully it may be readable enough to capture much needed interest. Support for loose generalizations and assertions will in all instances be found in the suggested reading list that follows. This evident frustration can only be corrected by acceptance of these concepts and by implementations that should potentiate achievements and achieve the potential.

More than thirteen years have elapsed since we began to talk about *counterpulsation* to change the heart's pressure work to flow work. Sarnoff and associates and many since them have demonstrated that the myocardial metabolism for pressure work requires much more oxygen than in flow work. For even more years it has been appreciated that most coronary artery flow is during diastole, and that flow is a function of the *caliber of the vessels,* the *pressure at the aortic base* in diastole, and the duration of diastole.

More than a decade ago we established the fact that by aspirating blood in systole and returning it during diastole one could reduce the pressure against which the left ventricle contracted (reduce pressure work), and return that aliquot of blood in diastole to sustain body perfusion and augment coronary perfusion (thus providing more coronary flow with less need). Pressure work was changed to flow work via "counterpulsation," as the term was coined to suggest. The timing of the aspiration and return of blood was effected by a bellophragm pump timed with the "R" wave of the electrocardiogram. That first successful laboratory counterpulsation device was created by engineer Birtwell and conducted in our laboratory. Publication with him, Clauss, and our group took place in 1961!

Early work in our laboratory with Jacobey and Taylor, endlessly repeated, showed that in controlled Agress microsphere myocardial ischemia the intercoronary communications could be opened within minutes by counterpulsation.

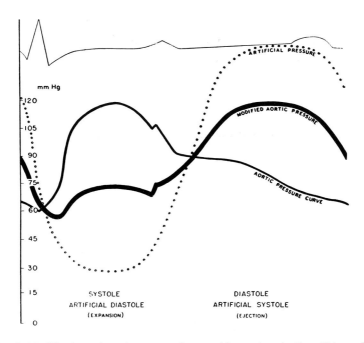

mm Hg

120
105
90
75
60
45
30
15
0

SYSTOLE
ARTIFICIAL DIASTOLE
(EXPANSION)

DIASTOLE
ARTIFICIAL SYSTOLE
(EJECTION)

Fig. 1. Modification of aortic pressure by arterial counterpulsation. Triggered by the ECG "R" wave, the intra-aortic balloon is deflated in systole (effect of aspirating blood) reducing resistance against which heart contracts (*dotted line* in systole). In diastole the balloon is inflated with the effect of injecting blood. Modified pressure curve (*heavy line*) indicates the resultant high diastolic perfusion pressure for body perfusion and increased coronary perfusion.

Two hours of counterpulsation *reversed* an animal mortality rate of 75% to a *survival* rate of 75% in identical matched series. Coronary blood flow was found to be greatly increased and myocardial necrosis decreased in carefully controlled experiments by us, by Soroff, by Braunwald, and by others.

Soroff, Birtwell, and then Moulopoulos showed that such timing clued to the R wave of the electrocardiogram could be accomplished by inflating and deflating an intra-aortic balloon with helium. Hemolysis could be reduced by means of intra-aortic balloon counterpulsation with helium without sacrificing (indeed enhancing) the pressure phase shift.

Kantrowitz and Kantrowitz (Adrian, a surgeon, and his brother Arthur, an engineer) advanced the concept by extensive laboratory experimental work and by the design and development of fine equipment for laboratory, then clinical application. They spearheaded and continue to foster cardinal clinical work that indicates significant improvement and survival in cardiogenic shock by means of balloon counterpulsation (or as they designate it "phase-shift diastolic augmenta-

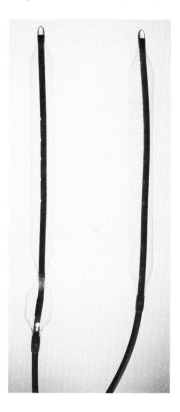

Fig. 2. The standard sausage-shaped single intra-aortic nonocclusive balloon (*right*). The double balloon (*left*) with small occlusive caudad balloon enhances the cephalad nonocclusive efficacy. When used with Datascope activator, limited quantities of carbon dioxide can be used, affording great safety.

tion"). Adrian Kantrowitz, in a national cooperative seven-center study of cardiogenic shock, has shown that the great majority of interventions have been after multiple organ death. Thus shock can be temporarily relieved, but failure to survive is inevitable with such patient selection. On the other hand, even in otherwise fatal cardiogenic shock there can be better than 10% salvage. Arthur Kantrowitz, working with Austen, Mundth, Daggett, Buckley, DeSanctis, and their colleagues at the Massachusetts General Hospital, has stressed the use of counterpulsation as a means of supporting the patient, who would otherwise die in shock, until angiographic studies can define and allow appropriate surgical intervention. This intervention has comprised saphenous vein bypass, correction of an interventricular septal defect, and myocardial resection.

Goetz, with Bregman and Datascope engineers, has improved the balloon design to utilize a small caudad occlusive balloon combined with a cephalad larger nonocclusive sausage-shaped balloon. This equipment improves coronary perfusion and uses a limited volume of carbon dioxide, which is a safer gas than helium should there be balloon leak or rupture.

Soroff and Birtwell pioneered, then Messer, Banas, and Mueller expanded the use of external counterpulsation, some with and some without a negative pressure phase. Soroff and Birtwell have conducted a community hospital rescue system that has study limitations, but nonetheless has impressive salvage. Messer has conducted a matched controlled prospective study that has shown statistically significant improved survival for patients in cardiogenic shock. Banas has clearly afforded consistent temporary relief from angina. Mueller has compared external compression assist with intra-aortic balloon counterpulsation, clarifying some advantages of each method in well defined and different circumstances.

All of these concepts, techniques, and accomplishments have been so endlessly repeated (with precious little evident response from our colleagues who treat coronary artery disease), that in frustration I record ten defensible assertions. All of these are abundantly supported by laboratory and clinical work detailed in the references that follow.

1) Myocardial oxygen demands are much greater for *pressure* work than for *flow* work.

2) Hemodynamic and pharmacologic factors within the control of the clinician may increase or decrease the extent of heart muscle damage by coronary occlusion (e.g., vasopressors, vasoconstrictors, glucagon, isoproterenol).

3) Pressure work can be reduced by counterpulsation.

4) Coronary blood flow can be increased by counterpulsation.

5) Myocardial infarction may reduce cardiac output, lower systemic pressure, increase heart rate, and by any or all of these reduce coronary flow. Reduced coronary flow in turn can extend myocardial ischemia, dysfunction, and necrosis. Such circumstances can become a lethal, self-aggravating spiral process. This is particularly likely where there is diffuse coronary artery disease.

6) The mortality rate from experimental coronary occlusion can be reduced by early counterpulsation. Early counterpulsation—within three hours—can reduce the size of the necrotic zone from experimental coronary occlusion. Early multilead precordial electrocardiographic screening suggests that this is also true clinically.

7) Counterpulsation can consistently reverse, at least temporarily, some consequences of low-flow states in experimental and human cardiogenic shock.

8) In otherwise irreversible cardiogenic shock, counterpulsation can constitute a holding action until the occluded vessel and infarcted areas can be defined angiographically and corrected surgically. Such surgery may involve either saphenous vein bypass or resection, or both.

9) Counterpulsation techniques seem safe, simple, and effective. The late utilization of counterpulsation in cardiogenic shock after extensive, even lethal brain, myocardial, gastrointestinal, liver, or renal damage appears to constitute abuse rather than use of the technique.

10) Use of early counterpulsation, even in minor infarctions, probably would reduce the zone of necrosis. This might in some patients with infarction reverse an otherwise self-aggravating spiral and reduce both morbidity and mortality.

Additionally, I offer suggestions regarding *potential* that may illustrate some areas of my confidence in one of the most exciting, unexplored (or at least grossly inadequately explored) horizons in the treatment of coronary artery disease.

1) There is promising *potential* in the use of counterpulsation therapeutically, even prophylactically, in chronic coronary low-flow states. This involves both patients with angina and catastrophe-prone candidates for coronary occlusion.

2) The use of counterpulsation by means of the intra-aortic balloon will become widely used (instead of rarely used) as a means of assisting the circulation in refractory cardiac resuscitation following open heart surgery.

3) Counterpulsation will become a form of standard (routine) early therapy in many forms of myocardial infarction—before necrosis, to salvage the bordering zones of necrosis and before the infarct can set up the self-aggravating cycle of ischemic hypokinesis, then necrosis.

4) All patients in cardiogenic shock will be offered *immediate* counterpulsation, *and* simultaneously the usual volume replacement and medical supportive programs. The "waiting to see" if medical methods avail will be replaced by a more aggressive attitude of simultaneous utilization of effective treatments. There should evolve synergism that could save much heart muscle mass yearly.

5) *Simplified* angiographic and hemodynamic measurement methods will augment the use of early study and early surgical intervention with counterpulsation as the holding mechanism.

6) While the "noninvasive" technique of external counterpulsation (with or without negative pressure cycle) will be more readily accepted by physicians, the lesser value of the *positive pressure only* technique will lead to acceptance of the relatively minor invasion of the double balloon, CO_2 counterpulsation advocated by Bregman and Goetz with Datascope.

REFERENCES

1. Albertal, G. A., Clauss, R. H., Fosberg, A. M., Taylor, W. J., and Harken, D. E. 1961. An improved electromagnetic flowmeter for extracorporeal circulation. J. Thorac. Cardiov. Surg. 41:368.
2. Agress, C. M., Rosenberg, M. J., Jacob, H. I., Binder, M. J., Schneiderman, A., and Clark, W. G. 1952. Protracted shock in closed chest dog following coronary embolization with graded microspheres. Amer. J. Physiol. 170:536.
3. Banas, J. S., Brilla, A., Soroff, H. S., and Levine, H. J. 1972. Evaluation of external counterpulsation for the treatment of severe angina pectoris. American Heart Association, 45th Scientific Sessions. Dallas, Texas, November 16-19, 1972 (in press).
4. Birtwell, W. C., Giron, R., Ruiz, U., Norton, R. L., and Soroff, H. S. 1970. The regional hemodynamic response to synchronous external pressure assist. Trans. Amer. Soc. Artif. Intern. Organs 16:462.
5. Braunwald, E. 1969. Bowditch lecture: the determinants of myocardial oxygen consumption. Physiologist 12:65.
6. Braunwald, E., Covell, J. W., Maroko, P. R., and Ross, J., Jr. 1969. Effects of drugs and counterpulsation on myocardial oxygen consumption: observations on the ischemic heart. Circulation 440:220.
7. Braunwald, E. 1971. Control of myocardial oxygen consumption: physiologic and clinical considerations. Amer. J. Cardiol. 27:416.
8. Bregman, D., Kripke, D. C., Cohen, M. N., Laniado, S., and Goetz, R. H. 1970. Clinical experience with the undirectional dual-chambered intra-aortic balloon assist. Circulation 41 (Suppl. III):76.
9. Buckley, J. J., Leinbach, R. C., Kastor, J. A., Kantrowitz, A. R., Laird, J. D., and Austen, W. G. 1969. Hemodynamic evaluation of intra-aortic balloon pumping (IAP) in man. Circulation (Suppl. 340):52.
10. Buckley, M. J., Craver, J. M., Gold, H. K., Mundth, E. D., Daggett, W. M., and Austen, W. G. 1972. Intra-aortic balloon pump assist for cardiogenic shock after cardiopulmonary bypass. American Heart Association, 45th Scientific Sessions, Dallas, Texas, November 16-19, 1972 (in press).
11. Clauss, R. H., Missier, P., Reed, G. E., and Tice, D. 1962. Assisted circulation by counterpulsation with intra-aortic balloon: methods and effects. Presented at Annual Conference on Engineering in Medicine and Biology, Chicago, November 5-7, 1962.
12. Corday, E., Swan, H. J. C., Lang, T., Goldman, A., Matloff, J. M., Gold, H., and Meerbaum, S. 1970. Physiologic principles in the application of circulatory assist for the failing heart; intra-aortic balloon circulatory assist and veno-arterial phased partial bypass. Amer. J. Cardiol. 26:595.
13. Daggett, W. M., Burwell, L. R., Lawson, D. W., and Austen, W. G. 1971. Resection of acute ventricular aneurysm and ruptured interventricular septum after myocardial infarction. New Engl. J. Med. 283:1507.
14. Dilley, R. B., Ross, J., and Bernstein, E. F. 1972. Serial hemodynamics during intra-aortic balloon counterpulsation for cardiogenic shock. American Heart Association, 45th Scientific Session, Dallas, Texas, November 16-19, 1972 (in press).
15. Harken, D. E. 1967. First Laurence Brewster Ellis lecture; heart surgery . . . legend and a long look. Amer. J. Cardiol. 19:393.
16. Harken, D. E. 1968. Arthur M. Master lecture, March 28, 1968. J. Mount Sinai Hosp. N.Y. 35:541.
17. Harken, D. E., Soroff, H. S., and Birtwell, W. C. 1972. Assisted circulation: counterpulsation and coronary artery disease. In P. Cooper, ed. Surgery annual, p. 165. Appleton, New York.
18. Jacobey, J. A., Taylor, W. J., Smith, G. T., Gorlin, R., and Harken, D. E. 1962. A new therapeutic approach to acute coronary occlusion. I. Production of standardized coronary occlusion with microspheres. Amer. J. Cardiol. 9:60.
19. Jacobey, J. A., Taylor, W. J., Smith, G. T., Gorlin, R., and Harken, D. E. 1963. A new therapeutic approach to acute coronary occlusion. II. Opening dormant coronary collateral channels by counterpulsation. Amer. J. Cardiol. 11:218.

20. Jacobey, J. A. 1971. Results of counterpulsation in patients with coronary artery disease. Amer. J. Cardiol. 27:137.
21. Jaron, D., Tomecek, J., Freed, P. S., Welkowitz, W., Fich, S., and Kantrowitz, A. 1970. Measurement of ventricular load phase angle as an operating criterion for in series assist devices: hemodynamic studies utilizing intra-aortic balloon pumping. Trans. Amer. Soc. Artif. Intern. Organs 16:466.
22. Kantrowitz, A., Tjonneland, S., Krakauer, J. S., Phillips, S. J., Freed, P. S., and Butner, A. N. 1968. Mechanical intra-aortic cardiac assistance in cardiogenic shock: hemodynamic effects. Arch. Surg. 97:1000.
23. Kennedy, J. Assisted circulation, an extended concept of cardiopulmonary resuscitation in man. J. Assoc. Adv. Med. Instrum. 4:237.
24. Killip, T., Scheidt, S., and Fillmore, S. 1971. Left ventricular function in acute myocardial infarction. Proceedings of Association of University Cardiologists, January 21, 1971.
25. Lefemine, A. A., Low, H. B. C., Cohen, M. L., Lunzer, S., and Harken, D. E. 1962. Assisted circulation. III. The effect of synchronized arterial counterpulsation on myocardial oxygen consumption and coronary flow. Amer. Heart J. 64:789.
26. Maroko, P. R., Bernstein, E. F., Covell, J. W., Ross, J., Jr., and Braunwald, E. 1971. The effects of intra-aortic counterpulsation on the severity of myocardial ischemic injury following experimental coronary occlusion. Circulation 43:67.
27. Matloff, J. M., Parmley, W. W., Manchester, J. H., Berkovits, B. V., Sonnenblick, E. H., and Harken, D. E. 1970. Hemodynamic effects of glucagon and intra-aortic balloon counterpulsation in canine myocardial infarction. Amer. J. Cardiol. 25:675.
28. Moulopoulos, S. D., Topas, S., and Kolff, W. L. Diastolic balloon pumping (with carbon dioxide) in aorta: mechanical assistance to failing circulation. Amer. Heart J. 63:669.
29. Mueller, H., Ayers, S. M., Gregory, J. J., Giannelli, S., Jr., Grace, W. J., and Nealon, W. 1970. Hemodynamics, coronary blood flow and myocardial metabolism in coronary shock; response to l-norepinephrine and isoproterenol. J. Clin. Invest. 49:1885.
30. Mueller, H., Ayers, S. M., Grace, W. J., and Giannelli, S., Jr. 1973. External counterpulsation—a noninvasive method to protect ischemic myocardium in man? American Heart Association, 45th Scientific Sessions, Dallas, Texas, November 16-19, 1972 (in press).
31. Mundth, E. D., Buckley, M. J., Leinbach, R. C., DeSanctis, R. W., Sanders, C. A., Kantrowitz, A. R., and Austen, W. G. 1971. Myocardial revascularization for the treatment of cardiogenic shock complicating acute myocardial infarction. Surgery 70:78.
32. Osborn, J. J., Russi, M., Salil, A., Bramson, M. L., and Gerbode, F. 1962. Diastolic augmentation by external pulsed pressure. Presented at the Annual Conference on Engineering in Medicine and Biology, Chicago, November 5-7, 1962.
33. Peel, A. A. 1962. Prognosis after myocardial infarction. Brit. Heart J. 24:745.
34. Rosensweig, J., Borromeo, C., Chatterjee, S., Sheiner, N., and Mayman, A. 1966. Treatment of coronary insufficiency by counterpulsation: experimental study. Ann. Thoracic Surg. 2:706.
35. Salisbury, P. F. 1966. Physiology of assisted circulation in mechanical devices to assist the failing heart. Washington, D. C., National Academy of Sciences-National Research Council. Publication 1283, pp. 3–19.
36. Sarnoff, S. J., Braunwald, E., Welch, G. J., Jr., Case, R. B., Stainsby, W. N., and Macruz, R. 1958. Hemodynamic determinants of oxygen consumption of the heart, with special reference to the tension-time index. Amer. J. Physiol. 192:148.
37. Soroff, H. S., Levine, H. J., Sachs, B. F., Birtwell, W. C., and Deterling, R. A., Jr. 1963. Assisted circulation. II. Effects of counterpulsation on left ventricular oxygen consumption and hemodynamics. Circulation 27:722.
38. Soroff, H. S., Cloutier, C. T., Birtwell, W. C., Banas, J. S., Brilla, A. H., Begley, L. A., and Messer, J. V. 1973. Clinical evaluation of external counterpulsation in cardiogenic shock. American Heart Association, 45th Scientific Sessions, Dallas, Texas, November 16-19, 1972 (in press).

PROGRESSIVE ALTERATIONS IN CARDIAC FUNCTION DURING CORONARY OCCLUSION AND REPERFUSION

SAMUEL MEERBAUM, TZU-WANG LANG, SHIGERU HIROSE,
COSTANTINO COSTANTINI, MARIA DALMASTRO,
HERBERT GOLD, and ELIOT CORDAY

Knowledge is still lacking of the progressive and detailed effects of coronary occlusion on cardiac function. Correlations of regional and global measurements of cardiac electrical, mechanical, and metabolic function, combined with morphologic study, are needed to provide insight into ischemic phenomena. Such data could bring about a better understanding of the progressive effects of myocardial ischemia secondary to coronary occlusion and lead to the development of better patient care. Unfortunately, human data do not supply adequate information because they lack a preocclusion base line control, which is an essential element in the analysis of occlusion mechanisms. The complex measurements which are required to define adequately metabolic and mechanical function of the heart clearly are difficult to accomplish in patients because of the extensive nature of the invasive procedures. Therefore, such comprehensive technical studies can be accomplished only in the experimental animal. It has been possible, in animal preparations, to achieve a satisfactory physiologic simulation of a number of clinical events which characterize ischemic disease.

In a new closed-chest model developed in the dog (1, 2), preocclusion control data serve as a base line for subsequent postocclusion measurements of regional and overall mechanical, electrical, and metabolic myocardial function. Measurements of left ventricular and aortic pressure, along with cardiac output, are used to derive indices of cardiac performance. Unique blood sampling provides myocardial arterio-venous (A-V) differences, which can be used to evaluate the state of myocardial metabolism, including oxygen consumption, lactate balance, and flux of electrolytes from both ischemic and nonischemic areas simultaneously. Also, electrocardiographic recordings and serum enzyme determinations are correlated with histopathologic determinations on the excised myocardium so as to evaluate the progressive damage to cardiac tissue (3). Differing anatomic sites and degrees of coronary occlusion may be chosen for study. Reperfusion, pharmacologic interventions, or circulatory assistance can be investigated. These comprehensive studies are designed to resolve specific questions, to verify or refute hypotheses, and to elucidate further the physiologic mechanisms.

This study was supported by Contract PH-43-68-1333 of the Myocardial Infarction Program, National Heart and Lung Institute, U.S. Public Health Service Grant HL-14644-01-02, and by Mrs. Anna Bing Arnold and the Jules Stein Foundation.

A NEW CLOSED-CHEST INTRACORONARY
BALLOON OCCLUSION-REPERFUSION MODEL

The primary features of the new closed-chest model are: 1) the intracoronary balloon occlusion of specific coronary arteries or their branches; 2) measurement of hemodynamic function; and 3) temporary balloon separation of venous compartments to permit simultaneous measurements of A-V differences representing regional as well as global myocardial metabolism and blood flow. The basic tool is a double-lumen intracoronary balloon catheter, which is maneu-

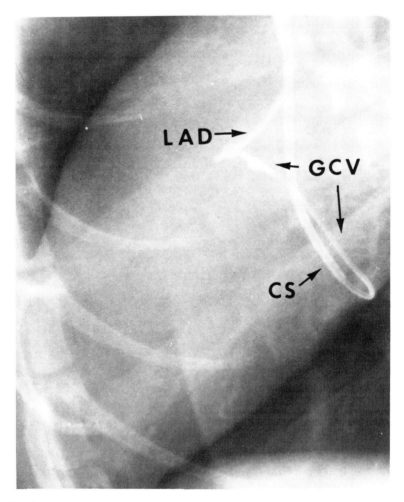

Fig. 1. Double-lumen balloon catheter positioned within the proximal LAD coronary artery and the great cardiac vein.

vered under fluoroscopic control into a segment of a specific artery selected for study. The balloon is located 1 cm from the tip of the catheter and can be positioned at any site within a coronary artery or its branches. Total or partial occlusion of the artery is performed under fluoroscopic control through infla- tion at a preselected time and chosen location. Partial or complete deflation of the balloon serves to reperfuse the previously occluded artery. It is relatively easy to perform the above maneuvers rapidly for single or sequential occlusion of the coronary arteries.

Figure 1 is a coronary angiogram which demonstrated complete occlusion of the proximal left anterior descending coronary artery (LAD) by means of the balloon. In Figure 2, contrast material was injected through the central lumen of

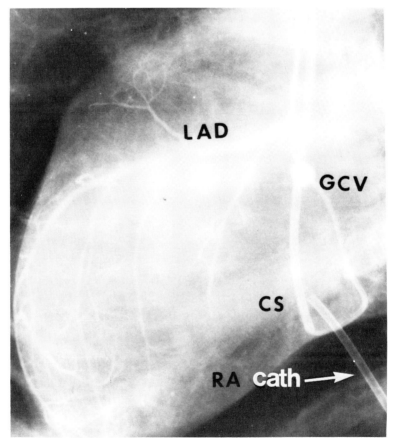

Fig. 2. Coronary angiography outlining the regional coronary vasculature distal to balloon occlusion of the LAD.

this catheter, and the photograph delineates the normally perfused region of the LAD which has been effectively cut off by proximal LAD occlusion. Similar occlusions now have been carried out in more than 100 dogs at different levels of the LAD and left circumflex coronary arteries, as well as of their smaller branches. Additional experiments using implanted electromagnetic flow probes proved that the intracoronary catheters (with balloon deflated) do not interfere with normal flow in the coronary arteries. Postmortem inspection of the coronary arteries in the excised hearts showed no damage to the vessel intima as long as the balloon is not excessively inflated.

A significant feature of the model is the ability to communicate through the central lumen of the intracoronary catheter with the region distal to the occlusion for measurements of coronary pressure, assessment of collateral flow, and blood sampling. Infusion of a variety of drugs into the occluded segment represents a novel approach to pharmacologic studies.

A major innovation is the use of a second double-lumen balloon catheter, which is inserted alongside a coronary sinus (CS) catheter into the great cardiac vein (GCV). Figure 3 is a schematic representation of the position of three catheters, one within the LAD coronary artery for proximal LAD occlusion, one in the CS, and one inserted through the latter catheter to lie deep within the GCV, draining the occluded area. Temporary inflation of the balloon within the GCV effectively separates venous drainages from the occluded and nonoccluded

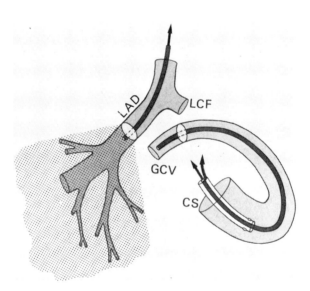

Fig. 3. Experimental methodology for coronary occlusion and temporary separation of venous compartments.

myocardium for both blood sampling and measurement of coronary flows. Following coronary artery occlusion, a significant difference in metabolic measurements from the ischemic and nonischemic regions of the heart is being observed, confirming that the technique is separating blood samples from distinct venous beds.

An intracoronary electrocardiogram is obtained from the epicardial surface in the occluded region of the myocardium by advancing a platinum wire through the central lumen of the intracoronary artery balloon catheter into the zone beyond the point of occlusion. The value of this promising new method is being assessed.

METABOLIC AND HEMODYNAMIC MEASUREMENTS FOLLOWING CORONARY OCCLUSION AND REPERFUSION

Methodology

Our new model was applied to study the progressive changes in myocardial metabolism and hemodynamics after LAD occlusion and reperfusion. Measurements were obtained of left ventricular pressure, left ventricular end-diastolic pressure (LVEDP), left ventricular dP/dt (LV dP/dt), aortic root pressure, and coronary pressure distal to the point of occlusion. Cardiac output and venous flows from the coronary sinus and regional myocardium were measured by thermodilution. The CS measurement was performed prior to and during inflation of the balloon within the GCV, thus measuring total coronary sinus drainage and flow from the nonoccluded myocardium, respectively. Great cardiac vein flow from the occluded zone of the left ventricle could then be deduced by difference. Damming up of the pressure in the temporarily occluded GCV was avoided by simultaneous syringe aspiration through the central lumen of the double-lumen balloon catheter.

Occasional direct retrograde blood collection was performed through the central lumen of the intracoronary artery balloon catheter to assess coronary collateral flow beyond the point of occlusion and to analyze blood samples which were found to be equally oxygenated arterial blood.

Separation of blood samples from the occluded and nonoccluded regions of the myocardium was achieved by the temporary inflation of the balloon within the great cardiac vein. Comparison of these two venous blood specimens with aortic blood samples permitted computation of A-V differences. These blood samples were collected at regular intervals during the preocclusion control, during the occlusion period, and subsequent to reperfusion. These samples were analyzed for oxygen, pH, lactic acid, potassium, and creatine phosphokinase.

Standard precordial V_4 and intracoronary electrocardiograms were recorded simultaneously along with hemodynamic data.

RESULTS

Hemodynamic Function

Hemodynamic recordings obtained during the preocclusion control, after coronary occlusion, and during reperfusion are shown in Figure 4. Figure 5 is a bar chart representing the average level of hemodynamic data of a series of 14 closed-chest dog experiments with statistical data presented as mean percentage of change from its preocclusion control and corresponding standard error of mean. Preocclusion control levels of all the hemodynamic parameters were

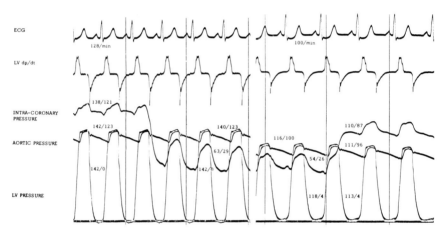

Fig. 4. Hemodynamic recording of LAD occlusion and reperfusion. Note the intracoronary pressure distal to the balloon, which drops sharply during the occlusion period and rises to systemic levels upon reperfusion.

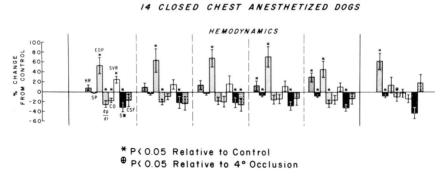

Fig. 5. Statistical summary of hemodynamics in 14 normotensive dogs following coronary occlusion and reperfusion.

measured after achieving 15–30 min of stabilization in the fully instrumented preparations. Measurements then were performed at five minutes, 30 minutes, one, two, three, and four hours following acute LAD coronary artery occlusion. These measurements were repeated immediately following reperfusion and at the end of a 30 minute reperfusion period.

First 30 minutes after proximal LAD occlusion

Heart rate rose about 10% and peak systemic aortic pressure was maintained near control, while systemic vascular resistance increased significantly (about 20%). At the same time, LVEDP rose approximately 50% above its control level, and there was a 20–30% drop in LV dP/dt_{max}, cardiac output, and left ventricular stroke work. Total coronary sinus flow was reduced about 15% relative to preocclusion control, reflecting the LAD occlusion.

From one to four hours postocclusion

Over this period, there are no further striking changes in the hemodynamic findings. Heart rate increased until it was 30% above control at four hours of the occlusion period. Systemic vascular resistance increased further to about 20% above control two hours after occlusion, and then in the third and fourth hour diminished to about 10%. Left ventricular end-diastolic pressure rose slightly and was 70% above control at three hours; at the end of four hours, it diminished to 45%. LV dP/dt and cardiac output remained at about the same diminished level as at 30 minutes after occlusion.

Thirty minute reperfusion

Shortly after the intracoronary balloon was deflated, the heart rate increased to 60% above preocclusion control. Systemic pressure dropped about 10%. LVEDP, LV dP/dt, and cardiac output returned to normal levels, and there was a 10% drop in systemic vascular resistance. Stroke work diminished further to about 45% below its control level.

Metabolic Function

Figure 6 presents the statistical data averaged in 14 dogs and illustrates the progressive alterations in metabolism from base line control levels, through four hours of proximal LAD occlusion, and through 30 minutes of reperfusion. A feature of these measurements is that blood samples were obtained simultaneously in the ascending aorta and in both the coronary sinus as well as in the great cardiac vein during temporary separation of the venous compartments by means of the GCV catheter balloon. Thus, myocardial A-V differences in concentration are obtained across the occluded and nonoccluded regions of the left ventricle.

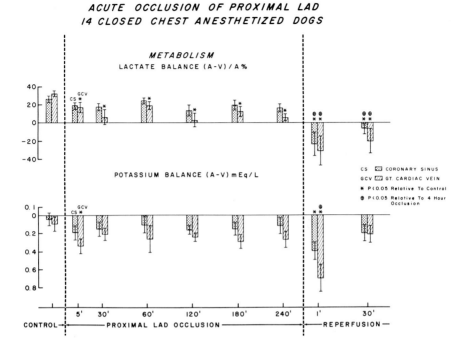

Fig. 6. Statistical summary of myocardial lactate metabolism and potassium losses in 14 normotensive dogs following coronary occlusion and reperfusion.

Occasional blood sampling from the LAD coronary artery distal to the occlusion established that this blood is fully saturated and reflects the oxygen tension seen in the aorta.

Myocardial lactate balance

First 30 minutes following occlusion: Blood samples collected in the first five minutes revealed a slight drop in myocardial lactate extraction; however, 30 minutes after occlusion, there was a significant drop in the GCV lactate balance to about 5% [(A-V)/A], indicating that abnormal lactate metabolism is taking place in the occluded region.

From one to four hours postocclusion: One hour after occlusion, the lactate balance returned toward control levels, but when the blood was sampled two hours after occlusion, the CS balance decreased to 14%, while the GCV dropped to 3%. At three hours, the lactate balance improved in both the CS (19%) and the GCV (12%). At four hours, the CS balance declined to 16% and the GCV was down to 5%.

Thirty minute reperfusion: Immediately following reperfusion, the CS lactate balance was −24%, and that of the GCV was −32%. After 30 minutes of reperfusion, the CS balance was −8% and the GCV was −21%.

Potassium balance

First 30 minutes following occlusion: Five minutes after coronary occlusion, there was a marked loss in potassium from both the coronary sinus and the great cardiac vein. A-V balance was about −0.2 mEq/l for the CS and −0.34 mEq/l for the GCV. Thirty minutes after occlusion, the values for the CS and GCV were −0.15 and −0.21 mEq/l, respectively.

From one to four hours following occlusion: A-V differences at one hour of occlusion were −0.1 mEq/l in the CS and −0.26 mEq/l in the GCV. The potassium loss from the CS and GCV continued at about these levels for the entire four-hour period.

Reperfusion: One minute following reperfusion, the CS balance was −0.39 mEq/l and the GCV (A-V) was −0.69 mEq/l. Thirty minutes following reperfusion, the CS and GCV (A-V) balances were −0.2 and −0.21 mEq/l, respectively.

Oxygen studies

Limited data were obtained for A-V oxygen saturation. During occlusion, this A-V difference appears elevated in the nonoccluded zone. Initial reperfusion, after four hours of occlusion, resulted in a sharp drop in the A-V differences, but 30 minutes later, there was a return to preocclusion control A-V oxygen levels. The coronary sinus flows were measured in five of the 14 dogs. Such measurements performed during temporary separation of the great cardiac vein provide data on regional myocardial oxygen consumption.

DISCUSSION

Almost all of the animal models of coronary occlusion used to date have been criticized, either because they do not properly mimic coronary occlusions in the human or because opening of the pericardial sac and other surgical interventions destroy a physiologic simulation. Open-chest experiments are characterized by greatly depressed cardiac function and coronary flow artifacts. Hence, there has been urgent demand for models which would permit extensive instrumentation and allow selective and reversible coronary occlusions in the closed-chest animal.

Sophisticated preparations have been developed in which instruments and externally controlled coronary occluders are first implanted in the open chest and pericardium, following which the chest is closed (4, 5). After a recuperative period of days or weeks, experimental coronary occlusion, reperfusion, or other interventions can be studied in anesthetized or conscious states.

To avoid the need for prior surgery, several experimental techniques have been explored. These include microsphere embolization of the left coronary artery (6) or selective embolization of one or two of its major branches (7). A modification consists of injection of a bolus of mercury into coronary arteries (8). Such techniques provide effective embolization of the microvasculature, leading to early and severe depression of myocardial function. Particles often are introduced inadvertently into other locations of the peripheral vasculature, causing an artificial increase in systemic resistance. Mercury has toxic effects on the myocardium, which may be significant in experiments of longer duration. Embolization precludes reversal of the coronary occlusion.

A series of ingenious methods of performing local coronary occlusion in the closed chest recently have been proposed. Among these methods is an intra-coronary wire electrical cauterization leading to local coronary thrombosis (9); insertion into the coronary artery of a spiral wire to promote thrombosis (10); and placing within the coronary artery a full or hollow cylinder or a large glass bead (11–13). These techniques have been employed to simulate acute and gradual occlusions; but they are not reversible, do not provide easy control of the site of occlusion, and the degree of coronary occlusion may be questioned. It has been suggested that intracoronary occlusion may have an advantage in that it is less likely to interrupt veins and sympathetic innervation accompanying coronary arteries which are often disrupted by external occlusion devices (14).

A closed-chest model that would permit measurements during control and occlusion periods and allow complete reversal of the occlusion was developed by us (1, 2). It also permits measurements and infusions distal to the occlusion. In addition to providing simultaneous studies of the global electrocardiographic, metabolic, and mechanical indices, the model is designed to measure regional metabolic function of the occluded segments of the myocardium.

Difficulties of interpreting myocardial metabolism during regional ischemia and revascularization solely on the basis of coronary sinus blood sampling have led to attempts to segregate the venous blood draining ischemic from that draining nonischemic myocardium (15). Coronary sinus catheterization and blood sampling have been used in recent clinical studies of myocardial ischemia metabolism (16, 17). In contrast to normal aerobic lactate extraction from the coronary blood supply, interruption or major reduction of coronary flow often results in lactate production by the ischemic myocardium. However, local anaerobic metabolism could not always be demonstrated, and one of the presumed reasons was the mixing within the coronary sinus of venous drainages derived from both the ischemic and nonischemic portions of the heart (18).

Myocardial ischemia, secondary to coronary occlusion, also is associated with a loss of electrolytes, such as serum potassium, which is believed to be related to the genesis of ventricular arrhythmias. Nonselective sampling of mixed blood from the coronary sinus does not permit full evaluation of the consequences of regional anaerobic myocardial metabolism or potassium loss. The nonischemic myocardium may itself participate in the altered regional state by hypercontraction or other compensatory mechanisms, and these results may affect the metabolic function of the ischemic zone. Thus, if we are to learn more about the nature of ischemic process, it is important to be able to separate out and simultaneously measure the regional venous drainage from both the occluded and nonoccluded segments of the myocardium (18).

Recent attempts to carry out the above venous separation of coronary sinus and great cardiac vein blood following LAD occlusion have been reported in the open-chest dog (19, 20). Our data were obtained in 14 dogs by use of the closed-chest model with intracoronary balloon occlusion of the LAD and intermittent balloon separation of the CS and GCV during the sampling (18). This method is not subject to artifacts in cardiac function generally associated with thoracotomy and pericardiotomy.

Progressive Alterations of
Cardiac Function during Ischemia

Hemodynamic alterations which were seen 30 minutes following LAD occlusion remained relatively unchanged throughout four hours of occlusion. The heart rate increased about 25%, and systemic vascular resistance first rose and then gradually diminished. Relative to preocclusion control, LV dP/dt and cardiac output were reduced by 20–30%, signifying a drop in global cardiac mechanical function. However, no significant hypotension was experienced in these animals. Because of the rise in heart rate, stroke volume and stroke work diminished progressively during the occlusion period. Upon reperfusion, there was a further increase in heart rate to 60% of control, which might have been caused by anesthesia or stimulation of the adrenergic innervation. There was a return of LVEDP, LV dP/dt, and cardiac output toward normal, but stroke work dropped further because of increasing heart rate. Systemic vascular resistance diminished.

Metabolic measurements indicated that the simultaneous and separate sampling of the CS and GCV provided striking differences between the venous drainage of occluded and nonoccluded segments. Within the first 30 minutes following LAD occlusion, lactate extraction dropped from 26% to 17% in the nonoccluded zone and from 32% to 6% in the occluded zone of the myocardium. The latter represents a change from aerobic to anaerobic lactate metabolism in the occluded region. During the four hours of occlusion, there were fluctuations in the lactate balance, the most striking dysfunction being at two hours when CS and GCV showed lactate balances of 13.6% and 2.8%, respectively. The data suggest that metabolic function of both the nonoccluded and occluded myocardium were affected at that time by the occlusion, when severe anaerobic metabolism supervened in the occluded segment. Upon reperfusion, lactate balances dropped further to markedly negative levels, probably indicating a washout of accumulated metabolites from the interstitial spaces of both the occluded and nonoccluded segments. At 30 minutes of reperfusion, long after the washout should have been completed, there was still a marked negative lactate balance, indicating that both segments of the myocardium were functioning in an anaerobic state. It is significant that at this time, the hemodynamic measurements exhibited a return toward control levels, but the heart rate was accelerated.

Immediately following the onset of arterial occlusion, there was a marked loss in potassium in both occluded and nonoccluded segments. There was some fluctuation in potassium balance over the four-hour period of occlusion, but a significant loss of potassium resulted, particularly from the occluded segment. Upon reperfusion, there was a marked washout of potassium from both segments. This implies accumulation of potassium in the interstitial spaces during occlusion which was subsequently washed out when the intracoronary balloon was deflated as a result of increased coronary flow. However, a negative potassium balance persisted 30 minutes following reperfusion, suggesting a significant continuing potassium loss 30 minutes following reperfusion.

We are impressed that the progressive derangement in lactate metabolism, often denoting extensive anaerobic metabolic function, and the marked myocardial potassium loss during four hours of occlusion and 30 minutes of reperfusion, were not accompanied by serious alterations in hemodynamic function.

While there exist separate studies of hemodynamics and limited data on myocardial metabolism, we are not aware of comprehensive simultaneous measurement and correlation of global and regional hemodynamic and metabolic data in the intact preparation. Such a correlation is attempted in our forthcoming publication (18). We also attempt to correlate the hemodynamic and metabolic derangements which occurred when shock or arrhythmias supervened and those factors which might have led to such complications (21, 22). Our observations of the progressive hemodynamic alterations which occur following occlusion are similar to those noted in the human; however, progressive alterations in metabolic function have not as yet been reported in the human.

A striking observation of this study, that the nonoccluded segment often also revealed serious metabolic dysfunction in terms of abnormal lactate metabolism and potassium loss, requires an explanation. This could be attributable to reflex angiospasms of the arteries nourishing the nonoccluded segments. It is also possible that the increased left ventricular afterload caused by the observed rise in peripheral vascular resistance, or the attempt of the myocardium to compensate for dyskinesia of the occluded segment, might inordinately increase the nutritional demands placed upon the normal myocardium.

Jennings (23) has reported that myocardial ischemia and consequent cessation of function cannot be equated with cell death. In dogs, if the coronary blood flow was restored within 19 minutes, the structure and function of the affected cells returned to normal. However, cell death is believed to occur after 20 minutes of coronary occlusion. He noted that not all ischemic cells die simultaneously. Between 20 and 60 minutes after occlusion, most of the cells in an area of maximum ischemia become irreversibly injured. He based his studies on electron microscopy because routine histologic techniques such as light microscopy do not show the changes until about 12–24 hours after occlusion (23). In our studies, the LAD occlusion lasted for four hours, well beyond what Jennings believed to be the period of irreversibility.

During the occlusion period, the nonoccluded myocardium already appeared to compensate for the reduced contraction of the LAD occluded myocardial segment. Regional metabolic and mechanical function are seriously depressed after four hours of occlusion. It might return toward normal after longer reperfusion. This leads to the currently contested theories and data regarding the duration and extent of myocardial viability following coronary occlusion. Ventriculography and hemodynamic measurements in humans tend to confirm a return of mechanical function to all segments of the heart after revascularization (24). The fact that mechanical function appeared quite normal in our studies, despite apparent anaerobic metabolism, suggests that the heart is capable of adequately contracting even with severe metabolic dysfunction of the myocardium. We must question whether our new technique really reflects the mechanical function of the local myocardium, which is seriously deranged metabolically after occlusion and reperfusion. Further studies are needed to focus on mechanical alterations taking place within an occluded segment.

A common observation in our experiments has been a slight but distinct drop in overall cardiac function occurring shortly after the acute occlusion of the proximal LAD. This is particularly reflected in a reduced LV dP/dt and cardiac output, while LVEDP and systemic vascular resistance are increased. The increased peripheral resistance, which appears to occur almost immediately, probably represents a sympathoadrenal compensatory reflex aimed at cutting off less vital circulation while maintaining perfusion of more critical areas. On the other hand, the metabolite derangements persisted throughout the occlusion and for a short period during reperfusion. These changes were not related directly to the global hemodynamic measurements, which tend to mask regional effects. It is also possible that there is a time lag between the metabolic and mechanical alterations in cardiac function.

REFERENCES CITED

1. Corday, E., Lang, T. W., Crexells, C., and Meerbaum, S. 1972. Intracoronary balloon—A new model for induction of myocardial ischemia (Letter to Editor). Amer. J. Cardiol. 29:301.
2. Corday, E., Lang, T. W., Meerbaum, S., Gold, H. et al. 1973. A closed chest intracoronary occlusion model for the study of regional cardiac function. Amer. J. Cardiol. (In press).
3. Maroko, P. R., Kjekshus, J. K., Sobel, B. E., Watanabe, T., Covell, J. W., Ross, J., Jr., and Braunwald, E. 1971. Factors influencing infarct size following experimental coronary artery occlusion. Circulation 43:67.
4. Chimoskey, J. E., Szentivanyl, M., Zackheim, R., and Barger, A. C. 1967. Temporary coronary occlusion in conscious dogs: Collateral flow and electrocardiograms. Amer. J. Physiol. 212:1025.
5. Pasyk, S., Bloor, C. M., Khouri, E. M., and Gregg, D. W. 1971. Systemic and coronary effects of coronary artery occlusion in the unanesthetized dog. Amer. J. Physiol. 220:646.
6. Agress, C. M., Rosenberg, M. J., Jacobs, H. I., Binder, M. J., Schneiderman, A., and Clark, W. G. 1952. Protracted shock in the closed-chest dog following coronary embolization with graded microspheres. Amer. J. Physiol. 170:536.
7. Palmer, J. D., O'Rourke, R. A., Olson, M. S., and Pickard, R. N. 1971. Experimental myocardial infarction. Amer. Heart J. 81:729.
8. Lluch, S., Moguilevsky, H. C., Pietra, G., Shaffer, A. B., Hirsch, L. J., and Fishman, A. P. 1969. A reproducible model of cardiogenic shock in the dog. Circulation 39:205.
9. Blair, E., Nygren, E., and Cowley, R. A. 1964. A spiral wire technique for producing gradually occlusive coronary thrombosis. J. Thorac. Cardiov. Surg. 48:476.
10. Kordenat, R. K., Kezdi, P., and Stanley, E. L. 1972. A new catheter technique for producing experimental coronary thrombosis and selective coronary visualization. Amer. Heart J. 83:360.
11. Nakhjavan, F. K., Shedrovilzky, H., and Goldberg, H. 1968. Experimental myocardial infarction in dogs: Description of a closed chest technique. Circulation 38:777.
12. Khomazyuk, A. I., Nescheret, A. P., and Kuzminsky, N. P. 1965. Some new ways of experimental research of myocardial infarction. Kardiologiia 5(4):19.
13. Ribeilima, J. 1964. Selective embolization of the coronary arteries. A hemodynamic, metabolic and radiologic study. Proc. Soc. Exp. Biol. Med. 117:367.
14. Oliver, M. F., and Lassers, B. W. 1972. Relevance of studies with experimental models to the effect of ischaemia on myocardial metabolism in man. Cardiology 57:66.
15. Gorlin, R. 1972. Assessment of hypoxia in the human heart. Cardiology 57:24.
16. Herman, M. V., Elliott, W. C., and Gorlin, R. 1967. An electrocardiographic, anatomic and metabolic study of zonal myocardial ischemia in coronary heart disease. Circulation 35:834.
17. Parker, J. O., Chiong, M. A., West, R. O., and Case, R. B. 1969. Sequential alterations in myocardial lactate metabolism, S-T segments, and left ventricular function during angina induced by atrial pacing. Circulation 40:113.
18. Meerbaum, S., Lang, T. W., Corday, E., Rubins, S. et al.: Progressive alterations of cardiac hemodynamic and regional metabolic function following acute coronary occlusion. Amer. J. Cardiol (in press).
19. Obeid, A., Smulyan, H., Gilbert, R., and Eich, R. H. 1972. Regional metabolic changes in the myocardium following coronary artery ligation in dogs. Amer. Heart J. 83:189.
20. Owen, P., Thomas, M., Young, V., and Opie, L. 1970. Comparison between metabolic changes in local venous and coronary sinus blood after acute experimental coronary arterial occlusion. Amer. J. Cardiol. 25:562.
21. Lang, T. W., Corday, E., Gold, H., Meerbaum, S. et al.: Consequences of reperfusion following coronary occlusion: effects on hemodynamic and regional myocardial metabolic function. Amer. J. Cardiol. (in press).

22. Corday, E., Lang, T. W., Meerbaum, S. 1973. Precursors of shock state: Alterations of metabolic and hemodynamic function secondary to coronary occlusion. (In preparation.)

23. Jennings, R. B., and Reimer, K. A. 1973. The fate of the ischemic myocardial cell. Page 13 *in* E. Corday and H. J. C. Swan, eds. Myocardial infarction. Williams & Wilkins, Baltimore.

24. Chatterjee, K., Swan, H. J. C., Sustaita, H., Matloff, J., and Parmley, W. W. 1973. Impending infarction and direct myocardial revascularization. Page 362 *in* E. Corday and H. J. C. Swan, eds. Myocardial infarction. Williams & Wilkins, Baltimore.

DETERMINANTS OF MORTALITY IN ACUTE
MYOCARDIAL INFARCTION

SYLVAN LEE WEINBERG, HUASCAR E. JESSEN,
and JACQUES J. COL

The development during the past few years of relatively low risk and apparently highly effective surgery for occlusive coronary disease has made mandatory a more accurate delineation of the natural history and prognosis of acute myocardial infarction. The surgical alternatives to classical forms of treatment have thus stimulated a great deal of research into the history and factors affecting mortality in acute myocardial infarction.

We have previously presented data from our institution describing the significance of three factors in assessing mortality in acute myocardial infarction (1–3). These are location, presence of previous infarction, and intraventricular conduction disturbances. The current presentation expands these observations to a series of 426 patients with acute myocardial infarction treated in the Coronary Care Unit at the Good Samaritan Hospital in Dayton, Ohio. These patients comprised two consecutive series of approximately equal numbers treated in 1967–1968 and a second group in 1971.

A comprehensive data code sheet was completed on each patient for future computer analysis. In addition, the records of the 426 patients were reviewed in detail in compiling the data for this presentation. Information from a larger series beginning with 1966 and comprising 1,013 cases, which also will be alluded to, was taken directly from computer printouts. All patients were treated in the Good Samaritan Hospital's coronary care complex which includes a 10-bed acute care unit and an adjacent 28-bed intermediate care unit (4–6) capable of monitoring an additional 20 patients by wire and telemetry. Each patient was under the care of his individual physician. The results, therefore, reflect the use of similar facilities, nursing and house staff, but not necessarily a unified therapeutic philosophy.

Table 1 illustrates the magnitude of the problem of mortality in acute myocardial infarction. The 50% mortality indicated for the pre-hospital phase of myocardial infarction is assumed from impressions gained in the literature and is

We express great appreciation to Mrs. Sylvia Stevens, Research Assistant, Coronary Care Unit, Good Samaritan Hospital, for invaluable assistance in preparation of this manuscript. This research is supported in large part by a grant from the Arthur Beerman Foundation, Dayton, Ohio.

Table 1. Mortality Rates in
Acute Myocardial Infarction

Phase	Rate
Pre-Hospital	50%
C.C.U.	15%
Post C.C.U.	5%
30 months post-hospital	15%

Table 2. Projected 30-Month Mortality,
Acute Myocardial Infarction

Total mortality	65%
Mortality for patients reaching hospital	32%

not documented specifically. The 15% coronary care unit (CCU) mortality, 5% post-CCU mortality, and 15% mortality 30 months after leaving the hospital, are taken from our own observations (1–3). Thus the projected 30-month total mortality in acute myocardial infarction is 65%. For patients reaching the hospital it is 32% (Table 2).

DETERMINANTS OF MORTALITY

Table 3 lists the determinants of mortality which will be analyzed. Not included are such obviously unfavorable factors as overt congestive failure where the mortality in our series approximates 30%, and shock where mortality is generally considered to range from 85% to 95% or even higher.

Table 3. Analyzed Determinants of Mortality

Anterior location
Previous infarction
Intraventricular conduction defects
Atrioventricular block
Increasing age
Cardiac enlargement
Tachyarrhythmias

Anterior Location

Among the 426 patients studied in this series, anterior location was an important determinant of mortality. Anterior location is related to a mortality almost twice that of inferior location during the in-hospital phase (Table 4).

Table 4. Effect of Location of Infarction on Survival

Location	No.	Mortality (%)
Inferior	182	14
Anterior	217	26
Indefinite	27	19
Total	*426*	*20.4*

Previous Infarction

As might be expected, previous infarction also contributes heavily to increased in-hospital mortality (Table 5). During the in-hospital phase, where previous infarction exists, the mortality is almost twice that for an initial episode.

Table 5. Effect of Previous Myocardial Infarction on Survival

Type	No.	Mortality (%)
No previous infarct	291	16
Previous infarct	135	30
Total	*426*	*20.4*

Intraventricular Conduction Defects

An even more striking determinant in mortality is the presence of intraventricular conduction defects. A threefold increase in mortality occurs with such defects in the presence of acute infarction. This factor was emphasized in a previous communication (3) based on approximately half of the series shown in Table 6. In this group, analysis of patients with conduction disturbances and a series matched for age showed that the higher mortality associated with intraventricular conduction defects was not a function of increasing age. The mean age of death for the intraventricular conduction disturbance group is actually lower than that of the matched controls (3).

Table 6. Intraventricular Conduction Defects Increase
Mortality Threefold

Type	No.	Mortality (%)
No intraventricular conduction defect	327	14
Intraventricular conduction defect	99	42
Total	*426*	*20*

Among the 426 cases of myocardial infarction analyzed in this series there were 99 cases of intraventricular conduction disturbances. This 23% incidence is somewhat higher than most observers have reported, because we have included left anterior hemiblock, which is the most commonly encountered intraventricular conduction disturbance and also the most benign.

Among our 31 cases with left anterior hemiblock there were 9 deaths with a mortality of 29%, as compared with a mortality of 20% for the entire series. If these cases are omitted from the bundle branch block series, a group of patients is identified with an exceedingly high mortality. In Table 7 these patients are referred to as having "major bundle branch block." The overall mortality for this group is approximately 49%. Bifascicular block is numerically the largest group among the major bundle branch blocks. This group includes left anterior hemiblock with right bundle branch block which comprises 29 of the cases of bifascicular block. Other forms of bifascicular block in this series include four cases of right bundle branch block with left posterior hemiblock, three instances of combined right and left bundle branch block, and other combinations involving bundle branch block and atrioventricular conduction disturbances.

Table 7. The High Mortality of Major Bundle Branch Block

Type	No.	Deaths	%
Total myocardial infarcts	*426*	*87*	*20*
RBBB	12	5	42
LBBB	19	13	68
Bifascicular BBB	36	15	42
LPHB	1	0	0
Total MBBB	*68*	*33*	*49*

There were 42 deaths among the 99 patients with bundle branch block in acute myocardial infarction; 25 of these deaths occurred with congestive heart failure. Eleven patients died suddenly. While the exact mechanism could not be defined in each instance, ventricular fibrillation did occur in 6 patients. Among the 68 cases of major bundle branch block, anterior location predominated by a ratio of 2.4 to 1. A similar ratio of 2.3 to 1 of anterior to inferior location occurred in the bundle branch block group who died. Pump failure occurred two times more frequently than sudden death among patients with anterior infarction who died. Pump failure and sudden death occurred equally among fatal instances of inferior infarction. Thus, in general, anterior location predisposed more toward pump failure than did inferior location. The incidence of ventricular arrhythmias was 40% in patients with major bundle branch block and much lower in patients with left anterior hemiblock as an isolated conduction disturbance (19%). Major bundle branch block causes an increased propensity to high grade atrioventricular block. The incidence of the latter defect was 28% among the 68 cases of major bundle branch block, and only 5% in those without major bundle branch block (Table 8).

Table 8. Major Bundle Branch Block (MBBB) Increases Risk of High Grade Atrioventricular (A-V) Block

Type	No.	High grade A-V block	%
No MBBB	358	19	5
MBBB	68	18	28
Total	*426*	*37*	*9*

Atrioventricular Block

Table 9 shows the specific breakdown for the development of high grade atrioventricular (A-V) block with the various kinds of major bundle branch block. The presence of bifascicular block offers a 39% incidence of high grade A-V block, as compared with 5% for those patients without major bundle branch block. The overall mortality of high grade A-V block is approximately 50%, with or without the use of pacemakers. The 68 cases of major bundle branch block contributed half of the cases of complete A-V block in the whole series of 426 patients, as illustrated in Table 9.

The combination of an intraventricular conduction disturbance and an anterior or inferior myocardial infarction increases mortality from 19% to 42% and from 9% to 50%, respectively (Table 10). The mortality of anterior infarction occurring as a second episode increases mortality from 21% to 37%; in inferior infarction the increase for a previous episode is from 10% to 24% (Table 11).

S. L. Weinberg, H. E. Jessen, and J. J. Col

Table 9. High Grade Atrioventricular (A-V) Block is
Frequent in Major Bundle Branch Block

Type	No.	High grade A-V block	%
RBBB	12	1	8
LBBB	19	3	16
Bifascicular BBB	36	14	39
LPH	1	0	0
Total	*68*	*18*	*26*

Table 10. Intraventricular Conduction Defects Increase Mortality Sharply
in Both Anterior and Inferior Myocardial Infarction

Type	Incidence		Deaths	Mortality (%)
	No.	(%)		
Anterior and no conduction defect	151	35	28	19
Anterior and conduction defect	66	16	28	42
Inferior and no conduction defect	160	38	15	9
Inferior and conduction defect	22	5	11	50
Total	*426*	*100*	*87*	*20.4*

Table 11. Previous Myocardial Infarction Increases Mortality
in Anterior More than in Inferior Infarction

Type	No.	Deaths	Mortality (%)
Anterior and no previous myocardial infarct	149	31	21
Anterior and previous myocardial infarct	68	25	37
Inferior and no previous myocardial infarct	128	13	10
Inferior and previous myocardial infarct	54	13	24
Total	*426*	*87*	*20.4*

A synthesis of the three risk factors is shown in Table 12, which illustrates the very high mortality of the combination of anterior or inferior infarction, a history of previous episode, and presence of intraventricular conduction disturbance (55%). A relatively low mortality of 8% occurs in inferior infarction without a previous lesion or intraventricular conduction disturbance (Table 12).

In a preliminary survey of 136 patients followed for approximately 30 months after discharge from the hospital, the differential mortality of anterior and inferior location and for patients with previous infarction which was so striking in the hospital phase was no longer apparent. Thus, the mortality for these three categories in the 30-month post-hospital period was 15%. Intraventricular conduction defects, however, continued to have the relatively high mortality of 24% (Table 13). During the 30-month post-hospital survey, sudden death occurred 15 times among the 21 patients who died. There were 4 instances of progressive pump failure and in 2 the mode of death was not known (Table 14). Interestingly, the 34 patients with intraventricular conduction defect, who represented 25% of the patients followed after discharge from the hospital, contributed more than 33% of the total deaths and more than 50% of the sudden deaths (Table 13).

Thus, intraventricular conduction disturbances emerge as one of the major determinants of mortality in myocardial infarction during the hospital phase and for at least 30 months thereafter. There is also the suggestion of increased propensity to sudden death among those with intraventricular conduction disturbances.

Table 12. Combined Effect of Anterior Location, Previous Myocardial Infarction (MI), and Intraventricular Conduction Defects Increases Mortality Fourfold Over Anterior Infarction

Type	No.	Mortality (%)
Anterior, no previous MI, no conduction defect	112	17
Anterior, previous MI, conduction defect	29	55
Inferior, no previous MI, no conduction defect	118	8
Inferior, previous MI, conduction defect	12	58
Total	*426*	*20.4*

190   S. L. Weinberg, H. E. Jessen, and J. J. Col

Table 13. Isolated Effect of Localization, Previous Myocardial
Infarct (MI), and Intraventricular (IV) Conduction Defect 30 Months after
Acute MI

Type	No.	Incidence (%)	Deaths	Mortality (%)
Anterior	72	53	11	15
Inferior	64	47	10	15
No previous MI	110	81	17	15
Previous MI	26	19	4	15
No IV conduction defect	102	75	13	13
IV conduction defect	34	25	8	24
Total	*136*	*100*	*21*	*15.4*

Table 14. Types of Deaths Among 21 (15.4%) of 136 Survivors
Followed for 30 Months

Type	Progressive pump failure	Sudden	Unknown
Localization			
anterior	2	8	1
inferior	2	7	1
IV conduction defect	1	7	
Previous MI	3	4	
Cause of death	1(recurrent MI) 1(post coronary vein graft)	10(?) 3(recurrent MI) 1(complete hemiblock) 1(ventricular rupture)	
Total	*4*	*15*	*2*

Increasing Age

Other factors associated with increased mortality in acute myocardial infarction are age, the presence of tachyarrhythmias and cardiac enlargement as shown by x-ray examination. In a study of 1,013 cases of myocardial infarction, a breakdown by decades shows a trend toward increasing mortality with age (Table 15).

Tachyarrhythmias

Tachyarrhythmias contribute to a higher mortality in acute myocardial infarction. Table 16 shows the incidence and mortality of some frequently encoun-

Table 15. Mortality in Acute Myocardial Infarction Tends to Increase with Age

Decade of life	No. of patients	No. of deaths	Mortality (%)
4th	144	16	11
5th	304	26	9
6th	266	37	11
7th	224	61	25
8th	44	15	34

Table 16. Tachyarrhythmias Increase Mortality in Acute Myocardial Infarction

Type	No.	No. of deaths	Mortality (%)
Atrial fibrillation	132	40	30
Ventricular fibrillation	70	46	65
Ventricular tachycardia	113	46	41
Supraventricular tachycardia	111	42	40
Total	1,013	165	16

Table 17. Cardiac Enlargement Shown by X-ray is Associated with a Major increase in Mortality in Acute Myocardial Infarction

Heart size	Total	No. of deaths	Mortality (%)
Normal	408	25	6
Enlarged	337	72	21

tered tachyarrhythmias. Perhaps the most interesting aspect of this information is the relatively high mortality of supraventricular tachycardia (40%), which is virtually the same as for ventricular tachycardia (41%).

Cardiac Enlargement

Cardiac enlargement, as shown by x-rays, was associated with a much higher mortality than that found in patients with normal heart size. Among the 1,013 patients for whom x-ray information on heart size was available, the mortality in the presence of enlargement exceeded that for patients with normal heart size by a factor of 3.5 to 1 (Table 17).

SUMMARY

It appears to be possible to select several determinants of mortality from which an approach to the in-hospital and post-hospital prognosis in acute myocardial infarction can be made. Perhaps the best prognosis for survival during the in-hospital phase occurs when an initial myocardial infarction is inferior in location and is not associated with an intraventricular conduction disturbance, an increase in heart size, or a tachyarrhythmia. The worst prognosis seems to be present when myocardial infarction is superimposed on a previous lesion and associated with an intraventricular conduction disturbance. We further note that a relatively high 30-month mortality occurs in patients with an intraventricular conduction disturbance.

Therapeutic approaches to acute myocardial infarction are changing rapidly. It may not be unreasonable to project that in the foreseeable future all patients with acute myocardial infarction may be subjected to coronary arteriography and the possibility of surgical intervention considered. At the present time there is increasing tendency to intervene in pre-infarction angina and in patients with acute infarction who experience shock, persistent pain, and intractable cardiac failure.

To the group of patients currently being studied by coronary arteriography with the hope of finding a surgically remedial lesion, perhaps we should add those whose prognosis is known to be highly unfavorable. The data we have presented suggest that patients with anterior infarction, recurrent episodes, and intraventricular conduction disturbances, singly or in combination, may have a highly unfavorable prognosis. Therefore, perhaps criteria for definitive study should be expanded to include these patients. We have drawn particular attention to the destructive effect of intraventricular conduction disturbances on the clinical course of myocardial infarction.

REFERENCES CITED

1. Weinberg, S. L., and Col, J. J. 1972. The changing coronary care unit. P. 204 *in* H. Russek and B. Zohman, eds. Cardiovascular therapy. Williams & Wilkins, Baltimore.
2. Col, J. J., and Weinberg, S. L. 1972. Factors affecting prognosis in acute myocardial infarction. Heart & Lung 1:74.
3. Col, J. J., and Weinberg, S. L. 1972. The incidence and mortality of intraventricular conduction defects in acute myocardial infarction. Amer. J. Cardiol. 29:344.
4. Weinberg, S. L. 1968. The current status of instrumentation systems for the coronary care unit. Prog. Cardiov. Dis. 11:1.
5. Weinberg, S. L. 1969. Complacency in coronary care. Chest 56:273.
6. Grace, W. J., Crockett, J. E., Weinberg, S. L., and Soffer, A. 1972. Intermediate care after myocardial infarction. Heart & Lung 1(6):818.

INDICATIONS AND CONTRAINDICATIONS FOR
MYOCARDIAL REVASCULARIZATION

STEVEN RUBINS, SHIGERU HIROSE,
and ELIOT CORDAY

Direct myocardial revascularization by aortocoronary bypass is probably the most significant advance in cardiovascular surgery in the past five years. However, it has already become obvious that the operation is not a panacea, because it is accompanied by a significant mortality; 20–30% of the vein grafts are closed within the first year, and if significant myocardial damage is present, results are often poor. Thus, such revascularization surgery should be employed only in highly selected cases of coronary artery disease.

The indications for surgery are still controversial because 1) results of long-term follow-up are lacking; 2) controlled, randomized studies are needed; 3) insufficient knowledge exists of the life history, prognosis, and life expectancy of various coronary artery disease subgroups; 4) there is need for further animal experimentation to provide data on the time factor which governs myocardial viability following ischemia (1).

Despite these gaps in knowledge, the clinical indications and contraindications for surgery appear to be gradually emerging. There are still many "gray" areas which may not be clarified until some of our deficits in knowledge are corrected.

GENERAL CONSIDERATIONS

Data are being accumulated which suggest that coronary artery bypass surgery may be indicated to 1) avert impending infarction; 2) protect and preserve myocardium when a coronary attack is imminent; and 3) relieve disabling angina symptoms unresponsive to treatment and thus improve the quality of life. Debate continues on whether such surgery extends life. The physician must decide whether the anticipated natural history of the disease in that individual might warrant the risk of surgical mortality and morbidity. Moreover, the decision must be made with incomplete knowledge of long-term surgical follow-up in similar patients and of the natural life course of various subsets of coronary artery disease.

Unfortunately, many decisions for or against surgery are now based on inadequate knowledge, bias, or emotionalism. The so-called widow maker (isolated lesion of left anterior descending [LAD] coronary artery), which was believed to be accompanied by an inordinate mortality rate, now has been found

193

to have a medical mortality rate of only 4%/year in the asymptomatic patient. It is not yet known whether these grafts will remain patent long enough to preserve or protect myocardium in a stable angina patient. There are convincing data emerging, however, that the surgical morbidity and mortality probably are justified in selected cases of unstable or "preinfarction" angina.

Why, after five years of this surgery, are the indications and contraindications not clear-cut? To date, there has not been a randomized, controlled, clinical study. Even the best-planned randomized studies inevitably introduce bias, because the private physician selects out certain patients. It may be more fruitful to set up prospective studies in which patients are classified into subsets based on their degree of disability, stress test, and the specific anatomy of the lesion based upon an angiogram and ventriculogram. There must be uniform cross-checks in such a study, as each physician has his own definition of what constitutes akinesis, dyskinesis, preinfarction angina, and cardiogenic shock. Mortality of the preinfarction angina patient followed medically is regarded to be anywhere from 18–40% (2,3). Obviously, this varied mortality rate reflects individual definition used in patient selection.

Because angiographers may differ tremendously in their interpretation of an individual angiogram and because the quality of angiograms is often substandard, the experts may differ considerably as to which arteries are significantly narrowed, which have adequate runoff, which are the predominant lesions, and the extent and nature of collateral blood vessels. Although techniques have become more sophisticated for analyzing ventriculograms by ventricular mapping, measurement of ejection fractions, and the use of multiple views, the cardiologist has difficulty distinguishing between surgically reversible ischemic myocardium and irreversible scar tissue, or the degree of temporary ischemic myocardium caused by the contrast medium itself. It is evident that if the patient is having angina during the radiographic procedure, it may cause temporary hypocontractility of localized areas which cause erroneous interpretation. It would seem foolhardy to bypass into an area which is already just fibrous tissue. For this reason, researchers are developing new radioisotopic scanning methods to identify areas of viable myocardium that would benefit from bypass surgery (4,5).

At the present time, patients who have sustained a myocardial infarction and are free of anginal symptoms should not be subjected to angiography or surgery. Certainly, the coronary angiograms of a person who has sustained an infarct usually will reveal significant coronary arterial narrowing or occlusion. If the patient has no symptoms, his expected mortality should be approximately 4–5%/year (6), which at present is as good as can be expected after coronary bypass surgery.

Postoperative angiography suggests that approximately 30% of vein bypass grafts occlude within two years (7). Early closures may be related to technical mishaps such as poor vessel selection, whereas late closure may be caused by degenerative changes occurring in the vein graft. We find that many proximal coronary lesions that were bypassed occluded completely because of lack of preferential flow. The patient's life may then be dependent upon the graft patency of that single vessel. Perioperative infarction appears to be quite significant, in both postoperative mortality and morbidity, with an incidence of 20–30% (7).

Most patients obtain relief of their angina, but when we realize the high rate of closure following bypass surgery, one may reasonably ask whether relief of symptoms is related to infarction of previously intermittently ischemic tissue. Also, the relief of angina may be psychological, because it was well established that 60–70% of patients obtain relief from a sham operation (8).

Bypass following the onset of a definite coronary occlusion has been advocated by some surgeons because it may preserve life of the tissue, but others have reported a prohibitive mortality. Our preliminary animal studies show little evidence that reperfusion 3–5 hours following infarction causes improvement in cardiac hemodynamics or myocardial metabolism. In fact, the microscopic changes of infarction often appear to be accelerated and are associated with reactive hyperemia or intramyocardial hemorrhage (9).

CONTRAINDICATIONS FOR SURGERY

Inadequate Myocardium

There must be sufficient contractile myocardium remaining that could benefit by augmenting the blood supply. Therefore, patients who have extensive ventricular damage, as evidenced by diffuse hypocontractility, akinesis, cardiomegaly, or elevated left ventricular end-diastolic pressure are poor candidates for bypass in terms of beneficial results and surgical mortality.

Accelerated Atherogenesis

Patients with severe lipid disturbances or diabetes mellitus are apt to have diffuse coronary arterial disease, and therefore are not ideal candidates for surgery. Accelerated atherosclerotic deposits are likely to occur in the bypass veins in these metabolic disorders.

Hypertension

Hypertension unresponsive to medical therapy is associated with a higher graft closure rate. Unless the cardiologist is assured that the hypertension can be controlled postoperatively, surgery may be contraindicated.

Medical Complications

Patients with severe associated vascular disease such as cerebrovascular or reno-vascular insufficiency may develop cerebral strokes or renal failure, and therefore are high risks for surgery. Although old age is not an absolute contraindication for bypass surgery, many elderly patients develop medical complications, such as postoperative stroke, pulmonary insufficiency, and prolonged confusional states.

CURRENT INDICATIONS FOR SURGERY

Preinfarction Angina (Impending Myocardial Infarction)

Crescendo or preinfarction angina is recognized by the sudden onset of chest distress or worsening of pre-existing coronary insufficiency. This is characterized by a change in the severity or character of the previous angina, angina at rest, nocturnal angina, or the fact that the angina is not relieved by nitroglycerin. This is usually accompanied by ECG changes (S-T segment depression or elevation; T wave inversion), which may be intermittent or persistent. The cardiac enzymes remain normal.

The electrocardiographic changes frequently give a clue to which vessel may be primarily involved (e.g., anterior wall LAD, inferior wall right coronary, etc.). It should be stated that not all patients go on to infarct, only a percentage of these infarcts are transmural, and the mortality rate without surgery is reported to be as low as 18%. This should be contrasted to the varied immediate surgical mortality of bypass surgery for these patients, quoted at between 5 and 25% (10,11). In evaluating a patient with the stated clinical syndrome, the cardiologist is influenced toward surgery if the ventricle has good function, even though it appears hypocontractile in the ischemic segment (ischemic myocardiopathy). Surgery often will cause return of mechanical function in the ischemic area (12). Runoff distal to the high-grade (>80%) stenotic lesions must be adequate to accept a graft flow in excess of 30 cc/min.

One is inclined toward surgery in the younger individuals who are free of medical complications such as severe hypertension, diabetes, or cerebrovascular, renal, or pulmonary disease. The presence of troublesome ventricular arrhythmias developing during ischemic episodes might influence toward surgical intervention. Anterior wall ischemia is perhaps more ominous than inferior wall ischemia, and the presence of intermittent ischemia-dependent atrioventricular or intraventricular block should indicate bypass surgery. Lack of clinical response to a therapeutic trial of nitrates and propranolol would lead the physician to consider early surgical intervention. The decision for surgery should be obtained by both cardiologist and surgeon together. The patient's consent must be given after he has been fully informed of all possible drawbacks. The patient should be aware of the possible alternative of medical therapy.

Disabling Angina

Patients who fail to respond to adequate medical treatment, including rest, nitrates, and beta-blockade, and who are unable to lead a nearly normal life because exertion or excitement cause angina, should be considered for bypass surgery. Clinical results are often gratifying, with improvement in angina occurring in up to 80% of patients who survive. Immediate hospital mortality varies according to many factors, especially the status of the ventricular myocardium. Congestive heart failure rarely is improved postoperatively. Perioperative infarct occurs in 20–30% of patients. Mechanical lesions such as localized aneurysm or significant mitral insufficiency should be corrected simultaneously, if possible. Unfortunately, those patients who need the operation most because they are disabled have the highest risk and poorest results of surgery.

Precarious Lesions

Symptomatic patients undergoing valve replacement or ventricular aneurysmectomy should be considered for simultaneous bypass of high-grade coronary lesions which are not adequately collateralized, even in the absence of disabling angina. Such surgery adds some time to the "pump run" but may prevent postoperative infarction or low-output failure. Angina patients with high-grade lesions of the main left coronary artery are particularly susceptible to sudden death; therefore, some surgeons urge bypass even though angina is not disabling.

POSSIBLE INDICATIONS

Extending Infarct

Patients who have recurrent pain at rest and are threatening to extend shortly after an acute myocardial infarction may be successfully operated upon. Animal studies suggest that the infarcted area may become hyperemic and develop hemorrhage after reperfusion. At present, this indication is controversial, as mortality may be as high as 30% (13).

Cardiogenic Shock

Some patients have been reported to survive bypass surgery following failure of medical treatment for cardiogenic shock (14). Medical treatment should include a trial of fluid loading, norepinephrine, afterload reduction, and, possibly, circulatory assist devices. One should not operate on a patient with long-standing ventricular failure and extensively scarred myocardium.

Intractable Ventricular Arrhythmias

Recurrent ventricular tachycardia caused by coronary insufficiency or occlusion may respond to successful bypass (15). Medical treatment should be exhausted before surgery is considered.

Other Precarious Lesions

Some authors urge bypass of a major artery if there is a positive stress test associated with a noncollateralized high-grade stenotic lesion of a major vessel such as the left coronary or LAD. One should not bypass into an area which is already completely scarred from previous infarction.

CONCLUSION

Coronary artery bypass surgery has been a major advance in the treatment of coronary insufficiency in selected cases. Restraint is urged, however, because long-term results are not known, and significant mortality and morbidity occur following surgery.

ACKNOWLEDGMENTS

This study was supported in part by grants from Mr. Berle Adams, Mrs. Anna Bing Arnold, Mr. Hal Wallis, and the Jules Stein Foundation.

REFERENCES CITED

1. Corday, E. 1972. Myocardial revascularization. Need for hard facts (Editorial). J.A.M.A. 219:507.
2. Yu, P. N. 1973. Preinfarction syndrome. Pages 210–214 *in* E. Corday and H. J. C. Swan, eds. Myocardial infarction. Williams & Wilkins, Baltimore.
3. Chatterjee, K., Swan, H. J. C., Sustaita, H., and Matloff, J. 1973. Impending infarction and direct myocardial revascularization. Pages 362–370 *in* E. Corday and H. J. C. Swan, eds. Myocardial infarction. Williams & Wilkins, Baltimore.
4. Judkins, M. 1973. Assessment of Myocardial Perfusion: Angiographic and Metabolic Approaches Presentation, American College of Cardiology convention, San Francisco, February 16.
5. Gorlin, R. 1973. Presentation, American College of Cardiology convention, San Francisco, February.
6. Kannel, W. B., and Feinlieb, M. 1972. Natural history of angina pectoris, The Framingham Study, Prognosis and Survival. Amer. J. Cardiol. 29:154.
7. Bourassa, M. G., Lesperance, J., Campeau, L., et al. 1972. Fate of left ventricular contraction following aorto-coronary venous grafts. Early and late postoperative modifications. Circulation 46:724.
8. Dimond, E. G., Kittle, C. F., and Crockett, J. E. 1960. Comparison of internal mammary artery ligation and sham operation for angina pectoris. Amer. J. Cardiol. 5:483.
9. Corday, E., Lang, T. W., Meerbaum, S., and Gold, H. 1973. Hemodynamic and metabolic alterations during coronary occlusion and reperfusion in the closed chest dog. Amer. J. Cardiol. (in press, Dec. 1973).
10. Sustaita, H., Chatterjee, K., Matloff, J. M., and Swan, H. J. C. 1973. The rationale for surgery in preinfarction angina [abstract]. Amer. J. Cardiol. 31:160.
11. Conti, R., Brawley, R., Pitt, B., and Ross, R. 1973. Unstable angina: Morbidity and mortality in fifty-seven consecutive patients evaluated angiographically [abstract]. Amer. J. Cardiol. 31:127.

12. Chatterjee, K., Swan, H. J. C., Parmley, W. W., Sustaita, H., Marcus, H., and Matloff, J. 1972. Depression of left ventricular function due to acute myocardial ischemia following aorto coronary saphenous vein bypass. New Engl. J. Med. 286:1117.
13. Hill, J. D., Kerth, W. J., Kelly, J. J., Selzer, A., Armstrong, W. Popper, R. W., Langston, M. F., Cohn, K. E., et al. 1971. Emergency aortocoronary bypass for impending or extending myocardial infarction. Circulation 32 (Suppl 1): 105.
14. Matloff, J., Don Michael, A., Swan, H. J. C., and Fields, J. 1973. Surgical management of cardiogenic shock. Pages 371–383 in E. Corday and H. J. C. Swan, eds. Myocardial infarction. Williams & Wilkins, Baltimore.
15. Nakhjavan, F. K., Morse, D. P., Nichols, H. T., and Goldberg, H. 1971. Emergency aortocoronary bypass. Treatment of ventricular tachycardia due to ischemic heart disease. J.A.M.A. 216:2138.

CRITICAL APPRAISAL OF THE QUALITY OF
MEDICAL CARE IN TODAY'S CORONARY CARE UNIT

OSLER L. PETERSON

To begin this discussion of effectiveness and efficiency of coronary care units, we can profitably start with the end results; that is, with death rates. Death rates for both males and females have been declining for many years in the economically advanced countries; the recent tendency is for the rate of decline to level off. The United States has participated in this general decline, for which medical science has often taken credit.

However, instead of following the trend to level off, male death rates in the United States unexpectedly increased between 1957 and 1968 (1). Vascular diseases are one of the many causes of increased death. For example, deaths from aneurysms, peripheral vascular disease, emboli, thrombosis, and peripheral gangrene all increased during this ten-year period. These deaths are probably not unrelated to the atherosclerotic process which underlies myocardial infarcts. Atherosclerotic heart disease deaths increased among white males aged 70 to 74 years, but remained stable among most age groups. Among nonwhite males the increase in atherosclerotic heart disease deaths, which includes myocardial infarcts, increased for most ages. Male death rates for a number of other diseases including emphysema and cirrhosis, and from accidents, suicides, and homicides also increased.

It is ironic that these death rate increases occurred at a time when knowledge of medical science was greater than ever before, and when this knowledge was being applied more intensively and skillfully to clinical problems than at any time in the past. Medical scientists must be careful in taking credit for improvements of death rates, because they may also be held accountable when death rates worsen.

If we take a conservative position, it is possible to say that there is no evidence from death rates that coronary care units have been effective. This evidence stands in interesting contrast to the drop in pneumonia death rates following the introduction of first sulfapyridine and then antibiotics. With use of these chemotherapeutic agents there was a sharp, dramatic change in the clinical course of lobar pneumonia, confirmed by a sharp diminution of pneumonia death rates.

Coronary care units are an example of the increasing application of technology to patient care problems. As so often happens, this new technology has proved considerably more expensive than the previous care. Before examining the economics and efficiency of coronary care units (CCU's), I would like to review briefly the evidence which supported this technological development.

A survey of the clinical studies of intensive care of patients with myocardial infarcts indicates that most published articles are unsatisfactory or, more plainly, worthless. Virtually all such studies are based upon experience before and after the institution of intensive care. In many of these articles the only evidence for the efficacy of the CCU is a case fatality rate in the unit of 15% or some similar result. Most reports give no information on the death rate in the prior year, and almost none supply any information on the number of patients treated.

The report on one hospital's experience from New Haven, Connecticut contains the following statistics (2):

	Number of patients	Case fatality rate
Year prior to CCU	202	27%
First CCU year	369	15%

The fact that the death rate dropped from 27% to 15% was of course attributed to the care given in the unit. The fact that the number of patients treated increased by 167, or 83%, between the time of comparison and the study year was not mentioned. A change of this magnitude in patient numbers immediately raises the question whether patients were selected according to different criteria—the bane of all "before and after" studies. Given this substantial increase, the most probable explanation for the decline in death rate was inclusion of more low risk patients during the study year.

Many investigators are becoming skeptical about the importance of coronary care units in treating atherosclerotic disease. A disease which begins in the second decade of life and progresses to dramatic visibility in the fifth, sixth, and seventh decades seems unlikely to be significantly altered by treatment during one of the many crises which it is capable of causing. Similarly, the fact that the atherosclerotic process involves not only the major coronary arteries but frequently is also found diffusely in the smaller arteries is a point which seems to argue that any specific episode-limited treatment is unlikely to have much effect upon its course.

The unsatisfactory state of the clinical evidence for the effectiveness of CCU's was punctuated in 1971 by Mather's report on a clinical trial in which home and hospital treatments of myocardial infarct patients were compared (3). This well conducted trial demonstrated a small but not important or technically significant advantage for home over hospital care, the latter in coronary care units.

Martin compared the treatment (4) of patients with myocardial infarcts and the outcomes in one of the better Boston community hospitals in 1939, 1949, 1959, and 1969. Since death rates are determined by severity of patient illness, he utilized a scale devised by Alexander Burgess and myself to calculate a severity-adjusted death rate for each year. When adjusted for severity there was a significant decline in deaths between 1939 and 1949 for which we could find no explanation. Between 1949, 1959, and 1969 the severity-adjusted death rate did not change in any important or significant manner. In 1969, patients received intensive care.

It was interesting to observe that in 1959 anticoagulants were administered to most patients. Rigorous clinical trials ultimately demonstrated the ineffectiveness of this treatment. Between 1939 and 1969 there was a massive increase in patient study and treatment. The use of blood chemistries, bacteriological tests, and x-rays increased quadratically. This means that the rate of increase in patient study and treatment was also increasing. Electrocardiograms and similar tests increased in a linear fashion. Since the money available to medical care is finite, it follows that it should not be spent on useless or dubious treatments, whether these are drugs, laboratory procedures, or intensive care.

The situation with respect to coronary care units stands in strange contrast to the regulations covering drugs. The introduction of a new drug must be based on evidence of its safety and effectiveness. Coronary care units have been widely replicated without any satisfactory evidence of effectiveness.

Coronary care units, the economists would say, are labor intensive. Like all medical care, they cannot readily be made more efficient by substitution of capital for personnel as is done in industry. Even though CCU's have not been demonstrated to be effective, I have no illusions that they will be closed. Since this is so, it is important to make them as economical as possible. *This is a second best solution.*

ECONOMICS OF CORONARY CARE UNITS

The following tables are taken from a standard representative sample of hospitals in New England (5). At the conclusion of the study when certain economies of scale became evident, it was decided to extend the study to other areas to obtain data on large CCU's (eight beds or more). One such unit from Connecticut was included, as well as a sample of units in New York City with eight or more beds.

Table 1 shows the number of patients and the proportion of myocardial infarcts treated in different hospitals. The selection of patients was clearly more discriminating, as measured by the proportion of myocardial infarct patients treated in university and other teaching institutions to those treated in nonteaching hospitals. These differences are statistically significant.

Table 1. Diagnosis of Patients Treated in Coronary Care Units

Hospital type	No.	No. of patients	Myocardial infarcts (%)	Other heart disease (%)	Other disease (%)
University	7	2,442	54.6	39.8	5.3
Other teaching	5	2,180	51.6	39.8	8.6
Nonteaching	20	3,393	46.8	47.5	5.7

Table 2. Deaths from Myocardial Infarcts and Other Causes

Hospital type	Myocardial infarct patients		All other patients	
	Deaths (%)	Range (%)	Deaths (%)	Range
University	16.3	14.3–29.0	0.6	0.6–0.8
Other teaching	19.2	10.0–24.2	0.6	0.5–0.7
Nonteaching	18.7	5.9–48.0	1.4	1.0–1.8
All hospitals	18.1 (N=683)		1.0 (N=40)	

Table 2 presents the death rates of patients with myocardial infarcts and other diseases who received intensive care. Myocardial infarct death rates vary from about 16% to 19% in the different hospital classes. The death rates of other patients (some of whom were admitted as "question MI's") from other heart diseases, other medical diseases, and a few with nonmedical diseases, were unusually low (overall about 1%) in all types of hospitals. Death rates in community hospitals usually are about 3% whereas in teaching hospitals where patients are sicker, death rates often are 6% to 8%. About half of the coronary care unit capacity is therefore being used by very low risk patients—patients whose risk of dying is less than the general hospital population. What appears to have happened is that a considerable excess of coronary care unit capacity has been provided, thus the units are being filled with patients suffering from a melange of cardiac and other diseases.

Figure 1 shows a frequency distribution of hospitals by death rates. The lowest rate in any institution was 6%, found in a small hospital. We can adduce no reason why this institution should have such a favorable rate. All three institutions with death rates below 10% were small and treated relatively few patients. At the other extreme we again find that the hospitals with high death rates are mostly small hospitals treating few patients. There is one exception— the highest rate, 48%, was found in a well known urban institution with an excellent medical staff. In general, the larger hospitals with more patients tended

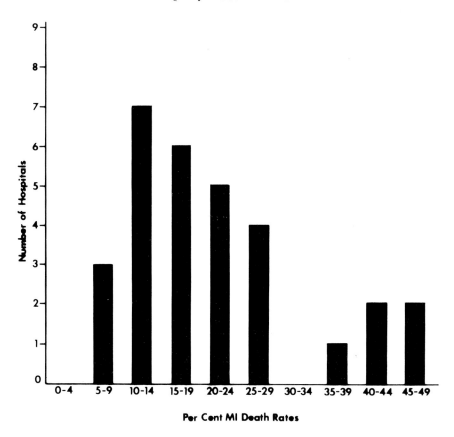

Fig. 1. Frequency of myocardial infarct death rates, by hospital.

to have rates that clustered about the mean death rate, strongly suggesting that patient selection rather than treatment effectiveness causes the unusual varia- tions. It seems evident that the reported hospital experiences are from institu- tions with more favorable rates, another example of how selected data may mislead.

The next few tables illustrate some of the economic measures that have been used to characterize efficiency. Table 3 shows the mean length of stay. The stay was shortest in the university hospitals and longest in the nonteaching institu- tions. Since the latter had fewer patients with myocardial infarcts, it might have been expected that their stays would actually have been shorter.

A second measure, efficient use of personnel, is illustrated in Table 4. Despite the fact that the number of discharges per nurse in university hospitals is impressively greater than in nonteaching hospitals, these results are not signifi-

Table 3. Length of Stay

Hospital type	Average length of stay (days)	Range
University	4.4	3.5–5.0
Other teaching	4.5	3.3–4.9
Nonteaching	5.1	2.9–8.8
All hospitals	4.7	

Table 4. Discharges per Nurse

Hospital type	Discharges per nurse	Range
University	34.3	21.2–42.8
Other teaching	29.8	20.5–46.6
Nonteaching	27.3	10.0–46.8
All hospitals	29.8	

cant. The explanation for this lies in the great variation within each hospital class. Some hospital coronary care units, university and nonteaching alike, were efficient by this measure, others were inefficient.

Discharges per bed, presented in Table 5, is another result related to efficient use of both personnel and other resources. The greater number of discharges per bed in the teaching hospitals was significantly different from the number from nonteaching hospitals ($P = < .05$). Large hospitals normally operate at higher occupancy rates than small ones, and from Table 6 this also seems true for coronary care units. The larger units found in university hospitals and other teaching institutions are occupied more of the time than are the beds in nonteaching hospitals. However, because of variation within classes, this statistic is of borderline significance. Although there are important differences in the group means, this is further evidence that not all university hospitals are run efficiently nor are all nonteaching hospitals inefficient.

Table 7 summarizes the daily cost of care in a coronary care unit in 1970. The right column shows the average daily cost for all patients—medical, surgical, pediatric, or other—treated in each type of hospital. The nonteaching hospitals clearly have the lowest costs in this category. The left column shows the calculated costs of treatment for all patients in coronary care units. Since about half of these patients do not have myocardial infarcts and since a large majority of this group seems to have no very compelling need for intensive care, a third calculation is shown in the middle column. Here the coronary care unit costs

Table 5. Discharges per Bed

Hospital type	Discharges per bed	Range
University	64.3	52.3–79.8
Other teaching	62.3	49.7–95.5
Nonteaching	48.5	16.0–95.5
All hospitals	56.0	

Table 6. Occupancy Rate

Hospital type	Occupancy (%)	Range
University	78.8	71.1–96.4
Other teaching	76.9	66.2–87.1
Nonteaching	70.6	27.6–92.6
All hospitals	74.3	

have been allocated to patients with myocardial infarcts and to others who probably represent the "question or probable MI" or the false positive diagnosis. This group should receive intensive care if the rationale for CCU's is accepted. When costs are allocated in this manner it can be seen that the average is very high. It is also clear that intensive care is particularly expensive in the smaller nonteaching hospitals and is least in the larger units in teaching institutions.

The above details represent the quantitative story obtained from an investigation of coronary care units. In addition, there are certain nonquantitative results which might be entitled "The Nurse's Tale." In visiting the units, many differ-

Table 7. Calculated Daily Costs for CCU and Other Hospital Inpatients

Hospital type	Costs in CCU		Costs for all hospital inpatients
	All patients	MI and "suspect MI" patients	
University	$104	$160	$96
Other teaching	$102	$171	$100
Nonteaching	$107	$232	$80

ences were uncovered. Nurses in some units volunteered that there was a lack of concordance between their responsibility and authority. Many doctors, they felt, did not understand the theory of intensive care; nurses, some added, were blamed for failures in the unit while doctors took credit for the successes. In retrospect it appears there were three types of units: units with full time directors which were well and efficiently run, units with part time directors which were competently directed, and units with part time directors that were not well managed. The nurses' complaints were heard mainly in the last type of unit.

Another nonquantitative result was exemplified by one large university CCU which had an occupancy rate of only 38%. The explanation for this uneconomic operation was that a few minutes away was a small coronary care unit with which it was sharing patients. One unit might have operated with acceptable efficiency, but with two, neither could.

In 1969 Duffy and Peterson published a study of coronary care units in the three-state area of Massachusetts, New Hampshire, and Rhode Island (6). They concluded there was a comfortable access of coronary care unit capacity sufficient to meet the expected demand for proved and probable myocardial infarcts. A second study in mid 1971 by Keairnes (7) uncovered the fact that there had been a 27% increase in capacity in the same area. The fact that every hospital in the study region had received the 1969 report did not deter the provision of more and more facilities.

It is clear that the type of technology represented by coronary care units has been applied uncritically, without adequate proof of effectiveness or without attention to the amount of facility needed. Obviously the question of whether a service can be provided economically or not is one that should be considered in planning for intensive care of patients with myocardial infarcts.

There are certain types of medical services, such as radiotherapy and intensive care of patients with myocardial infarcts, which should be rationed because they are costly, require specially trained technical and professional personnel, and serve relatively small patient populations. Physicians should be able to do this kind of rationing themselves; obviously they have not. This is one of the many weaknesses of medicine which has brought the government into the medical care system. Physicians who oppose government responsibility for medical care—and there are many—should recognize that the only possible alternative is effective organization and administration of medical care by the profession itself.

REFERENCES CITED

1. National Center for Health Statistics. 1971. Leading components of upturn in mortality for men, United States—1952–67. U. S. Department of Health, Education, and Welfare, Public Health Service, Publication No. (HSM) 72-1008.

2. 1968. Organization of a four-bed coronary care unit at the Hospital of St. Raphael (New Haven, Conn.). Conn. Med. 32:214.
3. Mather, H. G., et al. 1971. Acute myocardial infarction: Home and hospital treatment. Brit. Med. J. 3:334.
4. Martin, S. P. 1973. Inputs into coronary care over thirty years: A cost effectiveness study. (to be published)
5. Bloom, B. S., and Peterson, O. L. 1973. End results, cost and productivity of coronary-care units. New Engl. J. Med. 288:72.
6. Peterson, O. L., and Duffy, B. J. 1970. A report on coronary care in the Tri-State Region. Medical Care and Education Foundation, Inc., Boston.
7. Keairnes, H. W. 1972. Coronary care and intensive care units in New England: The geographic distribution of facilities, resources and personnel. Medical Care and Education Foundation, Inc., Boston.

Current Therapy:
"Capsule" Reports on Progress

THE SILENT CORONARY

ARTHUR M. MASTER*

What is silent coronary disease? It is a completely asymptomatic disease and the person who has it is usually unaware of its presence. He has no symptoms at all, no matter how much he exerts himself physically or to what unusual mental or emotional strain he is subjected. Because of this, and because of the increasing number of deaths caused by this disease, all physicians must be alerted to the problem.

Unless there is an acute myocardial infarction, the physical examination generally does not reveal any evidence of coronary artery disease. X-ray and fluoroscopic examinations may disclose an enlarged heart, left ventricular hypertrophy, ventricular aneurysm, calcification of the coronary arteries (in a relatively young man), and congested lungs. Fluoroscopic examination also may disclose paradoxical or absent pulsation of the left ventricle attributable to a previous infarction. (We were the first to report this finding in human subjects [1,2]; Tennant and Wiggers [3] initially observed it during their experiments on dogs.)

We have found the electrocardiogram to be the most useful agent in detecting silent coronary disease. In this regard, however, it must be borne in mind that even in classic angina pectoris the resting electrocardiogram is normal in 50–83% of the cases [4,5]. The fact that the electrocardiogram at rest is normal does not mean that coronary artery disease is not present. To rule out the possibility under these circumstances, it is necessary to determine the function of the heart. The regular double or "augmented" Master two-step test, which is completely safe, is ideal for this.

The value of the two-step test in detecting coronary artery disease has been confirmed by various investigators [5–7]. In their studies, the results of thousands of tests on industrial workers, life insurance applicants, and men in the armed forces have been analyzed. More important than the large number of people who performed this test, has always been a continuous, thorough follow-up. Robb and Marks [7] in a report on 2,224 male applicants for life insurance who were given the test, stated that "a long term follow-up of these cases disclosed: Ischemic S-T segment depression after exercise is pathognomonic of coronary insufficiency for all practical purposes." They found that deaths by coronary disease were 16 times greater among subjects with severe ischemic depression on exercise electrocardiograms than among those without a depression.

*Now deceased.

CORONARY ARTERIOGRAPHY AND THE TWO-STEP TEST

Coronary arteriography is also used to detect coronary artery disease. It is not, of course, an office procedure like the two-step test. In addition, coronary arteriography is not without danger. To date, mortality rates of 1% have been reported; complications have been observed in 7% of cases.

The two-step test is designed to study cardiac function, whereas the purpose of coronary cinearteriography is to delineate the anatomy of the blood vessels. Nevertheless, in the hands of experts, there is extraordinary and good correlation between the results obtained with cinearteriography and those obtained with the two-step test. Gorlin (8), in the lead article of the *Journal of the American Medical Association,* reported 82% correspondence between the positive Master two-step test and significant angiographic abnormalities.

PREVALENCE OF SILENT CORONARY ARTERY DISEASE

Postmortem Evidence

Just how prevalent is silent coronary artery disease? Let us first discuss the postmortem evidence of it in the young. Enos and co-workers (9) reported their autopsy findings in 300 American soldiers killed in battle in the Korean War. The mean age of these men was only 22.1 years. Nevertheless, 15% had plaques causing narrowing of one-half or more of the lumen in at least one coronary artery. Obviously these men had never complained of chest pain. Mason (10) reported a similar observation in 275 British male air crew personnel who died accidentally at the mean age of 27.3 years.

Clinical Evidence

Clinical evidence of silent coronary disease in the young has also been confirmed by various investigators (11–13). Mathewson and Varnam (11) reported evidence of this in 4,000 apparently healthy military and civilian pilots whose mean age was 27 years. Averill and Lamb (12) and Smith and Lamb (13) also reported their findings in 67,000 air force personnel in the United States, 90% of whom were under the age of 40 years. They observed ST segment depressions and T-wave abnormalities in 5.2 of every 1,000 men between the ages of 20 and 24 years, but this increased to 19 of every 1,000 men 45 years of age or more. What makes these figures so impressive is that these investigations were performed without the benefit of a two-step test; the diagnosis was made only on the basis of a resting electrocardiogram. Further testing probably would have shown an even greater number affected.

Silent Coronary Disease in the General Population

Postmortem evidence of silent coronary disease is tabulated in Table 1, which has been published previously (19).

In the three large series in Table 1, consisting of 792 subjects, evidence of silent healed infarctions was found in a total of 350 subjects. None of them had ever had any evidence or suspicion of previous myocardial involvement during life.

Clinical evidence of silent myocardial infarction in the general population, tabulated in Table 2, has also been presented before (19).

It has been found that 30% of all infarctions detected by electrocardiographic surveys are silent. In a study of 501 garment workers, Stokes and Dawber (17) and Price (18) found that 123 of them had silent or unrecognized myocardial infarction. This suggests that about 30% of all persons with electrocardiographic evidence of a myocardial infarction do not give a history of pain.

Clinical evidence of silent coronary disease without infarction has been demonstrated by the electrocardiogram and by the two-step or other functional tests of the heart. From 2 to 4% of persons do have asymptomatic heart disease. Of interest in this regard is that in 1951 we found coronary artery disease in at

Table 1. Postmortem Evidence of Silent Coronary Artery Disease (20) in the General Population

Author	Period of study	No. of cases	No. recognized	No. presumably silent
Achor et al. (14)	1945–50	227	108 (48%)	119 (52%)
Johnson et al. (15)	1953–54	113	57 (50%)	56 (50%)
Gould and Cawley (16)	1945–55	452	277 (61%)	175 (39%)

Table 2. Clinical Evidence of Silent Myocardial Infarction (20) in the General Population

Authors	Year of report	Total cases of infarction	Silent cases[a]
Stokes and Dawber (17)	1959	87	68 (33%)
Price (18)	1959	414	104 (30%)

[a]Actual plus probable cases

least 24 (5%) of 120 asymptomatic physicians examined over the age of 40 years. We have made many similar observations from which we concluded, conservatively, that no less than 4 to 6% of the general population in the United States, 35 years of age or more, are affected with silent coronary artery disease without infarction.

In previous studies in which we presented our estimate of silent myocardial infarction in the United States, we utilized two sources. From the United States Public Health Service report, in 1965 (19), we estimated that about 1,570,000 persons were affected with myocardial infarction. When this survey was made, only the electrocardiographic findings were utilized. It must be remembered that in many instances the electrocardiogram may be nondiagnostic and thus this figure may be even greater. In addition, after an acute infarction the electro-cardiogram may return to normal. On the basis of this and other studies, we concluded that nearly 2,000,000 people suffered a myocardial infarction in 1965 and that it was silent in about 600,000 of them (20).

In order to estimate the number of people with silent coronary artery disease without infarction, let us look at the 1970 U.S. Census Report which cites that there were 84 million people, 35 years of age and over, in the country. We have repeatedly presented evidence that from 4 to 6% of the people in this age group have silent coronary artery disease without infarction. If we take 4% and then 6% of 84 million people, we have from 3 to 5 million people in this category for the year 1970.

Why has the extent of silent coronary artery disease been generally ignored? We believe it is because the problem has not been stressed sufficiently. The existence and magnitude of the problem have to be proved again and again, before they are accepted.

Despite the evidence to the contrary, many physicians still assume that a normal resting electrocardiogram signifies a good heart and normal coronary arteries. Even lay people recognize this as a fallacy. They hear of heart attacks and sudden deaths in persons who had been reassured regarding their health by physicians because their resting electrocardiograms were normal. No physician can exclude the possibility of coronary artery disease in this way. He must determine the patient's cardiac function by utilizing either the two-step or treadmill test.

What if silent coronary artery disease is discovered? What can be done? We believe that much can be accomplished by taking the following measures: cessation of use of tobacco, reduction of excess weight, lowering of elevated blood pressure, treatment of diabetes, reduction of abnormally high cholesterol levels by diet and drugs, lowering of high serum uric acid levels, etc. Possible causes of arrhythmias should be removed and the administration of antiar-rhythmic drugs may be very helpful. We usually encourage the patient to exercise, but if he is quite sick he is advised to avoid undue emotional and physical stress. A serious attempt is made to engender a philosophic attitude; this can be accomplished in heart disease patients and it will prolong life.

REFERENCES CITED

1. Master, A. M., Gubner, R., Dack, S., and Jaffe, H. L. 1939. Form of ventricular contraction in cardiac infarction: Fluoroscopic studies. Proc. Soc. Exp. Biol. Med. 41:89.

2. Master, A. M., Gubner, R., Dack, S., and Jaffe, H. L. 1940. The diagnosis of coronary occlusion and myocardial infarction by fluoroscopic examination. Amer. Heart J. 20:475.

3. Tennant, R., and Wiggers, C. J. 1935. The effect of coronary occlusion on myocardial contraction. Amer. J. Physiol. 112:351.

4. Doyle, J. T., Heslin, A. S., Hilleboe, H. E., Formel, P. E., and Korns, R. F. 1957. A prospective study of degenerative cardiovascular disease in Albany: Report of 3 years' experience. I. Ischemic heart disease. Amer. J. Publ. Health 47:25.

5. Master, A. M., and Rosenfeld, I. 1961. Criteria for the clinical application of the "two-step" exercise test: Obviation of false-negative and false-positive responses. J.A.M.A. 178:283.

6. Robb, G. P., and Marks, H. H. 1964. Latent coronary artery disease: Determination of its presence and severity by the exercise electrocardiogram. Amer. J. Cardiol. 13:603.

7. Robb, G. P., and Marks, H. H. 1967. Two-step exercise electrocardiogram in arteriosclerotic heart disease. J.A.M.A. 200:918.

8. Cohn, P. F., Vohonas, P. S., Most, A. S., Herman, M. V., and Gorlin, R. 1972. Diagnostic accuracy of two-step postexercise ECG: Results in 305 subjects studied by coronary arteriography. J.A.M.A. 220: 501.

9. Enos, W. F., Holmes, R. H., and Beyer, J. 1953. Coronary disease among United States soldiers killed in action in Korea. J.A.M.A. 152:1090.

10. Mason, J. K. 1963. Asymptomatic disease of coronary arteries in young men. Brit. Med. J. 2:1234.

11. Mathewson, F. A. L., and Varnam, G. S. 1960. Abnormal electrocardiograms in apparently healthy people. II. The electrocardiogram in the diagnosis of subclinical myocardial disease: Serial records of 32 people. Circulation 21:204.

12. Averill, K. H., and Lamb, L. E. 1960. Electrocardiographic findings in 67,375 asymptomatic subjects. I. Incidence of abnormalities. Amer. J. Cardiol. 6:76.

13. Smith, G. B., and Lamb, L. E. 1960. Electrocardiographic findings in 67,375 asymptomatic subjects. IX. Myocardial infarction. Amer. J. Cardiol. 6:190.

14. Achor, R. W. P., Futch, W. D., Burchell, H. B., and Edwards, J. E. 1956. The fate of patients surviving acute myocardial infarction: A study of clinical and necropsy data in 250 cases. Arch. Internal Med. 98: 162.

15. Johnson, W. J., Achor, R. W. P., Burchell, H. B., and Edwards, J. E. 1959. Unrecognized myocardial infarction—A clinico-pathological study. Arch. Internal Med. 103:253.

16. Gould, S. E., and Cawley, L. P. 1958. Unsuspected healed myocardial infarction in patients dying in a general hospital. Arch. Internal Med. 101:524.

17. Stokes, J., and Dawber, T. R. 1959. The "silent coronary": The frequency and clinical characteristics of unrecognized myocardial infarction in the Framingham study. Ann. Internal Med. 50:1359.

18. Price, L. 1959. Severity of myocardial infarction in garment workers. J. Occup. Med. 1:150.

19. National Center for Health Statistics. 1965. Coronary Heart Disease in Adults, United States 1960–62. Vital Health Statistics, Publ. No. 1000, Series 11, No. 10, Public Health Service. U.S. Government Printing Office, Washington, D.C.

20. Master, A. M., and Geller, A. J. 1969. The extent of completely asymptomatic coronary artery disease. Amer. J. Cardiol. 23:173.

ANGINA PECTORIS WITH NORMAL
CORONARY ARTERIOGRAMS

WILLIAM LIKOFF

In most patients with angina pectoris, atherosclerosis is widely distributed throughout the major coronary arteries and seriously obstructs at least two main blood vessels. Electrocardiographic, hemodynamic, and myocardial metabolic abnormalities usually are observed in these individuals (1,2). Angina also occurs when the coronary vessels are normally patent. This takes place when a major anomaly of the coronary circulation, severe aortic valvular disease, idiopathic hypertrophic subaortic stenosis, or a cardiomyopathy is solely responsible for the clinical problem. In each of these instances, a mechanism other than blood vessel obstruction accounts for the imbalance between coronary flow and the nutritional needs of the myocardium.

In aortic stenosis, for example, the marked elevation of intraventricular pressure increases peripheral coronary resistance, thereby diminishing coronary blood flow during systole. At the same time, the thickened ventricular musculature, high intraventricular pressure, and prolonged ejection interval increase myocardial oxygen needs.

Subjects with aortic regurgitation may suffer from angina pectoris in spite of an overdeveloped and widely patent coronary arterial circulation. Factors responsible include the abnormally depressed aortic diastolic pressure accounting for diminished coronary blood flow, and the size and configuration of the dilated left ventricle resulting in increased myocardial oxygen consumption.

The mechanisms responsible for angina pectoris in idiopathic hypertrophic subaortic stenosis are identical with those in aortic stenosis. Those in restrictive and congestive cardiomyopathies are less certain but may include metabolic errors impeding oxygen utilization at a cellular level.

Since the advent of coronary arteriography, considerable interest has focused upon reports indicating that angina pectoris may be encountered in patients with normal arteriograms in the absence of other types of cardiovascular disease (3,4,5). The initial communications regarding this matter indicated that the majority of the individuals had classical angina. With some the pain occurred at rest as well as upon exercise and was not uniformly relieved by nitroglycerin. However, differences between the typical and atypical patterns were too subtle to suggest the latter was not the result of true coronary insufficiency.

The major electrocardiographic abnormalities reported consisted of ST segment depressions in bipolar and unipolar limb and precordial leads generally associated with flat or inverted T-waves. These changes were increased following stress tests.

A central issue among these patients was the fact that they did not have diabetes, hypertension, or hyperlipidemia. The vast majority were females in the fourth and fifth decades of life. The overall incidence of cigarette smoking was no greater than in a comparable population group.

Subsequent observations amply confirm the original reports (6). Indeed, experience recorded not only the clinical pattern of angina pectoris and electro-cardiographic signs of ischemia in patients with angiographically normal coronary arteries, but also myocardial infarction and death in subjects in whom post-mortem study confirmed patent coronary arteries (5,7).

There are a number of possible explanations for the appearance of clinical manifestations of coronary heart disease, angina, and electrocardiographic abnormalities involving the RST segment and T-wave in bipolar and unipolar leads, in individuals in whom cinearteriography reveals normal coronary vessels. There is the possibility that arteriography does not accurately detail vascular pathology. Although contrast study of the coronary circulation admittedly underestimates the severity of atherosclerosis, this failing is relatively small and cannot possibly account for diffusely diseased arteries being depicted as perfectly normal blood vessels.

It also does not seem reasonable to claim that vascular obstructions may have been present in these patients and recanalized prior to the arteriography. In individuals in whom recanalization of obstructing lesions has been recorded by serial cinearteriography the residual hallmarks of the basic vascular abnormality are still readily recognizable.

The possibility that functional constriction of the coronary arteries is responsible for the clinical manifestations of coronary insufficiency and the electro-cardiographic abnormalities is extremely remote, for when unusual vasomotor activity is present it is generally recognized at the time of coronary arteriography.

The view has been expressed that structural or functional disease of the peripheral coronary system logically explains the clinical findings in these patients. However, the peripheral coronary system is adequately visualized during cinearteriography. Abnormalities in form or function have not been reported. Furthermore, obstructive disease of peripheral vessels is exceptional unless major arteries are similarly involved.

Theoretically, an oxygen diffusion impairment at the level of the microcirculation or inappropriate oxygen utilization by the myocardial cell could account for the paradox of myocardial ischemia or necrosis in the presence of adequate arterial saturation and patent coronary arteries. However, evidence supporting this concept has not been presented to this point.

Neill, Kassebaum, and Judkins (8) demonstrated myocardial hypoxia and anaerobic metabolism during induced tachycardia in a female with angina pectoris, an abnormal exercise electrocardiogram, and normally patent coronary arteries. They postulated that myocardial hypoxia was responsible for the chest pain and the electrocardiographic changes, and included among the explanations for the hypoxia inadequate size of coronary arteries, abnormal distribution of the vessels, and inappropriate vasomotor reactivity of the coronary circulation to an increased metabolic need of the myocardium.

It has been suggested that the chest pain associated with normal coronary arteriographic findings can be clearly distinguished from the angina pectoris associated with large vessel obstructive atherosclerosis and that it usually is related to neurocirculatory asthenia (9). This is not consistent with the critical experiences of most investigators. Indeed, the central theme in most reports regarding this subject is that the differentiation between patients with obstructing coronary atherosclerosis and those with normally patent vessels is the absence of usual risk factors in the latter, rather than the modalities of the subjective discomfort or electrocardiographic abnormalities at rest and following stress testing.

The prognosis of patients with angina pectoris and normal coronary arteriograms has not been precisely defined. In the series of Elliott and Brat (7), 3 of 15 female patients with this syndrome died of myocardial infarction. By contrast, 86 patients were followed by Waxler, Kimbiris, and Dreifus (10) for periods varying from 6 months to 2.5 years and there was no instance of sudden death or myocardial infarction. Approximately one-half of the patients noted a decrease in the frequency and severity of chest pain during that interval.

Careful long-term observations of 37 patients were conducted by Bemiller, Pepine, and Rogers (10) over a mean of 4.8 years. Clinical, hemodynamic, and angiographic deterioration were not observed. There was a striking absence of complication in these patients. Basically, the observation suggested a nonprogressive disorder in no way related to coronary artery disease.

In brief, there now resides in the experiences recorded ample documentation that angina pectoris associated with abnormal resting and exercise electrocardiographic patterns may be found in patients with normal coronary vessels as seen by cinearteriography. These patients bear no relation to other subjects with chest pain and normal coronary arteries such as encountered in aortic valvular disease and idiopathic hypertrophic subaortic stenosis. Furthermore, there is every reason to believe that they should not be categorized as having an abnormal vasoregulatory syndrome, cardiac neurosis, or neurocirculatory asthenia.

Myocardial hypoxia has been implicated as the underlying pathophysiology. The cause for the hypoxia, however, remains obscure. Among the explanations, the possibility of a defective microcirculation or an abnormality in the enzyme activity of the myocardial cell are considered attractive hypotheses. Abnormal oxygen dissociation may be involved but apparently it is not a consistent default.

Treatment has not been defined. The natural history of the disease, however, appears to be benign and it is not marked by serious clinical or pathophysiologic deterioration.

REFERENCES CITED

1. Cohen, L. S., Elliott, W. G., Kline, D., and Gorlin, R. 1966. Coronary heart disease: Clinical cine arteriographic and metabolic correlation. Amer. J. Cardiol. 17:153.
2. Parker, S. O., DiGiorgio, S., and West, R. O. 1966. A hemodynamic study of acute coronary insufficiency precipitated by exercise. Amer. J. Cardiol. 17:470.
3. Likoff, W., Segal, B. L., and Kasparian, H. 1967. Paradox of normal selective coronary arteriograms in patients considered to have unmistakable coronary heart disease. New Engl. J. Med. 276:1063.
4. Kemp, H. G., Elliott, W. G., and Gorlin, R. The anginal syndrome with normal coronary arteriography. Trans. Assoc. Amer. Physicians 80:59.
5. Elliott, R. S., and Brat, G. 1969. The paradox of myocardial ischemia and necrosis in young women with normal coronary arteriograms. Amer. J. Cardiol. 23:633.
6. Neill, W. A., Judkins, M. P., Bkinbsa, B. S., Metcalfe, J., Kassebaum, D. G., and Kloster, F. E. 1972. Clinically suspected ischemic heart disease not collaborated by demonstrable coronary artery disease. Amer. J. Cardiol. 29:171.
7. Dwyer, E. M., Weiner, L., and Cox, W. J. 1969. Angina pectoris in patients with normal and abnormal coronary arteriograms. Amer. J. Cardiol. 23:639.
8. Neill, W. A., Kassebaum, B. G., and Judkins, M. P. 1968. Myocardial hypoxia is the basis for angina pectoris in a patient with normal coronary arteriogram. New Engl. J. Med. 279:789.
9. Waxler, E. B., Kimbiris, D., and Dreifus, L. A. 1971. The fate of women with normal coronary arteriograms and chest pain resembling angina pectoris. Amer. J. Cardiol. 28:25.
10. Bemiller, C. R., Pepine, C. J., and Rogers, A. K. 1973. Long term observations of patients with abnormal and normal coronary arteriograms. Circulation 47:36.

CAPSULE REPORT ON THE ANTICOAGULANTS

GEORGE C. GRIFFITH

The morbidity and mortality of thrombus formation and thromboembolism are well-documented facts; therefore, no elaboration is necessary.

HEPARIN

Heparin is a sulfonated mucopolysaccharide with a heavy negative electrostatic charge. Through its interference with the intrinsic normal coagulation mechanism, it prevents the activation of clotting factor IX (Christmas factor). The thrombin-mediated conversion of fibrinogen to fibrin is retarded (1). Heparin also lessens viscosity and the aggregation of platelets by thrombin. Thus, it is useful in preventing the white intra-arterial thrombus, the red intravenous thrombus, and the diffuse clotting in small vessels that is associated with consumption coagulopathy.

The indications and contraindications are well known. I emphasize that heparin does not cross the placental barrier and, therefore, may be used in pregnant states without affecting the fetus. Also, there is reason to believe in the anticarcinogenetic effect of heparin.

ORAL ANTICOAGULANTS

The oral anticoagulants are divided into four groups according to chemical structure: 1) dicoumarols (bishydroxycoumarin and ethylbiscoumacetate); 2) monocoumarols (phenprocoumon, acenocoumarin, and warfarin); 3) cyclocoumarols; and 4) indandiones (phenindione, diphenadione, anisindione, and chlorphenylindandione (2).

It is proposed that the action of an oral anticoagulant depends upon the irreversible inhibition of the transport of vitamin K_1 to its intracellular site of action in the liver (3). All oral anticoagulants act in the same manner, first by decreasing the activity of factor VII, followed by decreases in factors IX, X, and II. Variability in response to coumarin drugs depends upon absorption, vitamin K, rates of metabolism, prolongation of platelet survival, and decrease in platelet adhesiveness (4). Cancer cells contain an agent which induces fibrin formation (5). The beneficial effect of coumarin therapy in cancer patients has been documented in 1,569 patient/years by Michaels (6).

The indications for oral anticoagulation therapy are thrombophlebitis, thromboembolism, preinfarction angina, valvular heart disease, valvular prosthesis, atrial arrhythmia with embolization, vein bypass graft, acute myocardial infarction, recurrent myocardial infarction, congestive failure with embolism, prolonged bed rest in the elderly, increased platelet adhesiveness, and hypercoagulable states.

The contraindications are well known; however, one contraindication which is not familiar is the teratogenesis which occurs in pregnancy because warfarin crosses the placental barrier. Therefore, warfarin should not be used in the first and second trimesters of pregnancy.

UROKINASE AND STREPTOKINASE

Urokinase and streptokinase are new and useful therapeutic agents in lysing of thrombi, especially in acute thrombophlebitis and pulmonary embolism. The side-effects of hemorrhage can be avoided by care in patient selection, especially where those patients with lesions such as peptic ulcer and the blood dyscrasias are concerned (7). A cooperative study on the clinical effectiveness of the fibrinolytic agents in acute myocardial infarction is now in progress (8).

OTHER ANTICOAGULANTS

Malayan pit viper venom is a fibrinolytic agent, but has not been widely tested in clinical trials.

Arvin and Reptilase are agents under investigation.

Dipyridamole (Persantine) prevents platelet aggregation by blocking adenyl cyclase. Its disadvantages are that it must be administered in large dosages and that it is expensive.

Cyproheptadine hydrochloride (Periactin) is an antiaggregation substance which blocks serotonin release.

Aspirin is an effective agent which inhibits platelet aggregation by blocking adenyl cyclase. Its advantages are that it is safe and inexpensive.

The action of acetaminophen is similar to that of aspirin.

Clofibrate acts as an antiaggregation substance by potentiating circulating fibrinolysins.

Phenylbutazone (Butazolidin) is an anti-inflammatory agent which acts as an antiaggregation substance.

Allopurinol is an antiplatelet-aggregating agent.

ACUTE MYOCARDIAL INFARCTION

Three important studies have been reported and evaluated in recent years: the British Medical Research Council report (9); the Australian study by Lovell and associates (10); and the Veterans Administration Cooperative study report (11). All subjects were entered into the study only when the prothrombin time was at an effective level. Warfarin or phenindione (Hedulin) were used only in the British Medical Research Council trial (Table 1). The survival rates for men of all ages, expressed as a percentage of the numbers starting treatment, show a definite advantage in the treated groups in all three studies; that is, by 12, 7, and 4%, respectively.

When the survival rates are studied for men 55 years old and younger, a similarly favorable result may be observed (Table 2). In addition, a similarly

Table 1. Survival Rates for Men of All Ages, Expressed as a Percentage of the Number Starting Treatment*

| | | | Survival Rates (%) | |
| | | No. of patients | At 1 yr | At 2 yrs |
Trial				
Brit. Med. Res. Council	Control Group	160		78
	Treated Group	166		90
Veterans Admin. (1965)	Control Group	359	91	83
	Treated Group	388	94	90
Lovell et al. (1967)	Control Group	178	88	81
	Treated Group	172	90	85
	Heparin-treated Group	62	85	79

*Age ranges were: B.M.R.C., 40–69 yrs; Vet. Admin., 21–75 yrs; Lovell et al., 30–70 yrs.

Table 2. Survival Rates for Men Aged 55 Years and Under, Expressed as a Percentage of the Number Starting Treatment

| | | | Survival Rates (%) | |
| | | No. of patients | At 1 yr | At 2 yrs |
Trial				
Veterans Admin. (1965)	Control Group	233	91	86
	Treated Group	243	96	94
Lovell et al. (1967)	Control Group	94	90	83
	Treated Group	92	95	92

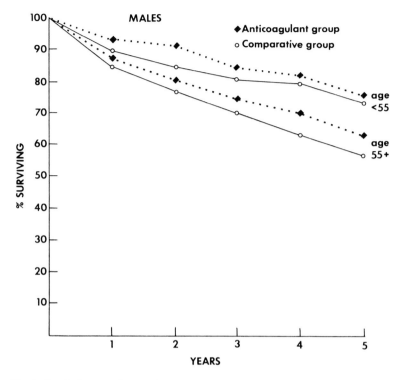

Fig. 1. Survival curves (international collaborative analysis).

favorable reduction in mortality is seen in the International Collaborative Analysis (12), as shown in Figure 1.

When age-specific death rates for males are considered, the increased survival rate in the treated group in all age categories may be compared to the survival rate in control group (Table 3).

MECHANISM OF ACTION

Decreased absorption of vitamin K results in potentiation of warfarin, with an increased prothrombin time measured in seconds.

A release of the circulating anticoagulant from its binding site, usually from albumin, causes potentiation. An increase in the metabolism of the drug results in a lowering of the prothrombin time. Finally, a delay in the metabolism increases the circulating anticoagulant and therefore increases the prothrombin time.

Other mechanisms probably exist but are ill defined.

Table 3. Age-specific Death Rates for Males
Included in International Collaborative Analysis

Patients' ages on entering trial (yrs)	Deaths per 100 man-months of exposure[a]	
	Control group	Treated group
15 to 24		0
25 to 34	0.65	0.12
35 to 44	0.52	0.36
45 to 54	0.65	0.54
55 to 64	0.85	0.76
65 to 74	1.16	0.90
75 to 84	2.01	1.51
55 yrs and under	0.60	0.46
More than 55 yrs of age	0.98	0.81
TOTAL	0.79[b]	0.63[b]

[a]Total number of man-months of exposure, 47,358
[b]The difference is significant (P < 0.01)

Table 4. Drugs Potentiating Warfarin Effect

Acetaminophen (Tylenol)	MAO inhibitors
Barbiturates	Meperidine (Demerol)
Carbon tetrachloride	Methandrostenolone (Dianabol)
Chloral hydrate	Mineral oil
Chlorpromazine (Thorazine)	Morphine sulfate
Chlorpropamide (Diabinese)	Neomycin
Clofibrate (Atromid-S)	Para-amino-salicylic acid
Dextrothyroxine (Choloxin)	Penicillin
Diphenylhydantoin (Dilantin)	Phenylbutazone (Butazolidin)
Disulfiram (Antabuse)	Quinine and quinidine
Ethacrynic acid (Edecrin)	Reserpine
Ethyl alcohol	Salicylates
Heparin	Sulfa compounds
Kanamycin	Tetracyclines

DRUGS POTENTIATING WARFARIN EFFECT

The drugs which potentiate the effect of warfarin and thus prolong the prothrombin time are given in Table 4.

DRUGS INHIBITING WARFARIN EFFECT

The drugs which inhibit the effect of warfarin and thus decrease the prothrombin time as measured in seconds are given in Table 5.

Table 5. Drugs Inhibiting Warfarin Effect

Antacids
Bile salts
Chloramphenicol (Chloromycetin)
Chlordiazepoxide hydrochloride (Librium)
Cholestyramine (Cuemid, Questran)
Colchicine
Diazepam (Valium)
Ethchlorvynol (Placidyl)
Glutethimide (Doriden)
Griseofulvin
Meprobamate (Miltown)
Vitamin K

Anticoagulants are useful agents that require patient education, a competent laboratory, and a physician with high interest in patient care.

REFERENCES CITED

1. Vieweg, W. V. R. 1972. The hazards of heparin in the elderly. Cardiol. Dig. 7:37.
2. Coon, W. W., and Willis, P. W., III. 1970. Some aspects of the pharmacology of oral anticoagulants. Clin. Pharmacol. Ther. 11:312.
3. Lowenthal, J., and Birnbaum, H. 1969. Vitamin K and coumarin anticoagulants: Dependence of anticoagulant effect on inhibition of vitamin K transport. Science 164:181.
4. Murphy, E. A., and Mustard, J. F. 1961. Dicumarol therapy and platelet turnover. Circ. Res. 9:402.
5. O'Meara, R. A. Q. 1958. Coagulative properties of cancers. Irish J. Med. Sci. (Series 6):474.
6. Michaels, L. 1964. Cancer incidence and mortality in patients having anticoagulant therapy. Lancet 2:832.
7. Sherry, S. 1972. Prospects in antithrombotic therapy. Amer. J. Cardiol. 29:81.
8. Mills, D. C. B. 1972. Effects of aggregating agents on platelet adenyl-cyclase [Abstr.]. Circulation 46 (Suppl. 2).
9. British Medical Research Council. 1964. An assessment of long-term anticoagulant administration after cardiac infarction. Brit. Med. J. 2:837.
10. Lovell, R. R. H. 1969. Rethinking coronary thrombosis: Lessons from experimental therapeutics with anticoagulants. Med. J. Austral. 2:425.
11. Veterans Administration Cooperative Study. 1965. Long-term anticoagulant therapy after myocardial infarction. J. Amer. Med. Assoc. 193:929.
12. International Anticoagulant Review Group. 1970. Collaborative analysis of long-term anticoagulant administration after acute myocardial infarction. Lancet 1:203.

THE CARDIOMYOPATHIES–PROGRESS IN MANAGEMENT

THOMAS W. MATTINGLY

A report of progress in any disease should be limited to a specific period of time. The seven-year period 1965–1972 has been selected for this progress report, primarily because a series of publications, symposia, and monographs that appeared in 1964 and 1965 (1–10) provides an excellent survey up to that time and constitutes an ideal baseline for this report.

Brief capsular reports of progress in therapy of cardiomyopathy (CM) are given under headings related to current classifications of the cardiomyopathies (1, 4, 11–13).

IDIOPATHIC CONGESTIVE CARDIOMYOPATHY

The therapy of idiopathic congestive cardiomyopathy is as unsatisfactory today as it was in the 1964–65 reports. Treatment remains chiefly symptomatic and supportive and is likely to remain as such until further progress is made in establishing specific etiologic factors, in identifying specific mechanisms of alteration of myocardial structure and function at the subcellular level, and in determining the relationship of associated clinical conditions (such as chronic alcoholism, virus infections, etc.) to the development of a CM.

Areas of knowledge have developed in this general field of ignorance which have resulted in progress, either in established therapeutic procedures or in potential approaches to therapy. In a few instances, they have provided progress in prevention.

Alcoholic Cardiomyopathy

The demonstration that alcohol can produce a CM in experimental animals (14) and significant alterations in myocardial function in acute experimental studies in man (15, 16) has strengthened support for alcohol as a specific etiologic agent even though all histochemical and ultrastructural studies have failed to identify changes which can be designated as being specific for an alcohol-induced injury (17). These observations, plus limited documentation of reversal of hemodynamic alterations in preclinical chronic alcoholics (18) and symptomatic chronic alcoholics (17), and improved myocardial function in the chronic alcoholic with a well developed CM upon the elimination of alcohol (17), have resulted in an almost universal opinion that abstinence from alcohol is beneficial in the management of alcoholic CM (11, 12, 17, 19). It is chiefly the chronic alcoholic himself who believes there should be further proof of a specific etiologic or "conditioning" relationship before he eliminates alcohol.

Toxic Cardiomyopathy (Beer-drinker's Cardiomyopathy)

The demonstration that cobalt can produce a CM in experimental animals (20) and the strong circumstantial evidence that cobalt, as an additive in beer, was responsible for the development of a CM in human consumers (21, 22), has not established whether the agent acts alone or is enhanced in its toxicity by synergistic action of an associated dietary deficiency (22) or by some other yet unrecognized "conditioning" effect (17, 23) of alcohol on human tissues (myocardium or liver). Nonetheless, these observations have provided preventive and possible therapeutic approaches to the management of this type of CM, which in various forms has puzzled clinicians since an initial description of the beer-drinker's heart by Bollinger in 1884 (24). The toxic or etiological factor may not have been the same in all these episodes, but the relationship to heavy beer drinking is common to all. An immediate preventive measure following the demonstration of the toxic effects of the additive, cobalt, was the removal from the market of beer containing the additive and its elimination in future beer production. Furthermore, the widely publicized deaths and cardiac disabilities resulting from these episodes of beer-drinker's CM (21, 22), presumably caused by the toxic effects of cobalt, have resulted in strengthening of the activities of the Food and Drug Administration relative to food additives in general. This may indirectly reduce the incidence of toxic CM, since there may be other toxic additives in use which have the capability of producing a CM, especially when consumed in large quantities, as happens with some beer drinkers. With the knowledge that a mineral, such as cobalt, is capable of producing a toxic injury to the myocardium, there exists a potential therapeutic approach in the administration of another less toxic mineral with a competitive action on myocardial enzymes, such as the one developed in the BAL (British anti-lewisite) therapy for mercury poisoning.

Toxic Cardiomyopathy (Drug Induced)

The demonstration that certain drugs now in clinical usage or under clinical trial and investigation are capable of producing structural and functional alterations in the myocardium, leading to the development of the features of a CM (cardiac hypertrophy, myocardial failure, and arrhythmias), extends the possibility that some of the currently classified idiopathic CM may be the result of unrecognized drug toxicity. The spectrum of such cardiotoxic drugs is increasing. In addition to the old antimony and arsenic compounds and emetine, the current list includes antidepression drugs such as the pentothiazines (25); antileukemic drugs such as Daunomycin, Adriamycin, and Daunorubicin (26); the commonly used antishock drugs such as the catecholamines (27); and antiobesity medications which are usually a combination of drugs (Strophanthin, digitalis, thyroid, etc.) (28). Cardiac failure from a recognized CM suspected as being induced by these drugs (25, 26) and supported by experimentally induced toxic lesions in animals (29) has resulted in caution in their use, introduction into trial studies, and final approval for clinical uses. These precautionary measures in the prevention of toxic CM are important, even though the need for a cure for leukemia, especially in childhood, for the control of severe mental depression, and for recovery from severe shock states is great. In such instances a limited risk of cardiac toxicity may be justified. On the other hand, since there are effective and safe methods for combating obesity, the use of toxic drugs is not justified. The publicized cardiac deaths and disabilities attributed to the use and abuse of "diet pills" consisting either of unapproved preparations or those improperly dispensed by poorly supervised obesity clinics have resulted in an increased public awareness of their hazards and tighter drug control.

Ultrastructural studies of the myocardium designed to determine the precise structural and functional alterations in the myocardium by these toxic drugs (30) and the development of studies designed to prevent such toxic effects (31) may provide benefits beyond that of safety in the use of these particular drugs. In most instances the site of injury has been traced to important membranes, allowing leakage of important enzymes or a direct inhibitory action on key myocardial tissue enzymes. It is interesting that recent ultrastructural and histochemical studies in diphtheritic CM (32) have indicated a marked abnormality in creatine phosphokinase enzyme activity, presumably from a "leak" of the enzyme from the myocardial fiber which in turn suggests localization of the toxic effect of the diphtheria toxin to membrane damage. The extension of similar molecular biologic studies as now applied to the study of drugs and toxins to other types of CM may provide new approaches to therapy.

Viral Cardiomyopathy (?)

The demonstration that a CM may follow an induced Coxsackie viral infection in the laboratory animal (33) has strengthened the long-standing suspicion that a similar but latent CM may follow as a sequella of Coxsackie and other cardiotrophic viral infections in man (34, 35). The precise mechanism for this latent CM of presumptive viral etiology remains to be established. An attractive autoimmune mechanism has been offered without complete substantiation at the present time (36). No specific therapeutic management has developed from this popular theory of viral etiology since presently developed antiviral agents as well as agents to block immunological responses are generally either not effective or, as in the case of immunosuppressive therapy, impractical for use as general preventive measures. Such therapy, moreover, is not without inherent problems of iatrogenic disease development. The high incidence of clinically suspicious viral infections, the impracticability of obtaining cultures and basic serology on each suspicious viral infection, the low incidence of even transient evidence of myocardial dysfunction in large series of adults having careful studies during the acute infection and convalescence, and the absence of documentation of sequential events in prospective studies (viral illness, cultural and serologic diagnosis of Coxsackie viral illness, recovery with or without transient clinical myocarditis, and latent cardiomyopathy) make it impractical at present to place all suspected postviral patients under long term surveillance. At best, surveillance and subsequent evaluations for myocardial damage must be limited to those individuals in whom there is some suspicion of slow recovery, or evidence of residual myocardial impairment beyond the usual period of recovery. The report of a five-year followup of cases suggestive of myocarditis has been disappointing (37). Retrospective serological evaluations in large groups of idiopathic CM, many with suspicious viral background histories, have provided only negative results. If overt or subclinical Coxsackie B viral infections were established as an important etiological factor in presently recognized idiopathic CM in either healthy adults or in those with "conditioning factors" such as chronic alcoholism or pregnancy, then protective immunization as now practiced against poliomyelitis, measles, and mumps would offer the greatest possibility of prevention and management. At present, a vaccine for effective protection against this virus has not been developed.

Peripartum Cardiomyopathy

In spite of continued reports of instances of peripartum CM, most investigators and clinicians cast doubt on the probability that pregnancy and the postpartum state itself is an etiologic factor (38). Emphasis continues to be placed on the importance of careful cardiovascular evaluations made before and during the earlier months of pregnancy in order to establish preexisting disease which may be aggravated or only recognized later. Recommendation for establishment of strict criteria for the placement of a CM in the category of a peripartum CM (39) provides a new approach for more careful investigation. The recent demonstration (40) that pregnancy enhanced the development of cardiac pathology in mice with induced viral infection suggests that pregnancy may be only a "conditioning factor" and not a basic etiologic factor: hence the recognition, management, and prevention of the basic factor in pregnancy may be the important measure as opposed to the virus factor being the only one of importance. The prognosis for good recovery from CM occurring in pregnancy remains poor, even with good management, and subsequent pregnancies definitely result in progression of the myocardial disease (39). The increase in the practice of contraception and more liberal abortion laws and practice should reduce instances of progression by reason of subsequent pregnancies.

Loeffler's Cardiomyopathy (Fibroplastic Myocarditis or Cardiomyopathy)

Observations that the so-called Loeffler's CM is part of the clinicopathologic spectrum of an eosinophilic leukemia or a definite myeloproliferative disorder, rather than being a simple association with eosinophilia or allergic states (41, 42), provide a new approach to the diagnosis and management of this long ill-defined entity. Unfortunately, the present status of therapy of leukemia, while promising, remains nonspecific and unsatisfactory.

Symptomatic and Supportive Therapy

Progress in symptomatic and supportive therapy of congestive CM has been confined to the improvements in the general management of congestive failure, to the limited progress in the management of severe pump failure in low cardiac output states, to significant progress in the management of complicating arrhythmias and conduction disorders, and to better management of thromboembolism.

The application of current therapeutic measures in management of congestive failure, utilizing an armentarium of modern cardiac drugs, diuretics, and their attenuating agents, combined with measures to maintain electrolyte stabilization, has resulted in a higher incidence of recovery from acute episodes of failure and longer periods of stabilization between episodes of failure *but* has not been successful in the prevention of eventual irreversible failure in the majority of chronic congestive cardiomyopathies. Early institution of these measures prior to the development of advanced hypertrophy and dilation is effective in increasing longevity but usually does not prevent ultimate deterioration in a well established CM. There continues to be a high mortality in long-term followup studies (43).

The application of modalities of therapy to support low cardiac output failure, such as intra-aortic balloon pumping (44, 45), has had only limited success but may have an occasional beneficial use, especially in those types of CM which have acute cardiac dilation and low cardiac output early in their clinical course. Such benefit was sometimes observed in the clinical course of the Quebec and Belgium beer-drinker's CM (21, 22), and may occur occasionally in the CM associated with postpartum states (39).

The admittance of a patient suffering from CM with overt or threatening fatal complications to intensive cardiac care units equipped with facilities for electro-cardiographic, hemodynamic, and chemical monitoring, electrical conversion and pacing, cardiac and pulmonary resuscitation, and staffed with trained personnel, has been a definite advancement in management. The application of the intensive care principle to this group of myocardial diseases has decreased mortali-

ty from arrhythmias, failure, and other complications as well as overall hospitalization time.

A greater appreciation of thromboembolism as a part of the clinical spectrum
of CM (especially with endomyocardial involvement, a low output state, and
arrhythmia), recognition of its frequent occurrence with the conversion of
arrhythmias, and the use of anticoagulants and other measures early in the
disease, during acute episodes of failure, and prior to conversion of arrhythmias,
have decreased mortality and disability from thromboembolism. The avoidance of
rapid diuresis and hemoconcentration is likewise important in the prevention of
thrombosis in low output failure. In spite of this progress, unexpected embolic
deaths continue to occur, including fatal embolism to the coronary arteries in
young adults (46).

Prolonged Bed Rest

Prolonged bed rest, introduced in the management of CM in 1960 (47), was
strongly recommended in a follow up report in 1963 (48) as a special form of
management in congestive cardiomyopathy deserving extensive study and widespread implementation. Its value continues to be inconclusive in subsequent
trials. Friedberg (49), in the introduction to a 1971 symposium on cardiomyopathies, stated that "bed rest was impractical and cannot be justified unless its
efficacy is unequivocally established." My personal observation has been that a
generous period of bed rest is usually beneficial in the early episodes of
congestive failure and cardiomegaly caused chiefly by dilation, but once advanced chronic hypertrophy and dilation develop, prolonged periods of bed rest
are not likely to alter significantly the subsequent clinical course from that
obtained with short periods of hospital bed rest, until recovery from the acute
congestion occurs, followed by good management and limitation of activities
outside a hospital environment.

Surgery in Congestive Idiopathic Cardiomyopathy

As irreversible failure has been observed as the terminal event in many individuals with idiopathic congestive CM, including children and young adults, it is
natural that clinical cardiac transplantation would be applied at least as a pilot
program in the category of clinical research, once transplantation of the heart
was surgically feasible. The following capsule of progress in this area of therapy
is reported from Stanford University Medical Center (50) where one-fourth of a
worldwide total of about 200 cardiac transplantations had been performed
through 1972. As of November 28, 1972, 14 of the 50 cardiac transplants
performed at Stanford had been on patients with congestive CM of the idiopathic type. Four patients were surviving as of that date, which represents a 30%
survival as compared to a 36% survival for the 50 operated upon. Criteria for

cardiac transplantation at Stanford are that the CM patient must be considered to be in terminal congestive failure and expected to die within three months. Transplant patients have experienced the same problems of rejection and have required suppressive therapy with all its inherent problems, as has been experienced with patients with coronary disease. The quality of life of the survivors has been largely determined by the limited success of surgery versus the difficulties in postoperative management which are not small or likely to be solved in the near future.

RESTRICTIVE CARDIOMYOPATHY

Fortunately, pure restrictive or constrictive CM continues to be rare, either the idiopathic type as represented by fibroelastosis or the secondary type as represented by amyloidosis or some forms of metastatic or invasive carcinomatosis. It is noteworthy that significant progress has been made in the clinical recognition of CM associated with amyloidosis (51) and in the differential diagnosis of restrictive CM from constrictive pericarditis (52), thus permitting more prompt and surgical management of the latter.

SECONDARY CARDIOMYOPATHY

(Primary Myocardial Disease or Heart Muscle Disease of Known Etiology or Association)

I consider that the greatest progress in the entire area of myocardial diseases has been the acceptance of the principle, and its practice, of making a *positive diagnosis* of primary myocardial disease based on the clinical manifestations, rather than eventually arriving at a late diagnosis by exclusion, often after many unnecessary diagnostic studies and therapeutic trials. Recent publications have emphasized this approach (13, 53). This has resulted in an early recognition that a CM exists as the main problem; and, with the increased knowledge of the etiologic types, a diligent search for a treatable form of disease often results in the application of specific therapy rather than resorting to symptomatic and supporting measures as the only management. Specific therapy often results in reversal of the CM.

Specific progress in therapy relating to each of the etiologic entities or associated diseases as contained in current classifications of secondary CM cannot be covered in these brief notes of progress. Comments are limited to a few entities in which progress in therapy, therapeutic approach, or prevention is considered important.

Metabolic Cardiomyopathy

Many of the metabolic cardiomyopathies that have been experimentally induced in laboratory animals (54) now have recognized clinical counterparts in human disease, either those that occur naturally or those iatrogenically induced. There has been progress in both diagnosis and effective therapy. Instances of pheo-chromocytomas masquerading initially as idiopathic CM have been appropriately recognized (55). These respond to both medical therapy (56) and to appropriate surgery which is now being accomplished without cardiovascular catastrophies as experienced in the past, and with reversal of metabolic cardiomyopathy (57). Recent investigative studies indicate that therapy with drugs that inhibit platelet aggregation may inhibit myocardial necrosis which may arise in either naturally occurring or drug-induced catecholamine CM (58).

There are increasing observations to indicate so-called diabetic CM is an appropriate classification for the CM associated with long standing diabetes. However, at this time it is not clear whether the mechanism involved is direct metabolic derangement of the myocardial tissues or is secondary to sclerosis in small coronary arteries or to the associated renal disease (59).

There have been additional reports of reversible CM associated with hemo-chromatosis when current therapeutic measures are instituted in the management (60).

Infective Cardiomyopathy

Infectious myocarditis and cardiomyopathy as a late residual are types of myocardial diseases not included in all classifications of CM. Some physicians accept only those instances of chronic myocarditis and residual damage from preexisting myocarditis as a secondary type of CM, but do not include the overt acute myocarditis with failure, arrhythmia, death, etc., as a form of infective CM of a secondary type if the etiology is established. These differences of inclusive-ness make this discussion difficult.

Chagasic CM is the model for this type of infective CM in that the etiologic agent is known, an early acute myocarditis occurs which can be recognized, and then after a latent period features of a classical CM appear. It is in this late stage that disability or death from the myocardial damage usually occurs. It has become a very important type of heart disease in certain parts of the world, especially in areas of South America. Therapy and prevention should ideally consist of the use of antimicrobial therapy directed against the etiologic agent of trypanosomiasis (*Trypanosoma cruzi*) in those patients with the disease and some form of preventive therapy directed toward those who are living in the area where they are exposed to the vectors of the disease. None of the antimicrobial drugs developed today has been found sufficiently effective to constitute real progress in the specific treatment of this disease. Vaccines and antitoxin which have been developed have also been ineffective. With the recent observation that there is irreversible damage to the neural elements of the myocardium in the late stages of the disease, it becomes all the more important to prevent these late stages of the CM.

Toxoplasmic Myocarditis and Cardiomyopathy

The recognition of *Toxoplasma gondii* infections in man as a cause of myocardial disease occurred only in recent years (61). Virus-like symptoms and glandular fever suggestive of infectious mononucleosis are now recognized as clinical manifestations of clinical infections in humans, and subclinical infections are common. Minimal pericardial and myocardial involvement is common; clinical pericarditis and myocarditis are less frequent; and severe and fatal acute myocarditis occasionally occurs, especially in the miliary form which has its highest incidence in immunologic deficiency states (individuals receiving immunosuppressive therapy or cytotoxic drugs). Chronic eye, cerebral, and myocardial involvement occurs and with the latter, all features of a cardiomyopathy have been reported (62). A diagnostic serologic pattern of increasing titer has been developed, resulting in an increased frequency in diagnosis as well as clinical surveillance for myocardial involvement. With the knowledge that subclinical forms of the disease are common, that clinical symptomatology may be vague, and that many individuals have a high antibody titer, a tendency has developed to make presumptive diagnoses of the disease as well as a presumptive diagnosis of toxoplasmic CM when confronted with a clinical CM. Since the disease is transmitted transplacentally, with congenital forms of the disease appearing in the offspring, such a presumptive diagnosis of either acute or chronic infection or CM in pregnancy has at times reached the proportions of a "scare disease" (63). Caution should be used in making such presumptive diagnoses. The current recommended therapy consists of the combined administration of pyrimethamine and triple sulfonamides (61, 63). All diagnosed infections should be treated as a preventive measure against acute and chronic myocardial involvement. Prevention of the initial infections consists of the avoidance of eating raw and partly cooked meat and care in washing hands after handling pets and their excreta, especially cats (63).

New Infective Agents in Cardiomyopathy

Special studies employed in the diagnosis and investigation of idiopahic CM, utilizing the technique of myocardial biopsy by cutaneous puncture of the left ventricle or other techniques and examinations of the myocardial tissues, have in general not provided significant new infective agents (64). Only occasionally is a definite infectious agent identified, such as tuberculosis or a nonspecific granulomatous infection or sarcoid. Results from a large series of patients having percutaneous biopsies, in association with hemodynamic and angiocardiographic studies, have provided only minor information which can be used in management (65). The information has been most useful when combined with the hemodynamic and angiocardiographic studies. Unfortunately, many of the reported biopsy studies have not included ultrastructural examinations. Paradoxically, percutaneous myocardial biopsies performed on the transplanted heart have been most helpful in following the myocardial changes resulting from rejection (50). An appreciation of their value in demonstrating the myocardial reaction in rejection has resulted in a revived interest in the use of this diagnostic procedure in the investigation and diagnosis of cardiomyopathies (50).

OBSTRUCTIVE CARDIOMYOPATHY

By 1965, the clinical, hemodynamic, and pharmacodynamic features of the hypertrophic obstructive cardiomyopathy, recognized only seven years earlier, had been well established (8, 9). A clinical diagnosis could be made with reasonable accuracy (66) and was well established with quantitation of the severity of the functional obstruction by existing laboratory procedures (9). Retrospective evaluations and a short period of prospective evaluations established basic ideas about natural history and the important differences in its clinical course as compared to the congestive type of CM. These early observations suggested a rather progressive deterioration with age, but by 1968 a more benign course was suggested (67, 68).

The use of beta adrenergic drug therapy and surgical therapy had been introduced by 1964 (69). The initial enthusiasm for surgical therapy was tempered by a lack of agreement as to the type and extent of surgery which should be performed. British surgeons at the Ciba conference in 1964 (70) described their approach as follows: "[we] have always been a little tentative in our acceptance of patients for surgery for obstructive cardiomyopathy and, like most surgeons, find ourselves in the undesirable position of performing an operation, the nature of which we do not fully understand, for a disease that is equally obscure." In spite of this obscurity of the disease and the early problems of surgical approach, it survived and became reasonably standardized in performance, but problems arose as to whether the clinical stage of the disease or the hemodynamic finding warranted surgery. This selection became even more difficult with changing concepts of the natural history to that of a more benign disease, by lack of establishment of a specific clinical or hemodynamic finding which heralded a rapid deterioration or a sudden death, and most of all, by a lack of information as to the effectiveness of the new drugs such as propranolol in management, especially in preventing ultimate deterioration. Recent reports from various centers (71–76) which have made careful evaluations of the results of management in series of well diagnosed patients, indicate that beneficial results have been obtained from both surgery and drug management. Even with the excellent clinical and surgical judgment provided in these centers, neither medical nor surgical therapy has produced consistently good results. Guidelines for management of a disease with such a wide spectrum of symptomatic and asymptomatic patients with variable hemodynamic features have been difficult to establish, especially when the natural history remains only partly known, its basic etiology obscure, its clinical features, disease mechanisms, and structural components constantly widening to include valvular insufficiencies and ischemic manifestations as components of its expanding disease spectrum. From this composite experience, the following guidelines have evolved (71):

Symptomatic Patients

Patients with mild symptoms and those with latent obstruction are managed with propranolol.

Patients with severe symptoms are given a trial of propranolol; if signs of deterioration develop, surgery is recommended.

Asymptomatic Patients

There is less uniformity in management of the asymptomatic patient with a clinical and hemodynamic diagnosis.

Prophylactic propranolol therapy is administered to some patients, especially intermittently during periods of increased physical activity.

Surgery is advised or performed in some asymptomatic patients with severe resting obstruction (gradients over 75 mm Hg).

Surgery is likewise advised if there is a family history of sudden death or if the physical activity of the individual cannot be curtailed.

A group of asymptomatic patients remains, with both congenital and acquired backgrounds, who continue stable with neither drug nor surgical therapy seemingly indicated. The natural history as revealed to date suggests at least some of these patients may be expected to deteriorate with increasing age, and further guidelines and decisions must be formulated as to whether drug or surgical therapy will be indicated in later life.

There are other patients who have associated lesions such as functional mitral insufficiency or associated congenital lesions, or coronary artery disease in older patients, in whom variations in drug and surgical procedures are indicated. Mitral valve replacements have been made in a small group with mitral insufficiency with beneficial results (72).

ISCHEMIC CARDIOMYOPATHY

The term and classification "ischemic cardiomyopathy" have been in medical usage since 1965. Burch (77) has given a somewhat limited definition while others use the term in such a loose manner as to include many instances of coronary disease with angina, myocardial failure, or cardiac enlargement.

This is very confusing in that Bridgen's (78) original definition of a cardiomyopathy was that it was "non-coronary disease." Fowler (13) states that cardiomyopathies may be defined as "diseases of the cardiac muscle in which the heart does not contract properly." This definition would include many instances of coronary disease, as abnormal contraction occurs with ischemia without infarction, is always present to some degree with myocardial infarctions, and is even more pronounced when complicated by congestive failure, myocardial aneurysmal formations, etc. Perhaps it would be more logical to classify the patients with angina, cardiac enlargement, and myocardial failure but with normal coronary arteriograms as described by Likoff in the past (79) and elsewhere in this volume (80) as ischemic cardiomyopathy. To add to the confusion, many individuals with obstructive CM have angina with normal coronary arteries on arteriograms while others at an older age develop associated coronary artery disease (81, 82). An increasing number of elderly individuals are being found to have obstructive CM (83). At present, progress in management of this confusing group of myocardial diseases is limited to the recognition that these confusing clinical conditions exist, to the application of diagnostic techniques to identify the various components, and to selection of the appropriate type of medical or surgical management. Propranolol, an effective drug for the relief of angina and obstructive symptoms in obstructive CM (84), is likewise effective in the relief of angina and abnormal myocardial contractility in obstructive coronary disease. However, nitroglycerin, which is effective in the relief of anginal symptoms in coronary disease, will in most cases aggravate the symptomatology in obstructive CM. There are specific indications for surgery in each type of myocardial disease.

DYSRHYTHMIC CARDIOMYOPATHY

Careful clinicopathological studies of deceased patients (85) and hemodynamic, angiocardiographic, and arteriographic studies in living patients with clinical features of recurrent tachyarrhythmias, bradyarrhythmias including the sick sinus syndrome (86), and atrioventricular and bundle branch blocks, initially considered to have coronary artery disease as the probable cause, have been found not to have significant coronary disease but to have structural and hemodynamic findings compatible with some form of idiopathic or secondary CM. The clinical recognition of this variant of CM has been an important advance in that management can be appropriately directed toward the control of the presenting problem, which includes utilization of intensive care units, electrical or drug conversion of arrhythmias, temporary or permanent pacemakers, or long term drug management. As many of this group are young (87) and do not have congestive failure (except secondary to the arrhythmias), significant hemodynamic alterations, or coronary disease, the appropriate management of the arrhythmia or conduction abnormality often provides relief of disability with a greater potential longevity than is found among those with similar problems but with significant occlusive coronary disease.

Occasionally, surgical procedures such as aneurysmectomy or myocardial resection of fibrotic or necrotic myocardium are successful in the control of life-threatening arrhythmias or conduction abnormalities in this type of non-coronary CM, as it is in coronary disease. Sarcoidosis has been reported as the etiologic agent in some instances (88).

PROGRESS IN PREVENTION OF CARDIOMYOPATHIES

Prevention was considered of paramount importance in the 1964 report (1). The only significant publication dealing with prevention of the cardiomyopathies since that time is the 1970 Report of the Committee on Cardiomyopathies, Inter-Society Commission for Heart Disease Resources (19). This report again enumerated many of the needs pointed out earlier in the 1964 report (1), indicating a lack of substantial progress. Some items of overt as well as subtle progress are briefly mentioned below.

Physician Education on Cardiomyopathies

Efforts toward widespread physician education and dissemination of available knowledge on cardiomyopathies, so important in recognition and prevention, are being accomplished by medical communications and cooperative efforts at national and international levels. Most national and international scientific programs in cardiology have included some aspects of these diseases in their programs. A plenary session of the 1970 World Heart Congress was devoted to this subject with contributions from many countries. The International Society of Cardiology has developed a Council on Cardiomyopathies within its scientific councils. Several highly successful meetings and seminars of this council have been held and a publication, *Introduction to Cardiomyopathies,* issued (89). The World Health Organization, recognizing the world-wide importance of this category of cardiac diseases, has supported a strong team of investigators since the mid-sixties. Essentially every textbook of medicine and cardiology has devoted space to this category of heart disease. A textbook entirely devoted to the subject of diseases of the myocardium has recently been published (90).

Epidemiological Studies and Investigation

An increasing awareness has developed of the potential involvement of the myocardium in infectious diseases, especially viral diseases; of myocardial damage in endocrine, metabolic, and nutritional diseases; of toxic effects on the myocardium by drugs, chemicals, additives to foods and beverages, or by alcoholic beverages themselves; and of myocardial damage from physical agents such as radiation to the thorax.

Early Diagnosis and Prompt Treatment

An increased utilization has been made of the cardiac consultant and of hemodynamic and other diagnostic studies, early in the evaluation when overt and suspected clinical features suggest a CM. Greater effort is being made to identify an etiological agent, an associated systemic disease amenable to treatment, a clinical association (e.g. alcoholism), or a specific mechanism of dysfunction (e.g. obstructive CM). While this is basically secondary prevention, it is important progress. Hopefully, the disease may be found curable or altered before the damage to the myocardium results in an irreversible cardiomyopathy.

The following advances may be listed as subtle progress in prevention:

1) Successful widespread vaccination and immunizations against infectious diseases, notably poliomyelitis, measles, mumps, and diphtheria.

2) Appropriate and prompt antibiotic therapy and chemotherapy in infections known to be responsive to specific therapy. While indiscriminate antibiotic therapy in nonspecific infections is generally not accepted as good medicine, there is probably a beneficial byproduct in that chance effectiveness in some instances may prevent myocardial damage.

3) Tighter food and drug control measures, resulting in removal from the market and thus from public consumption of substances known to be toxic to the myocardium. Hopefully, interest in human environmental control will extend beyond the eradication of polluted air and water to eradication of toxic substances currently taken into our bodies to satisfy our taste, appetites, and pleasure or applied to the exterior of our bodies to satisfy our vanity. With continued success in combating infections and other etiological agents, these external environmental agents may well become the important etiologic agents in diseases of man, including cardiomyopathies.

4) The increase in the number of qualified investigators and in support of research in myocardial structure, function, and metabolism in health and disease has resulted in better understanding of the nature of the myocardial dysfunction in the cardiomyopathies and should eventually provide greater progress in prevention, diagnosis, and management.

REFERENCES

1. Burch, G. E., Carlson, F. D., Davies, J. N. P., DePasquale, N., Ferrans, V., Fowler, N. O., Hibbs, R., Mattingly, T. W., Mogabgab, W., Sjoerdsma, A., and Walsh, J. 1964. Primary myocardial disease (heart muscle disease, cardiomyopathy). Pages 488–500 *in* E. C. Andrus and C. H. Maxwell, eds. [Second National Conference on Cardiovascular Diseases] The heart and circulation, Vol. 1 (Research). Federation of American Societies for Experimental Biology, Bethesda, Md.

2. Mattingly, T. W. 1964. Primary myocardial disease. Page 1073 *in* Encylopedia of medicine, Vol. 3. Davis, Philadelphia.
3. Mattingly, T. W. 1965. The clinical concept of primary myocardial disease. A classification and a few notes on management and prognosis. Circulation 32:845.
4. Mattingly, T. W. 1965. Changing concepts of myocardial disease. J.A.M.A. 191:33.
5. Harvey, W. P., Segal, J. P., and Gurel, T. 1964. The clinical spectrum of primary myocardial disease. Prog. Cardiov. Dis. 7:1.
6. Segal, J. P., Harvey, W. P., and Gurel, T. 1965. Diagnosis and treatment of primary myocardial disease. Circulation 32:837.
7. Harvey, W. P. 1965. Symposium: Clinical recognition and treatment of primary myocardial disease: Comments on Symposium. Circulation 32:857.
8. Wolstenholme, G. E. W., and O'Connor, M., eds. 1964. Cardiomyopathies, Ciba Foundation Symposium. Little, Brown, Boston.
9. Braunwald, E., Lambrew, C. T., Rockoff, S. D., Ross, J., and Morrow, G. M. 1964. Idiopathic hypertrophic subaortic stenosis: 1. Description of the disease based upon an analysis of 64 patients. American Heart Assn., Monograph No. 10. American Heart Association, New York.
10. Massumi, R. A., Rios, J. C., Gooch, A. S., Nutter, D., DeVita, V. T., and Datlow, D. W. 1965. Primary myocardial disease: Report of fifty cases and review of the subject. Circulation 31:19.
11. Goodwin, J. F., et al. 1972. The cardiomyopathies. Brit. Heart J. 34:545.
12. Brigden, W. 1971. Diseases of the myocardium. Pages 1089–1098 *in* P. B. Beason and W. McDermott, eds. Cecil-Loeb in Textbook of medicine. Saunders, Philadelphia.
13. Fowler, N. O. 1971. Differential diagnosis of cardiomyopathies. Prog. Cardiov. Dis. 14:113.
14. Burch, G. E., Colcolough, H. L., Harb, J. M., and Tsui, C. Y. 1971. The effect of ingestion of ethyl alcohol, wine and beer on the myocardium of mice. Amer. J. Cardiol. 27:522.
15. Regan, J. F., Levinson, G. E., Oldewurtel, H. A., Martin, J. F., Weisse, A. B., and Moschos, C. B. 1969. Ventricular function in noncardiacs with alcohol fatty liver: Role of ethanol in production of cardiomyopathy. J. Clin. Invest. 48:397.
16. Mitchell, J. H., and Cohen, L. S. 1970. Alcohol and the heart: Hemodynamic effects of alcohol. Mod. Concepts Cardiov. Dis. 39
17. Burch, G. E., and DePasquale, N. P. 1969. Alcoholic cardiomyopathy. Amer. J. Cardiol. 23:723.
18. Spodick, D. H., Pigott, V. M., and Chirie, R. 1972. Preclinical malfunction in chronic alcoholism: Comparison with matched control and with alcoholic cardiomyopathies. New Engl. J. Med. 287:677.
19. Burch, G. E., and DePasquale, N. P. 1970. Recognition and prevention of cardiomyopathy, Subcommittee on cardiomyopathy, Report of inter-society commission for heart disease resources. Circulation: 42:A47.
20. Mohiuddin, S. M., Tasker, P. K., Rheault, M., Paul, E. R., Chenard, J., and Morin, Y. 1970. Experimental cobalt cardiomyopathy. Amer. Heart J. 80:532.
21. Morin, W., and Daniel, P. 1967. "Quebec beer-drinkers" cardiomyopathy, etiological considerations. Can. Med. Assoc. J. 97:926.
22. Kesteloot, H., Roelandt, J., Williams, J., Claes, J. H., and Joossens, J. V. 1968. An inquiry into the role of cobalt in heart disease of chronic beer drinkers. Circulation 37:854.
23. Wuhrmann, F. 1970. Hepatogenic myocardosis. Scand. J. Gastraenal. 7(Suppl.):97.
24. Bollinger, O. von. 1884. Ueber die Haeugfigkeit und Ursachen der idiopathischem Herzhypertrophie in Muenchen. Dtsch. Med. Wochschr. 10:180.
25. Saint-Pierre, A., Perrin, A., Pouzeratte, J. P., et al. 1972. Chronic myocardiopathy induced by Impramine. Cour. Med. Interne 11:27.
26. Baledent, M., et al. 1972. Acute heart failure after a moderate dose of rubidomycin. Sem. Hosp. Paris 48:507.
27. Szakacs, J. E., and Mehlman, B. 1960. Pathologic changes induced by 1-norepinephrine. Quantitative aspects. Amer. J. Cardiol. 5:00.

28. Kattus, A. A., Briscoe, B. W., Dashe, A. M., and Davis, J. H. 1968. Spurious heart disease induced by digitalis-containing reducing pills. Arch. Internal Med. 122:298.
29. Herman, E., Mhatre, R., Lee, T. P., et al. 1971. A comparison of the cardiovascular actions of daunomycin, adriamycin, and N-acetyl daunomycin in hamsters and monkeys. Pharmacology 6:230.
30. Buja, M., Ferrans, V. J., and Roberts, W. C. 1973. Daunorubicin cardiomyopathy: An ultrastructural examination of a toxic cardiomyopathy. (In press).
31. Herman, E. H., et al. 1971. Prevention of cardiotoxic effects of adriamycin and daunomycin in the isolated dog heart. Proc. Soc. Exp. Biol. Med. 140:234.
32. Favara, B. E., and Franciosi, R. A. 1972. Diphtherial myocardiopathy. Amer. J. Cardiol. 30:423.
33. Abelman, W. H. 1971. Virus and the heart. Circulation 44:950.
34. Mattingly, T. W. 1963. Viral infections of the heart and circulation. Clinical manifestations and problems. New York Heart Association conference on infectious diseases of the heart and circulation, pp. 27-28. N.Y. Heart Association, New York.
35. Smith, W. G. 1970. Coxsackie B myocarditis in adults. Amer. Heart J. 80:34.
36. Kaplan, M. K., and Frengley, J. D. 1969. Autoimmunity to heart in cardiac disease: Current concepts of relation to autoimmunity to rheumatic fever, post cardiotomy and postinfarction syndromes and cardiomyopathies. Amer. J. Cardiol. 24:459.
37. Bengtsson, E., and Lomberger, B. 1966. Five year follow-up cases suggestive of acute myocarditis. Amer. Heart J. 72:751.
38. Brown, A. K., Dukas, N., Riding, W. D., and Jones, E. W. 1967. Cardiomyopathies in pregnancy. Brit. Heart J. 29:387.
39. Demakio, J. G., and Ruahimtoola, S. H. 1971. Peripartum cardiomyopathy. Circulation 44:964.
40. Farber, P. A., and Glasgow, L. A. 1970. Viral myocarditis during pregnancy. Encephalomyocarditis virus infections in mice. Amer. Heart J. 80:96.
41. Roberts, W. C., Liegler, D. G., and Carbone, P. P. 1968. Endomyocardial disease and eosinophilia—A clinical and pathological spectrum. Amer. J. Med. 46:28.
42. Flannery, E. P. Dillon, D. E., Freeman, M. V. R., Levy, J. D., D'Ambrosio, U., and Bedynek, J. L. 1972. Eosinophilic leukemia with fibrosing endocarditis and short Y chromosome. Ann. Internal Med. 77:223.
43. Goodwin, J. F. 1970. Congestive and hypertrophic cardiomyopathies. A decade of study. Lancet 1:732.
44. Moulopoulos, S. D., Topaz, S., and Kloff, W. J. 1962. Diastolic balloon pumping (with carbon dioxide) in the aorta—a mechanical assistance to the failing circulation. Amer. Heart J. 63:699.
45. Buckley, J. J., Leinbach, R. C., Kastor, J. A., Laird, J. D., Kantrowitz, A. R., Madras, P. N., Sanders, C. A., and Austen, W. G. 1970. Hemodynamic evaluation of intra-aortic balloon pumping in man. Circulation 41(Suppl. 2):130.
46. Parameswaran, R., Meadows, W. R., and Sharp, J. T. 1969. Coronary embolism in primary myocardial disease. Amer. Heart J. 78:682.
47. Burch, G. E., and Walsh, J. J. 1960. Cardiac enlargement due to myocardial degeneration of unknown cause: Preliminary report of prolonged bed rest. J.A.M.A. 172:207.
48. Burch, G. E., Walsh, J. J., and Black, W. C. 1963. Value of prolonged bed rest in management of cardiomegaly. J.A.M.A. 183:81.
49. Friedberg, C. K. 1971. Symposium on cardiomyopathy. Circulation 44:935.
50. Hancock, E. W. Personal communications.
51. Buja, L. M., Khoi, N. B., and Roberts, W. C. 1970. Clinically significant cardiac amyloidosis. Amer. J. Cardiol. 26:394.
52. Ramsey, H. W., Sbar, S., Elliott, L. P., and Elliott, R. S. 1970. Differential diagnosis of restrictive myocardiopathy and chronic pericarditis without calcification. Value of coronary arteriography. Amer. J. Cardiol. 25:635.
53. Perloff, J. K. 1971. The cardiomyopathies: Current perspectives. Circulation 44:942.
54. Bajusz, E. 1969. Experimental metabolic cardiomyopathies and their relationship to human heart disease. Ann. N. Y. Acad. Sci. 156:5.

55. Garcia, R., and Jenning, J. M. 1972. Pheochromocytoma masquerading as a cardio-myopathy. Amer. J. Cardiol. 29:568.
56. Engleman, K., and Sjoerdsma, A., 1964. Chronic medical therapy for pheochromocy-toma. Ann. Internal Med. 61:229.
57. Wiswell, J. G., and Crago, R. M. 1968. Reversible cardiomyopathy with pheochromocy-toma. Trans. Amer. Clin. Climat. Assoc. 80:185.
58. Haft, J. I., Gershengorn, K., Kranz, P. D., and Oestreicher, R. 1972. Protection against epinephrine-induced myocardial necrosis by drugs that inhibit platelet aggregation. Amer. J. Cardiol. 30:838.
59. Rubler, S., Dlugash, J., Yuseoglu, Y. Z., Humral, T., Branwood, A. W., and Grishman, A. 1972. New type of cardiomyopathy associated with diabetic glomerulosclerosis. Amer. J. Cardiol. 30:595.
60. Easley, R. M., Jr., Schreiner, B. F., Jr., and Yu, P. 1972. Reversible cardiomyopathy associated with hemochromatosis. New Engl. J. Med. 287:864.
61. Theologides, A., and Kennedy, B. J. 1969. Toxoplasmic myocarditis and pericarditis. Editorial. Amer. J. Med. 47: 169.
62. Arribada, A., and Escobar, E. 1968. Cardiomyopathies produced by *Toxoplasma gondii.* Amer. Heart J. 76:329.
63. Krogstad, D. J., Juranek, D. D., and Walls, K. W. 1972. Toxoplasmosis. Ann. Internal Med. 77:773.
64. Braimbridge, M. V., Parracott, S., Chayen, J., Bitensky, L., and Poulter, L. W. 1967. Possibilities of new infective etiological agent in congestive cardiomyopathy. Lancet 1:171.
65. Shirey, E. K., Hawk, W. A., Mukerji, D., and Effler, D. B. 1972. Percutaneous myo-cardial biopsy of the left ventricle. Experience with 198 patients. Circulation 46:112.
66. Burchell, H. B. 1963. Possible unrecognized forms of heart disease. Circulation 28:1153.
67. Frank, S., and Braunwald, E. 1968. Idiopathic hypertrophic substenosis. Clinical analy-sis of 126 patients with emphasis on natural history. Circulation 37:759.
68. Parker, B. M. 1969. The course in idiopathic hypertrophic muscular subaortic stenosis. Ann. Internal Med. 70:903.
69. Harrison, D. C., Braunwald, E., Glick, B., et al. 1964. Effect of beta adrenergic blockage on the circulation, with particular reference to observations in patients with hyper-trophic subaortic stenosis. Circulation 29:84.
70. Bentail, H. H. 1964. The technique of operation for obstructive cardiomyopathy. Page 272 *in* G. E. W. Wolstenholme and M. O'Connor, eds. Cardiomyopathies, Ciba Founda-tion Symposium. Little, Brown, Boston.
71. Adelman, A. G., Wigle, E. D., Ranganathan, N., Webb, G. D., Kidd, S. L., Bigelow, W. G., and Silver, M. D. 1972. The clinical course in muscular subaortic stenosis: A retrospective and prospective study of 60 hemodynamically proved cases. Ann. Internal Med. 77:515.
72. Cooley, D. A., Leachman, R. D., Hallman, G. L., Gerami, S., and Hall, R. J. 1971. Idiopathic hypertrophic subaortic stenosis. Surgical treatment, including mitral valve replacement. Arch. Surg. 103:606.
73. Morrow, A. G., Fogarty, T. J., Hannah, H., III, et al. 1968. Operative treatment in idiopathic hypertrophic subaortic stenosis. Techniques and the results of preoperative and postoperative clinical and hemodynamic assessments. Circulation 37:589.
74. Flamm, M. D., Harrison, D. C., and Hancock, E. W. 1968. Muscular subaortic stenosis. Prevention of outflow obstruction with propranolol. Circulation 38:846.
75. Adelman, A. G., Shah, P. M., Gramiak, R., et al. 1971. Long-term propranolol therapy in muscular subaortic stenosis. Brit. Heart J. 32:804.
76. Wolstenholme, G. E. W., and O'Connor, M., eds. Hypertrophic obstructive cardio-myopathy. Ciba Foundation Study Group No. 37. Churchill, London, and Williams & Wilkins, Baltimore.
77. Burch, G. E., Giles, T. D., and Colcolough, H. L. 1970. Ischemic cardiomyopathy. Amer. Heart J. 79:291.

78. Brigden, W. 1957. Uncommon myocardial diseases: Non-coronary cardiomyopathies. Lancet 273:1179, 1243.
79. Likoff, W., Segal, B. L., and Kasparin, H. 1967. Paradox of normal selective coronary arteriograms in patients considered to have unmistakable coronary disease. New Engl. J. Med. 276:1063.
80. Likoff, W. 1974. Angina pectoris with normal coronary angiograms. Pages 219–222 in H. I. Russek, ed. Cardiovascular disease, University Park Press, Baltimore.
81. Mattingly, T. W. 1967. Primary myocardial disease in middle age and older. Geriatrics 22:135.
82. Gulotta, S. J., Hamby, R. I., Aronson, A. L., and Ewing, K. 1972. Coexistent hypertrophic subaortic stenosis and coronary arterial disease. Circulation 46:890.
83. Whitney, R. B., Powell, W. P., Dinsmore, R. E., and Sanders, C. A. 1971. Idiopathic hypertrophic subaortic stenosis in the elderly. New Engl. J. Med. 285:196.
84. Cohen, L. S., and Braunwald, E. 1967. Amelioration of angina pectoris in idiopathic hypertrophic subaortic stenosis with beta-adrenergic blockage. Circulation 35:847.
85. Harris, A., Davies, M., Reedwood, D., Leatham, A., and Siddons, H. 1969. Etiology of chronic heart block. Clinicopathologic correlations in 65 cases. Brit. Heart J. 31:206.
86. Rubenstein, J. J., Schulman, C. L., Yurchak, P. M., and DeSanctis, R. W. 1972. Clinical spectrum of the sick sinus syndrome. Circulation 46:5.
87. Kaufmann, S. L., Chandra, N., Peress, N. S., and Rodriques-Torres, R. 1972. Idiopathic infantile cardiomyopathy with involvement of the conductive system. Amer. J. Cardiol. 30:648.
88. Lull, R. J., Dunn, B. E., Gregoratos, G., Cox, W. A., and Fisher, G. W. 1972. Ventricular aneurysm due to cardiac sarcoidosis with surgical cure of ventricular tachycardia. Amer. J. Cardiol. 30:282.
89. Shaper, A. G., ed. Introduction to cardiomyopathies. International Society of Cardiology. Karger, Basel.
90. Fowler, N. O., ed. 1973. Diseases of the myocardium. Grune & Stratton, New York.

Arterial Hypertension

THE MECHANISMS OF ACTION OF
ANTIHYPERTENSIVE AGENTS

WILLIAM B. ABRAMS

Approximately 20% of the North American population has hypertension (1) but in only about 10% of the patients with this disorder can an underlying causative disease process be identified (2). In the absence of a recognized etiology, it is not possible to apply specific therapy. Even in the minority with secondary hypertension, the most prominent specific therapy is surgical. Thus the current drug treatment of high blood pressure has been developed empirically. Despite this fact, drug treatment of hypertension has been quite successful. Deaths attributable to hypertension in the United States fell by more than 50% between the "before" period of 1950 and 1953 and a drug therapy period of similar duration ten years later (3). In the U.S. Veterans Administration Cooperative Study involving 143 men with moderately severe hypertension, those treated with a placebo suffered 27 severe complications and 4 deaths while an equally sized and matched drug-treated group experienced only 2 severe complications and no deaths (4). This group recently reported the results of a similar study with 380 individuals whose diastolic blood pressures averaged 90–114 mm Hg (5). The benefits of drug therapy were again clearly evident. The U.S. Public Health Service also documented the adverse impact of even mild hypertension on morbidity and mortality in a study of 390 subjects observed for up to 5 years (6). On the basis of these observations, and others (7–9), it now seems clear that it is the high blood pressure per se which is responsible for the clinical manifestations of hypertensive cardiovascular disease. It is also clear that lowering the blood pressure can favorably influence the course of this disease (3,4,10–13).

The drugs that are employed in the treatment of hypertension act on the homeostatic mechanisms that normally regulate blood pressure. These mechanisms are intact in hypertensive subjects and are responsive to physiologic and chemical interventions. This applies to baroreceptor activity (14), sympathetic nerve activity (15–17), and renin-aldosterone secretion (18–21). It is becoming increasingly apparent, however, that the net operation of these homeostatic mechanisms is not identical in individuals currently classified as having essential hypertension. Characteristically, subjects with essential hypertension have a normal cardiac output (15,16,22,23), increased basal heart rate (23), increased peripheral vascular resistance (15,16,22,23), slight reduction in plasma volume (24), and a normal plasma renin level (18,21,25). However, Eich and associates

(26) and Frohlich and associates (23) have identified a group of hypertensives with normal peripheral vascular resistance and increased cardiac output. Laragh and coworkers have noted that plasma renin levels may be low, normal, or high in hypertensive subjects and that individuals in the last category have a more severe clinical course (25,27). Finally, it has been observed that some hypertensive patients, in addition to those with primary hyperaldosteronism, have an expanded plasma volume (24,28). These important hemodynamic and biochemical observations suggest that the current empirical use of drugs in hypertension may soon give way to an approach in which drugs are selected for their applicability to individual patients. This approach, of course, requires a knowledge of the mechanisms of action of the drugs to be applied. In this chapter, antihypertensive agents will be classified according to the homeostatic mechanisms affected.

ANTIHYPERTENSIVE AGENTS AFFECTING THE SYMPATHETIC NERVOUS SYSTEM

Veratrum Alkaloids

The veratrum alkaloids are the only antihypertensive drugs which act on the afferent side of the sympathetic nervous system. These agents sensitize the pressure receptors, particularly in the heart and carotid sinus, so that a given level of blood pressure results in a larger amount of afferent nerve traffic (29,30). This is interpreted by the vasomotor centers in the brain stem as a higher than actual pressure, and sympathetic tone is decreased and vagal tone is increased. The result is a lowering of blood pressure and bradycardia. This is a desirable mechanism of action, but unfortunately the vagal afferent receptors for nausea and vomiting are also sensitized (31), and these side effects have greatly limited the clinical use of these agents.

Ganglionic Blocking Agents

Drugs which inhibit the cholinergic transmission in the autonomic ganglia are of great historical importance because they were the first substances of sufficient potency to establish the notion that medicines could indeed alter the clinical course of hypertensive cardiovascular disease. However, at this level sympathetic and parasympathetic impulses cannot be blocked separately, so their use is associated with an intolerable incidence of gastrointestinal and bladder side effects caused by the parasympathetic blockade. Other side effects include orthostatic hypotension, blurred vision, syncope, impotence, dry mouth, tremor, and mental aberrations. With the advent of more selective sympathetic inhibitors, the ganglionic blocking agents are seldom used at this time except in hypertensive emergencies. The routes of administration and dose range of three ganglion blocking agents are given in Table 1.

Table 1. Antihypertensive Drugs Affecting the
Sympathetic Nervous System

Generic name	*Trade name*	*Dosage range (mg)*
Rauwolfia derivatives		
Reserpine	Serpasil, Sandril, Reserpoid	oral: 0.1–0.5 once daily IM: 1–3
Alseroxylon fraction	Rauwiloid	oral: 2–4 once daily
Whole root	Raudixin	oral: 100–300 once daily
Methyldopa	Aldomet	oral: 250 b.i.d.→500 q.i.d.
Methyldopate hydrochloride	Aldomet ester	IV: 250–500 in 100 ml 5% dextrose solution infused in 30–60 min
Ganglion-blocking agents		
Pentolinium	Ansolysen	oral: 20 q.i.d.→100 q.i.d. IM: 1–10 IV: 10/20 ml given from syringe at 1 ml/min or 50–100/L as continuous infusion
Mecamylamine	Inversine	oral: 2.5 b.i.d.→25 b.i.d.
Trimethaphan camsylate	Arfonad	IV: 1,000/L as continuous infusion
Guanethidine sulfate	Ismelin	oral: 10–100 once daily
Pargyline	Eutonyl	oral: 10–100 once daily

Rauwolfia Alkaloids

Reserpine and the other rauwolfia alkaloids act at the distal end of the sympathetic postganglionic neuron to deplete this structure of norepinephrine (32,33). As the postganglionic neuron approaches the effector organ, it subdivides into a terminal network (34). Special staining techniques have demonstrated that the terminal network contains great numbers of norepinephrine-rich granules from which the norepinephrine is released in response to nerve stimuli (35). Norepinephrine gains access to the granules by means of biosynthesis and uptake from the circulation (35). The uptake mechanism has special importance because it is the major means of inactivating released norepinephrine, and it can involve certain drugs as well, leading to interactions which will be discussed subsequently. Biosynthesis involves the following steps: tyrosine, dihydroxyphenylalanine (DOPA), dopamine, norepinephrine. Norepinephrine is metabolized intraneuronally by monoamine oxidase in the mitochondria and extraneuronally by catechol-O-methyl transferase; both enzymes acting to produce vanillylmandelic acid (36). The rauwolfia alkaloids deplete norepinephrine by inhibiting its uptake into the storage sites (37). Blood pressure is lowered by this action because less norepinephrine is available for activation of adrenergic receptors in response to sympathetic nerve impulses. In the brain, the rauwolfia alkaloids deplete the neurons of all biogenic amines, i.e. serotonin and dopamine as well as norepinephrine. This probably accounts for the sedation and depression associated with their use and may contribute to the antihypertensive effect.

The routes of administration and dose range of commonly used rauwolfia derivatives are presented in Table 1. In addition to sedation and depression, other side effects associated with the use of these agents include nasal congestion, bradycardia, laxation, nightmares, and activation of peptic ulcer or bronchial asthma. When reserpine is given parenterally for hypertensive crises, profound somnolence may ensue which can interfere with neurologic evaluation.

Methyldopa

Methyldopa also reduces the content of norepinephrine in sympathetic nerve terminals and in the brain, but it does so by a different mechanism. Originally, this action was attributed to inhibition of the enzyme DOPA decarboxylase. It now appears, however, that methyldopa acts by replacing some of the norepinephrine with a "false transmitter" substance, alpha-methylnorepinephrine (38). Since alpha-methylnorepinephrine is released along with norepinephrine by sympathetic nerve activity (39), and since the former is a less potent pressor agent (40), the net effect is a lowering of blood pressure. An alternative explanation for the norepinephrine depletion is competition of alpha-methyldopamine, formed from alpha-methyldopa, with endogenous dopamine for the beta hydroxylating enzyme necessary to produce norepinephrine. There is some doubt whether the principal site of action relative to blood pressure lowering is the brain or the peripheral sympathetic nervous system. In any event, methyldopa reduces peripheral vascular resistance with little or no effect on cardiac output (41). Renal vascular resistance is decreased greater than in the general circulation (42), thus methyldopa is particularly useful in subjects with impaired renal function. The most common side effect is sedation which is probably related to interference with central adrenergic neurons. Other side effects include drug fever, skin rashes, headache, and fluid retention. Many subjects treated with this agent develop a positive Coombs test, but this is not usually associated with anemia (43). The dose range of methyldopa (oral) and methyldopate hydrochloride (intravenous) is given in Table 1.

Guanethidine

Guanethidine shares with the rauwolfia alkaloids and methyldopa the property of depleting catecholamine from sympathetic postganglionic neurons (44). However, its principal action at this site, relative to blood pressure lowering, appears to be a local anesthetic-like effect which inhibits nerve impulse transmission in the terminal rami (44). Guanethidine is accumulated at its site of action in adrenergic neurons and the degree to which it lowers blood pressure depends on its concentration in these nerves (45). The drug employs the same uptake pump mechanism as does norepinephrine to gain access to the neurons (46). Furthermore, guanethidine is released along with norepinephrine in response to nerve impulses (47). The uptake pump may be blocked by the tricyclic antidepressants (46). In this situation guanethidine cannot gain access to its site of action, and its antihypertensive effect is diminished or lost (48). Amphetamine has a similar effect (45). One must be careful to avoid this type of drug interference when the patient is being treated simultaneously for depression or obesity and hypertension. The elimination half-life of guanethidine is approximately 10 days (49). The fact that guanethidine must be accumulated in postganglionic sympathetic neurons before it can express its antihypertensive effect, has led to the suggestion that treatment begin with a loading dose of 125–525 mg given over 1–3 days; to be followed by a daily maintenance dose of 1/6 this amount (50). This quantity is considered that needed to "fill" the neuronal pool (50). The present dosage recommendation for initiating treatment calls for 10–25 mg daily. Under these circumstances, the neuronal pool is not "filled" and maximum blood pressure reduction may not be achieved for 5 half-lives or up to 50 days. The dosage range for maintenance is 10–100 mg given once daily (Table 1).

Bethanidine and Debrisoquin

Bethanidine and debrisoquin are similar to guanethidine in that they are accumulated by adrenergic neurons (44,51) and inhibit nerve transmission (44,52). They differ in not depleting the adrenergic neurons of norepinephrine (44,52). This difference may lie in the fact that the neuron membrane accumulating process concentrates these agents to a level where they are capable of inhibiting monoamine oxidase (44,51,53–55). Since the accumulating process does not take place in the liver, intestine, or kidney, these drugs do not cause adverse interactions when tyramine-rich foods are ingested (56). Guanethidine does not inhibit monoamine oxidase (MAO) even when concentrated (53). Bethanidine and debrisoquin are marketed in Europe, but are not yet available in the United States. Their clinical properties are similar to those of guanethidine except for a quicker onset and shorter duration of action (57,58). The major adverse effect of all of these drugs is orthostatic hypotension. Other side effects include diarrhea, bradycardia, weakness, and impotence.

Pargyline

Pargyline is a nonhydrazine monoamine oxidase inhibitor. Like other systemic MAO inhibitors, pargyline causes an accumulation of norepinephrine in the heart, brain, sympathetic nerves, and other tissues (59). The relationship of

MAO inhibition to blood pressure lowering is not clear. One hypothesis is that the blood pressure is lowered by the accumulation and release of a "false transmitter" substance, octopamine (60). This substance, like alpha-methyl-norepinephrine, is a less effective pressor agent than norepinephrine. Another suggestion is that norepinephrine accumulation produces a "negative feedback mechanism" with inhibition of the production of new norepinephrine (61).

Pargyline lowers blood pressure predominantly in the upright position and decreases peripheral vascular resistance (62). A decrease in the blood pressure and cardiac output responses to exercise also occurs (63).

Monoamine oxidase inhibitor activity, while producing the desired lowering of blood pressure, has inherent hazards. The general inhibition of MAO in liver and gut produces a marked sensitivity to tyramine-rich foods and beverages and to sympathomimetic drugs. As a result, paradoxical hypertensive crises may occur (64). Psychic stimulation varying from insomnia to the unmasking of a latent schizophrenia may also occur. The dose ranges from 10 to 100 mg given once daily (Table 1).

Clonidine

Clonidine (Catapres; ST 155) is a new drug which is still under investigation in the United States but is marketed in Europe. It is a derivative of imidazole, a class of drugs which includes tolazoline (Priscoline), an alpha adrenergic blocking agent with predominantly hypotensive effects, and tetrahydrozaline (Tyzine), a vasoconstrictor. Clonidine was, in fact, designed to be a vasoconstrictor for nasal decongestion, but when tried by this route in man it produced a lowering of the blood pressure, sedation, bradycardia, and dry mouth. Extensive pharmacologic studies have failed to clearly define its mechanism of action. Like other imidazole derivatives, it does have transient sympathomimetic effects followed by alpha adrenergic blockade (65). However, studies involving injection of the drug into the vertebral artery (66–68) and into the fourth ventricle (69,70) suggest its principal sites of action may be the vasomotor centers in the brain stem. It has also been proposed that stimulation of noradrenergic receptors in these centers is the specific cellular action involved (71,72). A central site of action is supported by the demonstration that clonidine reduces efferent sympathetic nerve activity after afferent stimulation (73). However, the high concentrations involved in these experimental studies detract from the clinical applicability of the results (68). The antisympathetic effects of clonidine have been found to include inhibition of renin release by the kidney (74,75) and decreased production of catecholamines and aldosterone (74).

Clinically, clonidine appears to be an effective antihypertensive agent of moderate potency (74–77). Its dose is in the range of 75–900 μg/day (75,77–79) and it can be given parenterally as well as orally (79). Side effects include sedation, dry mouth, and salt and water retention, the last of which can be overcome by the concurrent administration of a diuretic (75,77,78). Renal hemodynamic studies indicate that renal plasma flow and glomerular filtration rate are preserved while renal vascular resistance is decreased (75). The salt and water retention appear to be caused by enhanced tubular reabsorption of sodium stimulated by a decrease in renal perfusion pressure (75). A hypertensive rebound phenomenon when the drug is suddenly withdrawn has been described (74,76).

ANTIHYPERTENSIVE AGENTS AFFECTING ADRENERGIC RECEPTORS

Alpha Adrenergic Blocking Agents

Alpha adrenergic receptors mediate constriction in vascular smooth muscle in response to sympathetic agents such as epinephrine and norepinephrine. Thus alpha adrenergic blocking agents are useful when such substances are present in excess, as in pheochromocytoma. The two most commonly applied compounds are phentolamine and phenoxybenzamine. Although such drugs do indeed lower blood pressure, they are not useful in the treatment of essential hypertension. The hypotension produced by these drugs is associated with marked reflex cardiac overactivity because beta receptors are not blocked. In addition, the individual drugs in this group have toxic effects which limit their prolonged use.

Beta Adrenergic Blocking Agents

Beta adrenergic blocking agents are currently under investigation for a possible role in the treatment of hypertension. Such drugs have been used for this purpose in Europe for almost ten years and there seems little doubt they are effective antihypertensive agents (80–82). The mechanism or mechanisms of actions are not clear. Any one or all of the following may be operative: 1) diminution of cardiac output, 2) inhibition of central sympathetic activity, 3) reduction of plasma volume, and 4) inhibition of renin release.

The possible role of increased cardiac output in the genesis of certain types of hypertension has been the subject of several reports (83–85). Since beta blockers decrease output by inhibiting cardiac sympathetic activity, this is a logical mechanism for first consideration. It is also logical that such therapy would be effective in individuals with a hyperdynamic beta adrenergic circulatory state (86). Subsequent studies by these same investigators, however, indicated that response to beta blocker therapy by hypertensive subjects related more to a fall in peripheral vascular resistance than to reduction in cardiac output (81). The fall in peripheral vascular resistance was explained as a long term adaptation of the peripheral vascular tone to a chronic reduction of cardiac output. Furthermore, response to therapy could not be predicted from pretreatment hemodynamic values (81).

It is well established that vasomotor centers in the hypothalamus and medulla play a role in blood pressure regulation. There is also some evidence for a functional division of central adrenergic receptors into alpha and beta types (87–90). Furthermore, certain beta adrenergic blocking agents such as propranolol have been shown to cross the blood brain barrier and to concentrate in the appropriate areas of the brain (91–93). These observations have led to the possibility that inhibition of central beta receptors is one mechanism by which these drugs lower blood pressure. In support of this notion, blood pressure in dogs fell much more quickly after intracarotid or intravertebral artery injection of propranolol than after injection into the femoral artery (94). In cats, propranolol injected into the carotid artery blocked the pressor response to hypothalamic electrical stimulation (93). Studies in dogs involving intracerebroventricular injection and administration by cross circulation technique of alpha and beta agonists and antagonists, have suggested that both alpha and beta receptors in the brain can influence blood pressure (90). Other investigators have confirmed a central hypotensive action for propranolol, but suggest that beta blockade may not be the mechanism, since the dextro form, a very weak beta blocker, was equal in potency to the racemic form in lowering blood pressure when given into the cerebral ventricles of cats (95). In contrast to these studies, some beta blockers, such as practolol, enter the brain poorly yet have been shown to lower blood pressure (96,97). It remains possible that some beta adrenergic blocking agents exert at least part of their antihypertensive effect through central mechanisms.

Turning now to plasma volume, Dustan and associates (98) have noted that the success of long term treatment of hypertension seemed to depend on the ability of therapy to reduce plasma volume. These investigators (99) and Julius and associates (100) have recently reported that the administration of propranolol is associated with a substantial and prolonged contraction of the plasma volume. One explanation of how this might occur is constriction of the venous capacitance bed because of unopposed alpha adrenergic action (99,100).

Although the role of renin in the regulation of blood pressure and plasma volume is well defined, the question of its participation in the pathogenesis of essential hypertension is still open (2). However, the observations of Laragh and associates (27), referred to in the introduction to this chapter, that plasma renin levels seem to relate to the severity of the hypertensive disease process, suggest it may be important. For this reason, the related observations that renin release by the kidneys is mediated by adrenergic receptors (101,102), and its release is inhibited by beta blocking agents (101–103), provoked considerable interest (2). Numerous studies are underway to evaluate this relationship further.

ANTIHYPERTENSIVE AGENTS AFFECTING VASCULAR SMOOTH MUSCLE

Hydralazine

Hydralazine has been commercially available in the United States since 1953 and remains useful to this day. Extensive pharmacologic studies have shown it to be a nonspecific inhibitor of a variety of vasoconstrictor stimuli such as histamine, barium, vasopressin, pressor amines, and sympathetic tone (104). This evidence, plus the clinical behavior of producing hypotension and reflex tachycardia, indicates it produces direct vasodilation. The precise mechanism of the vaso-dilatation is not clear but may involve chelation of metal ions (105), monoamine oxidase inhibition (106), dopa decarboxylase inhibition (106), and/or catechol-amine depletion (107). Pharmacodynamic studies in man confirm that blood pressure is lowered by a decrease in peripheral vascular resistance caused by arteriolar vasodilatation (108). There is evidence that renal arterioles are espe-cially affected, thus renal blood flow is preserved unless the blood pressure fall is marked. For this reason hydralazine is often recommended for hypertensive individuals with renal vascular damage. Despite favorable pharmacodynamic properties, the clinical use of hydralazine is limited by side effects. These include headache, palpitations, nausea and vomiting, diarrhea, nasal congestion, conjunc-tivitis, drug fever, skin rash, peripheral neuropathy, and bone marrow suppres-sion. The cardiac stimulation responsible for the palpitations is attributed to beta mediated sympathetic reflexes but may involve direct stimulation as well. This effect may precipitate angina pectoris and ECG changes in atherosclerotic subjects. It has recently been proposed that the reflex side effects may be substantially reduced and the value of hydralazine enhanced, if it is used concomitantly with a beta adrenergic blocking agent (109). The most notorious side effect is a disseminated lupus erythematosis-like syndrome. It is of interest

Table 2. Antihypertensive Drugs Affecting
Vascular Smooth Muscle

General name	*Trade name*	*Dosage range (mg)*
Hydralazine	Apresoline	oral: 25 b.i.d.→75 q.i.d. IM: 10–50 IV: 10–20/20 ml given from syringe at 1 ml/min or 50–150/L as continuous infusion
Diazoxide	Hyperstat[a]	IV: 300–600 rapidly (within 20 seconds)

[a]Investigational drug

that one of the investigators who first described this syndrome has recently reported that the hydralazine-treated hypertensive patients who developed this syndrome had a better survival rate than those who did not receive hydralazine (110). It would appear from this and other evidence that this syndrome is not identical with the disease and is much more benign. The incidence of major side effects can be minimized by limiting the daily dose of hydralazine to 200 mg. Furthermore, it has recently been demonstrated that plasma levels of hydralazine are correlated to dose and both are correlated to the antihypertensive effect (111). Thus it may be possible to adjust dosage to a desired plasma level and avoid toxic concentrations. The usual dosage range and routes of administration are presented in Table 2.

Minoxidil

Minoxidil is a new direct vasodilator currently undergoing clinical investigation (112,113). It is chemically quite different from hydralazine, which means that only the pharmacodynamic type of side effects are likely to be in common. A unique adverse effect of this agent is hirsutism. An important advantage is its duration of action. Despite a plasma half-life of only 4.2 hours (114), antihypertensive effects persist for 24 hours or more (113). This suggests retention of the drug or metabolites at the site of action in arteriolar vascular tissue (115). Minoxidil has also been proposed for use in combination with beta adrenergic blocking agents in order to limit side effects and extend its range of action (112,113).

Diazoxide

Diazoxide is a benzothiadiazine analogue which produces salt and water retention by renal mechanisms, yet is a potent hypotensive agent (116). The oral or prolonged use of diazoxide leads to fluid retention and hyperglycemia (117,118), but when administered intravenously for short periods of time in subjects with severe hypertension, it is very effective, and the effects may persist long after treatment (119). Like hydralazine, diazoxide suppresses the vascular responses to a variety of vasoconstrictor stimuli (116) and reduces arteriolar tone in animals (120) and in man (118).

The precise mechanism of these effects is not clear but it may involve interference with calcium ions (121,122). Since diazoxide is rapidly bound to plasma protein, it must be given quickly as an intravenous bolus in order to obtain a hypotensive effect. The recommended dose is 300 mg delivered within 20 seconds. As would be expected, the fall in blood pressure is accompanied by an increase in heart rate and cardiac output (123). There is an immediate reduction in renal blood flow and glomerular filtration rate, but these parameters rise to levels above control within two hours after administration (123).

The marked and rapid fall in blood pressure which may be produced by diazoxide requires one to be cautious when treating patients with suspected cerebrovascular or coronary disease. The sodium-retaining and hyperglycemic effects of diazoxide can be moderated by the concomitant use of furosemide (124) or tolbutamide (125), respectively.

The routes of administration and dosage ranges of hydralazine and diazoxide are given in Table 2.

ANTIHYPERTENSIVE AGENTS AFFECTING PLASMA VOLUME

Thiazides and Related Drugs

The application of the oral diuretics to the treatment of hypertension is based on the clinical observation that dietary restriction of sodium is beneficial in this disorder. Despite the truth of this observation, and the natriuretic activity (by definition) of the oral diuretics, it is not clear that salt and water depletion is the only mechanism by which these drugs lower blood pressure. During the initial phases of treatment, the fall in blood pressure is associated with reductions in the plasma and extracellular fluid volumes and in total exchangeable sodium and potassium (126–129). These effects can be at least partially reversed by salt or volume replacement (126,127,129). After weeks and months of treatment, however, some investigators have reported that plasma volume and cardiac output return to normal levels (127,128,130), but peripheral vascular resistance is reduced (128,131) and the blood pressure remains lowered. At this stage the antihypertensive effects are not reversible by volume and sodium replacement (130) and the degree of blood pressure lowering appears unrelated to weight loss or diuresis (132). It has been demonstrated that thiazides diminish vascular resistance (132) and venous reactivity (133) in the forearm. The mechanism of this apparent direct effect on blood vessels is not clear. It has been suggested that thiazides diminish the contractile responses to norepinephrine (134,135) and angiotensin (136), but not all investigators have confirmed these findings (137). The advent of diazoxide provides evidence that drugs of this chemical class are capable of direct vascular actions. This benzothiadiazine analogue produces salt and water retention, yet is a potent hypotensive agent (116).

On the other side of the argument, it is true that the mercurials and other diuretics structurally unrelated to chlorothiazide, such as spironolactone, triamterene, and ethacrynic acid, are also antihypertensive. This suggests that the common property is diuresis. Furthermore, recent studies indicate that long term thiazide therapy is associated with a persistent contraction in plasma volume (138–140) despite an increased peripheral renin activity (138). In addition, the level of blood pressure has been observed to be directly related to plasma volume in a variety of treatment circumstances (98). At this time it would appear that contraction of plasma volume is an important mechanism by which the oral diuretics lower blood pressure, but direct vascular effects may operate as well.

All oral diuretic agents, including benzothiadiazines, phtalimidines, aldosterone antagonists, ethacrynic acid, and furosemide, are antihypertensive, and are about equally potent for this indication (141). The dose response curve for blood pressure lowering is maximum at approximately 150–200 mg of hydrochlorothiazide or its equivalent per day (142). There is no advantage to using the more potent diuretics ethacrynic acid and furosemide for this purpose, because they add no antihypertensive potency and have short durations of action.

In clinical use, normalization of blood pressure can be accomplished with oral diuretics alone only in some mildly hypertensive subjects. It is well established, however, that these agents potentiate the effects of more potent drugs and permit the latter to be used at lower doses and with less side effects. The probable mechanism of this potentiation is elimination of the fluid retention associated with most other antihypertensive drugs. The oral diuretics are extremely well tolerated in the usual hypertensive situation. Mild hypokalemia, hyperuricemia, and hyperglycemia are observed frequently but are rarely of clinical significance. Pre-existing renal insufficiency may be aggravated and the blood urea nitrogen levels increased. Hypersensitivity reactions are rare.

The nonkaliuretic diuretics, spironolactone and triamterene, may be used in combination with a thiazide-type drug to minimize and prevent hypokalemia.

Table 3. Diuretics Used in the Treatment
of Essential Hypertension

Generic name	Trade name	Usual daily dosage (mg)
Thiazides and related drugs:		
Bendroflumethiazide	Benuron, Naturetin	5–10
Benzthiazide	Exna	50–100
Chlorothiazide	Diuril	500–1,500
Cyclothiazide	Anhydron	2–4
Hydrochlorothiazide	Esidrix, Hydrodiuril, Oretic	50–150
Hydroflumethiazide	Saluron	50–150
Methyclothiazide	Enduron	5–10
Polythiazide	Renese	2–8
Trichlormethiazide	Metahydrin, Naqua	4–8
Chlorthalidone	Hygroton	50–100
Quinethazone	Hydromox	50–100
Potassium-sparing drugs:		
Spironolactone	Aldactone	100
Triamterene	Dyrenium	200

Spironolactone is, of course, specific in primary and secondary hyperaldosteronism. Diuretics used in the treatment of hypertension and their usual daily dosage are listed in Table 3.

SUMMARY

In summary, a system is developing for a more rational use of drugs in the treatment of hypertension. It is becoming evident that patients with essential hypertension have individual hemodynamic and biochemical characteristics. The proper application of drugs currently available or under development may make it possible to tailor therapy to the individual. For example, patients with an expanded plasma volume may require only a diuretic. Individuals exhibiting the characteristics of a hyperdynamic circulation may respond well to a beta adrenergic blocking agent. When the basic abnormality is an increased peripheral vascular resistance, a drug which inhibits sympathetic nerve transmission or a direct vasodilator would probably be required. Such drugs are best used in combination with a diuretic and possibly a beta adrenergic blocking agent. Finally, in those patients in whom plasma renin levels are primarily or secondarily elevated, a drug capable of inhibiting renin release might well improve the efficacy of the treatment program. It is clear that the proper application of drugs in this manner requires a knowledge of their mechanisms of action.

REFERENCES CITED

1. Report of Inter-Society Commission for Heart Disease Resources. 1971. Guidelines for the detection, diagnosis and management of hypertensive populations. Circulation 44:A237.
2. Laragh, J. M. 1972. Evaluation and care of the hypertensive patient. Amer. J. Med. 52:565.
3. Metropolitan Life Insurance States Bulletin. 45:3, 1964.
4. Veterans Administration Cooperative Study Group on Antihypertensive Agents. 1967. Effects of treatment on morbidity in hypertension. Results in patients with diastolic blood pressures averaging 115 through 129 mm Hg. J.A.M.A. 202:1028.
5. Veterans Administration Cooperative Study Group on Antihypertensive Agents. 1970. Effects of treatment on morbidity in hypertension. II: Results in patients with diastolic blood pressure averaging 90 through 114 mm Hg. J.A.M.A. 213:1143.
6. United States Public Health Service Hospitals Cooperative Study Group. 1972. Morbidity and mortality in mild essential hypertension. Circ. Res. 30, 31 (Suppl. II):110.
7. Smirk, F. H. 1967. The pathogenesis of hypertension. Page 1 in E. Schlittler, ed. Medicinal chemistry, Vol. 7. Academic Press, New York.
8. Pickering, G. 1972. Hypertension, definition, natural histories and consequences. Amer. J. Med. 52:570.
9. Kannel, W. B., Castelli, W. P., McNamara, P. M., McKee, P. A., and Feinleib, M. 1972. Role of blood pressure in the development of congestive heart failure. New Engl. J. Med. 287:781.
10. Page, I. H., and Dustan, H. P. 1962. Editorial: Persistence of normal blood pressure after discontinuing treatment in hypertensive patients. Circulation 25:433.

11. Breckenridge, A., Dollery, C. T., and Parry, E. H. O. 1970. Prognosis of treated hypertension. Quart. J. Med. 39:411.
12. Smirk, F. H. 1972. The prognosis of untreated and of treated hypertension and advantages of early treatment. Amer. Heart J. 83:825.
13. Freis, E. D. 1972. The treatment of hypertension, why, when and how. Amer. J. Med. 52:664.
14. Kezdi, P. 1953. Sinoaortic regulatory system. Arch. Internal Med. 91:26.
15. Peterson, L. H. 1961. Hemodynamic alterations in essential hypertension. In A. N. Brest and J. H. Moyer, eds. Hypertension: Recent advances. Lea and Febiger, Philadelphia.
16. Hoobler, S. W. 1961. Current concepts of the mechanisms of essential hypertension. Page 59 in A. N. Brest and J. H. Moyer, eds. Hypertension: Recent advances. Lea and Febiger, Philadelphia.
17. Wilson, C. 1961. Etiological considerations in essential hypertension. Page 64 in A. N. Brest and J. H. Moyer, eds. Hypertension: Recent advances. Lea and Febiger, Philadelphia.
18. Davis, J. O. 1965. Aldosteronism and hypertension. Progr. Cardiov. Dis. 8:129.
19. Cope, C. L., Harwood, M., and Pearson, J. 1962. Aldosterone secretion in hypertensive diseases. Brit. Med. J. 1:659.
20. Laragh, J. H., Ulick, S., Vlodzimierz, J., Deming, Q. B., Kelly, W. G., and Lieberman, S. 1960. Aldosterone secretion and primary malignant hypertension. J. Clin. Invest. 39:1091.
21. Helmer, O. M. 1965. The renin-angiotension system and its relation to hypertension. Progr. Cardiov. Dis. 8:117.
22. Freis, E. D. 1960. Hemodynamics of hypertension. Physiol. Rev. 40:27.
23. Frohlich, E. D., Tarazi, R. C., and Dustan, H. P. 1969. Re-examination of the hemodynamics of hypertension. Amer. J. Med. Sci. 257:9.
24. Tarazi, R. C., Dustan, H. P., Frohlich, E. D., Gifford, R. W., Jr., and Hoffman, G. C. 1970. Plasma volume and chronic hypertension. Relationship to arterial pressure levels in different hypertensive diseases. Arch. Internal Med. 125:835.
25. Laragh, J. H., Baer, L., Brunner, H. R., Buhler, F. K., Sealey, J. E., and Vaughan, E. D., Jr. 1972. Renin, angiotensin and aldosterone system in pathogenesis and management of hypertensive vascular disease. Amer. J. Med. 52:633.
26. Eich, R. H., Cuddy, R. P., Smulyan, H., and Lyons, R. H.: Hemodynamics in labile hypertension. A follow up study. Circulation 34:299.
27. Brunner, H. R., Laragh, J. H., Baer, L., Newton, M. A., Goodwin, F. T., Krakoff, L. R., Bard, R. H., and Buhler, F. R. 1972. Essential hypertension: renin and aldosterone, heart attack and stroke. New Engl. J. Med. 286:441.
28. Dustan, H. P., Tarazi, R. C., and Bravo, E. L. 1972. Physiologic characteristics of hypertension. Amer. J. Med. 52:610.
29. Dawes, G. S., and Comroe, J. H., Jr. 1954. Chemoreflexes from the heart and lungs. Physiol. Rev. 34:167.
30. Borison, H. L., Fairbanks, V. F., and White, C. A. 1955. Afferent reflex factors in veriloid-induced hypotension. Arch. Int. Pharmacodyn. Ther. 101:189.
31. Borison, H. L., and Fairbanks, V. F. 1952. Mechanism of veratrum induced emesis in the cat. J. Pharmacol. Exp. Ther. 105:317.
32. Abrams, W. B., Pocelinko, R., Moe, R. A., Bates, H., Hanauer, L., and Camacho, S. 1965. The clinical pharmacology of postganglionic sympathetic blocking agents. Dis. Chest 48:178.
33. Costa, E., Boullin, D., Hammer, W., Vogel, W., and Brodie, B. B. 1966. Interactions of drugs with adrenergic neurons. Pharmacol. Rev. 18:577.
34. Hillarp, N.-Å. 1959. The construction and functional organization of the autonomic innervation apparatus. Acta Physiol. Scand. 46 (Suppl. 157).
35. Potter, L. T. 1967. Role of intraneuronal vesicles in the synthesis, storage and release of noradrenaline. Circ. Res. 11 (Suppl. 3):13.
36. Kopin, I. J., and Gordon, E. K. 1963. Metabolism of administered and drug released norepinephrine-7-H^3 in the rat. J. Pharmacol. Exp. Ther. 140:207.

37. Von Euler, U. S., and Lishajro, F. 1967. Mechanisms of drug-induced catecholamine release from adrenergic nerve granules. Circ. Res. 21 (Suppl. III):63.
38. Day, M. D., and Rand, M. J. 1963. A hypothesis for the mode of action of alpha-methyldopa in relieving hypertension. J. Pharm. Pharmacol. 15:221.
39. Muscholl, E., and Maitre, L. 1963. Release by sympathetic stimulation of alpha-methylnorepinephrine stored in the heart after administration of alpha-methyldopa. Experimentia 19:658.
40. Day, M. D., and Rand, M. J. 1964. Some observations on the pharmacology of alpha-methyldopa. Brit. J. Pharmacol. 22:72.
41. Sannerstedt, R., Varnauskas, E., and Werkö, L. 1962. Hemodynamic effects of methyldopa (Aldomet) at rest and during exercise in patients with arterial hypertension. Acta Med. Scand. 171:75.
42. Mohammed, S., Haneson, I. B., Magenheim, H. G., and Gaffney, T. E. 1968. The effects of alpha-methyldopa on renal function in hypertensive patients. Amer. Heart J. 76:21.
43. Croft, J. D., Swisher, S. N., Jr., Gilliland, B. C., Bakemeier, R. F., Leddy, J. P., and Weed, R. I. 1968. Coombs'-test positivity induced by drugs. Mechanisms of immunologic reactions and red cell destruction. Ann. Internal Med. 68:176.
44. Boura, A. L. A., and Green, A. F. 1965. Adrenergic neuron blocking agents. Ann. Rev. Pharmacol. 5:183.
45. Brodie, B. B., Chang, C. C., and Costa, E. 1965. On the mechanism of action of guanethidine and bretylium. Brit. J. Pharmacol. 25:171.
46. Mitchell, J. R., and Oates, J. A. 1970. Guanethidine and related agents. I. Mechanism of the selective blockade of adrenergic neurons and its antagonism by drugs. J. Pharmacol. Exp. Ther. 172:100.
47. Boullin, D. J., Costa, E., and Brodie, B. B. 1966. Discharge of tritium-labeled guanethidine by sympathetic nerve stimulation as evidence that guanethidine is a false transmitter. Life Sci. 5:803.
48. Mitchell, J. R., Arias, L., and Oates, J. A. 1968. Antagonism of the antihypertensive action of guanethidine sulfate by desipramine HCl. J.A.M.A. 202:973.
49. McMartin, C., Rondel, R. K., Vinter, J., Allan, B. R., Humberstone, P. M., Leishman, A. W. D., Sandler, G., and Thirkettle, J. L. 1970. The fate of guanethidine in two hypertensive patients. Clin. Pharmacol. Ther. 11:423.
50. Shand, D. G., Nice, A. S., McAllister, R. G., and Oates, J. A. 1972. An improved method for treating severe hypertension with guanethidine. Clin. Res. 20:413.
51. Giachetti, A., and Shore, P. A. 1967. Monoamine oxidase inhibition in the adrenergic neuron by bretylium, debrisoquin, and other adrenergic neuronal blocking agents. Biochem. Pharmacol. 16:237.
52. Moe, R. A., Bates, H. M., Palkoski, Z. M., and Banziger, R. 1964. Cardiovascular effects of 3,4-dihydro-2 (1H) isoquinoline carboxamidine (Declinax). Curr. Ther. Res. 6:299.
53. Kuntzman, R., and Jacobson, M. M. 1963. The inhibition of monoamine oxidase by benzyl and phenethylguanidines related to bretylium and guanethidine. Ann. N.Y. Acad. Sci. 107:945.
54. Medina, M. A., Giachetti, A., and Shore, P. A. 1969. On the physiological disposition and possible mechanism of the antihypertensive action of debrisoquin. Biochem. Pharmacol. 18:891.
55. Malmfors, T., and Abrams, W. B. 1970. The effects of debrisoquin and bretylium on adrenergic nerves as revealed by fluorescence histochemistry. J. Pharmacol. Exp. Ther. 174:99.
56. Pettinger, W. A., Korn, A., Spiegel, H., Solomon, H. M., Pocelinko, R., and Abrams, W. B. 1969. Debrisoquin, a selective inhibitor of intraneuronal monoamine oxidase in man. Clin. Pharmacol. Ther. 10:667.
57. Bath, J., Pickering, D., and Turner, R. 1967. Clinical experience with bethanidine in treatment of hypertension. Brit. Med. J. 4:519.
58. Gupta, N., and McNay, J. L. 1972. Rapid control of hypertension with oral bethanidine. Europ. J. Clin. Pharmacol. 4:217.
59. Schoepke, H. G., and Wiegand, R. G. 1963. Relation between norepinephrine accumu-

lation or depletion and blood pressure responses in the cat and rat following pargyline administration. Ann. N.Y. Acad. Sci. 107:924.

60. Kopin, I. J., Fischer, J. E., Musacchio, J. M., Horst, W. D., and Weise, V. K. 1965. False neurochemical transmitters and the mechanism of sympathetic blockade by monoamine oxidase inhibitors. J. Pharmacol. Exp. Ther. 147:186.

61. Spector, S., Gordon, R., Sjoerdsma, A., and Udenfriend, S. 1967. End product inhibition of tyrosine hydroxylase as a possible mechanism for regulation of norepinephrine synthesis. Molec. Pharmacol. 3:549.

62. Onesti, G., Hovack, P., Ramirez, O., Brest, A. N., and Moyer, J. H. 1964. Hemodynamic effects of pargyline in hypertensive patients. Circulation 30:830.

63. Goldberg, L. I., Horwitz, D., and Sjoerdsma, A. 1962. Attenuation of cardiovascular responses to exercise as a possible basis for the effectiveness of monoamine oxidase inhibitors in angina pectoris. J. Pharmacol. Exp. Ther. 137:39.

64. Horwitz, D., Lovenberg, W., Engelman, K., and Sjoerdsma, A. 1964. Monoamine oxidase inhibitors, tyramine and cheese. J.A.M.A. 188:1108.

65. Hoefke, W., and Kobinger, W. 1966. Pharmakologische Wirkungen des 2-(2,6-dichlorphenylamino)-2-imidazolin-hydrochlorids, einer neuen, antihypertensiven Substanz. Arzneimittel-Forsch. 16:1038.

66. Sattler, R. W., and Van Zwieten, P. A. 1967. Acute hypotensive action of 2-2,6-dichlorophenylamino)-2-imidazoline hydrochloride (ST 155) after infusion into the cat's vertebral artery. Europe J. Pharmacol. 2:9.

67. Constantine, J. W., and McShane, W. K. 1968. Analysis of the cardiovascular effects of 2-(2,6-dichlorophenylamino)-2-imidazoline hydrochloride (Catapresan). Europ. J. Pharmacol. 4:109.

68. Katic, F., Lavery, H., and Lowe, R. D. 1972. The central action of clonidine and its antagonism. Brit. J. Pharmacol. 44:779.

69. Kobinger, W. 1967. Über den Wirkungsmechanismus einer neuen antihypertensiven Substantz mit imidazolinstructur. Arch. Pharmakol. Expt. Pathol. 258:48.

70. Kobinger, W., and Walland, A. 1972. Evidence for a central activation of a vagal cardiodepressor reflex by clonidine. Europ. J. Pharmacol. 19:203.

71. Schmitt, H., and Schmitt, H., Mme. 1969. Localization of the hypotensive effect of 2-(2,6-dichlorophenylamino)-2-imidazoline hydrochloride (ST 155, Catapresan). Europ. J. Pharmacol. 6:8.

72. Bolme, P., and Fuxe, K. 1971. Pharmacological studies on the hypotensive effects of clonidine. Europ. J. Pharmacol. 13:168.

73. Schmitt, H., Schmitt, H., Mme., Boissier, J. R., and Giudicelli, J. F. 1967. Centrally mediated decrease in sympathetic tone induced by 2(2,6-dichlorophenylamino)-2-imidazoline (S.T. 155, Catapresan). Europ. J. Pharmacol. 2:147.

74. Hökfelt, B., Hedeland, H., and Dymling, J.-F. 1970. Studies on catecholamines, renin and aldosterone following Catapresan (2-(2,6-dichlor-phenylamine)-2-imidazoline hydrochloride). Europ. J. Pharmacol. 10:389.

75. Onesti, G., Schwartz, A. B., Kim, K. E., Paz-Martinez, V., and Swartz, C. 1971. Antihypertensive effect of clonidine. Circ. Res. 28, 29 (Suppl. II):II–53.

76. Conolly, M. E., Briant, R. H., George, C. F., and Dollery, C. T. 1972. A crossover comparison of clonidine and methyldopa in hypertension. Europ. J. Pharmacol. 4:222.

77. Mroczek, W. J., Davidov, M., and Finnerty, F. A. 1972. Prolonged treatment with clonidine: comparative antihypertensive effects alone and with a diuretic agent. Amer. J. Cardiol. 30:536.

78. Davidov, M., Kakaviatos, N., and Finnerty, F. A., Jr. 1967. The antihypertensive effects of an imidazoline compound. Clin. Pharmacol. Ther. 8:810.

79. Iisalo, E., and Laurila, S. 1967. A clinical trial with a new antihypertensive drug. ST-155 (Catapresan). Curr. Ther. Res. 9(7):358.

80. Prichard, B. N. C., and Gillam, P. M. S. 1969. Treatment of hypertension with propranolol. Brit. Med. J. 1:7.

81. Tarazi, R. C., and Dustan, H. P. 1972. Beta adrenergic blockade in hypertension. Amer. J. Cardiol. 29:633.

82. Zacharias, E. J., Cowen, K. J., Prestt, J., Vickers, J., and Wall, B. G. 1972. Propranolol in hypertension: A study of long-term therapy, 1964–1970. Amer. Heart J. 83:755.
83. Lund-Johansen, P. 1967. Hemodynamics in early essential hypertension. Acta Med. Scand. 482 (Suppl.):8.
84. Julius, S., and Conway, J. 1968. Hemodynamic studies in patients with borderline blood pressure elevation. Circulation 37:282.
85. Conway, J. 1970. Labile hypertension: the problem. Circ. Res. 46 (Suppl. I):43.
86. Frohlich, E. D., Tarazi, R. C., and Dustan, H. P. 1969. Hyperdynamic beta-adrenergic circulatory state. Arch. Internal Med. 123:1.
87. Bertler, A. 1961. Occurrence and localization of catecholamines in the human brain. Acta Physiol. Scand. 51:97.
88. Carlsson, A. 1964. Functional significance of drug-induced changes in brain monoamine levels. Prog. Brain Res. 8:9.
89. Gagnon, D. J., and Melville, K. I. 1969. Alteration of centrally mediated cardiovascular manifestations by intraventricular pronethalol and phentolamine. Int. J. Neuropharmacol. 8:587.
90. Bhargava, K. P., Mishra, N., and Tangri, K. K. 1972. An analysis of central adrenoceptors for control of cardiovascular function. Brit. J. Pharmacol. 45:596.
91. Masouka, D., and Hansson, E. 1967. Autoradiographic distribution studies of adrenergic blocking agents, II ¹⁴ C-propranolol, a β-receptor-type blocker. Acta Pharmacol. Toxicol. 25:447.
92. Laverty, R., and Taylor, K. M. 1968. Propranolol uptake into the central nervous system and the effect on rat behaviour and amine metabolism. J. Pharm. Pharmacol. 20:605.
93. Garvey, H. L., Ram, N., Woodhouse, B. L., and Booker, W. M. 1972. Centrally mediated antihypertensive effects of propranolol. Fed. Proc. 31:382.
94. Stern, S., Hoffman, M., and Braun, K. 1971. Cardiovascular responses to carotid and vertebral artery infusions of propranolol. Cardiov. Res. 5:425.
95. Kelliher, G. K., and Buckley, J. P. 1970. Central hypotensive activity of dl- and d-propranolol. J. Pharm. Sci. 59:1276.
96. Scales, B., and Cosgrove, M. B. 1970. The metabolism and distribution of the selective adrenergic beta blocking agent, practolol. J. Pharmacol. Exp. Ther. 175:338.
97. Barrett, A. M. 1971. The pharmacology of practolol. Postgrad. Med. J. 47 (Suppl.):7.
98. Dustan, H. P., Tarazi, R. C., and Bravo, E. L. 1972. Dependence of arterial pressure on intravascular volume in treated hypertensive patients. New Engl. J. Med. 286:861.
99. Tarazi, R. C., Frohlich, E. D., and Dustan, H. P. 1971. Plasma volume changes with long-term beta-adrenergic blockade. Amer. Heart J. 82:770.
100. Julius, S., Pascual, A. V., Abbrecht, P. H., and London, R. 1972. Effect of beta-adrenergic blockade on plasma volume in human subjects. Proc. Soc. Exp. Biol. Med. 140:982.
101. Winer, N., Chokshi, D. S., Yoon, M. S., and Freedman, A. D. 1969. Adrenergic receptor mediation of renin secretion. J. Clin. Endocr. 29:1168.
102. Michelakis, A. M., and McAllister, R. G. 1972. The effect of chronic adrenergic receptor blockade on plasma renin activity in man. J. Clin. Endocr. 34:386.
103. Ueda, H., Yasuda, H., Takabatake, Y., Iizuka, M., Iizuka, T., Ihori, M., and Sakamoto, Y. 1970. Observations on the mechanism of renin release by catecholamines. Circ. Res. 26, 27 (Suppl. II):II–195.
104. Druey, J., and Tripod, J. 1967. Hydralazines. Page 223 in E. Schlittler, ed. Antihypertensive agents. Academic Press, New York.
105. Perry, H. M., and Schroeder, H. A. 1954. Studies on the control of hypertension by Hypex. III: Pharmacological and chemical observations on 1-hydrazinophthalazine. Amer. J. Med. Sci. 228:396.
106. Schroeder, H. A. 1959. In J. H. Moyer, ed. Hypertension, First Hahnemann Symposium on Hypertensive Disease. Saunders, Philadelphia.
107. Bygdeman, M., and Stjärne, L. 1960. Animal physiology: Effects of 1,4-dihydrazinophthalazine on the catecholamine. Nature 186:82.

108. Rowe, G. G., Huston, J. H., Maxwell, G. M., Crosley, A. P., Jr., and Crumptom, C. W. 1955. Hemodynamic effects of 1-hydrazinophthalazine in patients with arterial hypertension. J. Clin. Invest. 34:115.

109. Zacest, R., Gilmore, E., and Koch-Weser, J. 1972. Treatment of essential hypertension with combined vasodilation and beta-adrenergic blockade. New Engl. J. Med. 286:617.

110. Perry, H. M. 1969. Possibly increased survival of hydralazine toxic patients. J. Lab. Clin. Med. 74:994.

111. Zacest, R., and Koch-Weser, J. 1972. Relation of hydralazine plasma concentration to dosage and hypotensive action. Clin. Pharmacol. Ther. 13:420.

112. Gilmore, E., Weil, J., and Chidsey, C. A., III. 1970. Treatment of essential hypertension with a new vasodilator in combination with beta-adrenergic blockade. New Engl. J. Med. 282:521.

113. Gottlieb, T. B., Katz, F. H., and Chidsey, C. A., III. 1972. Combined therapy with vasodilator drugs and beta adrenergic blockade in hypertension. Circulation 45:571.

114. Gottlieb, T. B., Thomas, R. C., and Chidsey, C. A. 1972. Pharmacokinetic studies of minoxidil. Clin. Pharmacol. Ther. 13:436.

115. Pluss, R. G., Orcutt, J., and Chidsey, C. A. 1973. Tissue distribution and hypotensive effects of a new vasodilator, minoxidil. J. Lab. Clin. Med. In Press.

116. Rubin, A. A., Roth, F. E., Taylor, R. M., and Rosenkilde, H. 1962. Pharmacology of diazoxide, an antihypertensive, nondiuretic benzothiadiazine. J. Pharmacol. Exp. Ther. 136:344.

117. Hutcheon, D. E., and Barthalmus, K. S. 1962. Antihypertensive action of diazoxide. Brit. Med. J. 2:159.

118. Wilson, W. R., and Okun, R. 1963. The acute hemodynamic effects of diazoxide in man. Circulation 28:89.

119. Finnerty, F. A., Davidov, M., and Kakaviatos, N. 1967. Hypertensive vascular disease. The long term effect of rapid repeated reductions of arterial pressure with diazoxide. Amer. J. Cardiol. 19:377.

120. Rubin, A. A., Zitowitz, L., and Hausler, L. M. 1963. Acute circulatory effects of diazoxide and sodium nitrite. J. Pharmacol. Exp. Ther. 140:46.

121. Wohl, A. J., Hausler, L. M., and Roth, F. E. 1967. Studies on the mechanisms of antihypertensive action of diazoxide: In vitro vascular pharmacodynamics. J. Pharmacol. Exp. Ther. 158:531.

122. Ramaswamy, D., and Richardson, D. W. 1968. Mechanisms of hypotensive action of intravenous diazoxide. Circulation 38:160.

123. Hamby, W. M., Jankowski, G. J., Pouget, J. M., Dunea, G., and Gantt, C. L. 1968. Intravenous use of diazoxide in the treatment of severe hypertension. Circulation 37:168.

124. Finnerty, F. A., Jr. 1968. Hypertensive encephalopathy. Amer. Heart J. 75:559.

125. Wolff, F. W., Grant, A. M., and Wales, J. K. 1967. Reversal of diazoxide effects by tolbutamide. Lancet 1:1137.

126. Dustan, H. P., Cumming, G. R., Corcoran, A. C., and Page, I. H. 1959. A mechanism of chlorothiazide-enhanced effectiveness of antihypertensive ganglioplegic drugs. Circulation 19:360.

127. Wilson, I. M., and Freis, E. D. 1959. Relationship between plasma and extracellular fluid volume depletion and the antihypertensive effect of chlorothiazide. Circulation 20:1028.

128. Conway, J., and Lauwers, P. 1960. Hemodynamic and hypotensive effects of long term therapy with chlorothiazide. Circulation 21:21.

129. Winer, B. M. 1961. The antihypertensive action of benzothiadiazines. Circulation 23:211.

130. Hollander, W., Chobanian, A. V., and Wilkins, R. W. 1960. The role of diuretics in the management of hypertension. Ann. N.Y. Acad. Sci. 88:975.

131. Villarreal, H., Exaire, J. E., Revollo, A., and Soni, J. 1962. Effects of chlorothiazide on systemic hemodynamics in essential hypertension. Circulation 26:405.

132. Conway, J., and Palmero, H. 1963. The vascular effect of the thiazide diuretics. Arch. Internal Med. 11:203.
133. Ogilvie, R. I., and Schlieper, E. 1970. The effect of hydrochlorothiazide on venous reactivity in hypertensive man. Clin. Pharmacol. Ther. 11:589.
134. Aleksandrow, D., Wysnacka, W., and Gajewski, J. 1959. Influence of chlorothiazide upon arterial responsiveness to norepinephrine in hypertensive subjects. New Engl. J. Med. 261:1052.
135. Zsotér, T. T., Hart, F., and Rodde, I. C. 1970. Mechanism of antihypertensive action of prolonged administration of hydrochlorothiazide in rabbit and dog. Circ. Res. 27:717.
136. Gillenwater, J. Y., Scott, J. B., and Frohlich, E. D. 1962. Effect of chlorothiazide on response of renal vascular bed to vasoactive substances. Circ. Res. 11:283.
137. Silah, J. G., Jones, R. E., Bashour, F. A., and Kaplan, N. M. 1965. The effect of acute administration of chlorothiazide upon the pressor responsiveness to angiotensin and norepinephrine. Amer. Heart J. 69:301.
138. Tarazi, R. C., Dustan, H. P., and Frohlich, E. D. 1970. Long-term thiazide therapy in essential hypertension. Evidence for persistent alteration in plasma volume and renin activity. Circulation 41:709.
139. Leth, A. 1970. Changes in plasma and extracellular fluid volumes in patients with essential hypertension during long-term treatment with hydrochlorothiazide. Circulation 42:479.
140. Lund-Johansen, P. 1970. Hemodynamic changes in long-term diuretic therapy of essential hypertension. Acta Med. Scand. 187:509.
141. Wolf, R. L., Mendlowitz, M., Roboz, J., and Gitlow, S. 1966. Treatment of hypertension with antihypertensive diuretic drugs. Amer. Heart J. 72:692.
142. McLeod, P. J., Ogilvie, R. I., and Ruedy, J. 1970. Effects of large and small doses of hydrochlorothiazide in hypertensive patients. Clin. Pharmacol. Ther. 11:733.

COMPARATIVE RESPONSES TO BLOOD PRESSURE-LOWERING AGENTS USED DURING THE PAST TWO DECADES

JOHN H. MOYER

Effective antihypertensive drugs have been available for approximately 20 years. It is worth reviewing the effectiveness of the various categories of drugs that have been used during this period of time and evaluating some of their virtues and defects.

METHOD

Unselected hypertensive patients have been treated with different drugs over the past 20 years, using essentially the same technique for evaluation (1–7). After a thorough history and physical examination, routine laboratory studies were obtained. The patients were then placed on placebo medication and their blood pressures were recorded in the upright and supine positions, usually at weekly intervals. At least four control readings were obtained for each patient over a period of four or more weeks. In order to get a single figure for the arterial blood pressure as a control or baseline observation, the mean arterial blood pressure was used, employing the diastolic pressure plus one-third of the pulse pressure as the calculated value. Patients with diastolic pressures of less than 100 mm Hg were excluded from the study.

After the control observations were made, the patients were placed on various antihypertensive medications throughout the years, as recorded in Table 1. Those who required sequential dose titration were evaluated after maximum dosage had been employed, rather than during the dose titration period. The patients were followed for a minimum of three months after either the maximum tolerated dosage was reached or the blood pressure was reduced below 150/100 mm Hg in the standing position. Repeated observations were made during this period of time, following which the mean blood pressure was calculated in the same manner as during the control period. (All blood pressure observations reported in this study were made with the patient in the upright position.)

RESULTS

The results of our observations are summarized in Tables 1, 2, and 3. Table 1 is a summary of the antihypertensive response to the various drugs employed. A

Table 1. Blood Pressure Response to Antihypertensive
Drugs Studied Chronologically (% of Number Treated)

Drug or combination of drugs	No. of cases	Normo-tensive[a] (%)	Significant response[b] (%)
Placebo	110	2	10
Veratrum	31	3	19
Hydralazine (Apresoline)	54	11	35
Phenoxybenzamine (Dibenzyline)	32	47	72
Hexamethonium	58	47	81
Mecamylamine (Inversine)	40	50	84
Mecamylamine and rauwolfia	80	62	91
Pentolinium (Ansolysen) and rauwolfia	75	56	81
Chlorothiazide	50	24	46
Rauwolfia and chlorothiazide and mecamylamine	125	75	94
Rauwolfia and chlorothiazide and pentolinium	75	80	92
Guanethidine (Ismelin)	30	43	90
Guanethidine and chlorothiazide	30	54	94
(Alpha) methyldopa (Aldomet)	38	24	42
Methyldopa and chlorothiazide	50	36	62
Pargyline	33	45	82
Clonidine (Catapres)	16	0	37
Clonidine and chlorothiazide	20	10	80

[a] Normotensive: arterial pressure less than 150/100 mm Hg.

[b] Significant response: mean arterial blood pressure reduced more than 20 mm Hg.

group of patients receiving placebo medication only is included for comparative purposes. This group was followed for the usual control period of one month, and then again for an additional three months while receiving a placebo. The placebo group was not used as a correction factor but merely as a comparable group of patients to show the incidence of blood pressure response without antihypertensive medication. A small number of patients did obtain an antihypertensive response to placebo. However, the low incidence of responsiveness indicates that the patients in these control studies had relatively severe disease.

Efficacy

Veratrum

The usefulness of veratrum was limited by the side effect of nausea and vomiting. If it had been possible to titrate the dose to an effective antihypertensive level without producing the adverse effects, this would have been a valuable drug. Veratrum is a very physiological agent, since the reduction in pressure achieved with it is approximately the same in the supine as in the upright position. However, nausea and vomiting occur at about the same dose of the drug as does the antihypertensive effect, and therefore adequate antihypertensive doses cannot be attained.

Hydralazine

The blood pressure response to hydralazine (Apresoline) was greatest during the initial phase of dose titration (2). After a period of three months, tolerance frequently developed; consequently the rate of maintained response to hydralazine alone was rather low after continued use. Furthermore, in addition to these limitations, it has since been shown that doses in excess of 200 mg a day are more often associated with a lupus-like syndrome (hydralazine disease) than are lower doses. Therefore substantial reduction of the blood pressure with this drug can be anticipated less frequently than is indicated in Table 1. With the concurrent administration of a diuretic, however, the development of tolerance is greatly reduced.

Phenoxybenzamine

Factors limiting the use of phenoxybenzamine (Dibenzyline) were the marked orthostatic effect of the drug as compared to its effect in the supine position, and a related acute tachycardia in the upright position (3). Although phenoxybenzamine blocks the impulses carried by sympathetic nerve fibers to the blood vessel (Fig. 1), it does not block such impulses to the heart. Therefore, when the patient stands up and the blood pressure drops, there is a sharp reflex tachycardia together with excessive hypotension, which limits the usefulness of this drug.

PHARMACODYNAMICS AT THE NEUROEFFECTOR SITE OF THE BLOOD VESSEL

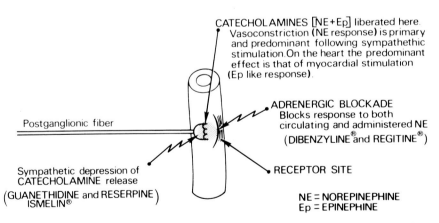

Fig. 1. General diagrammatic schema of the action of various groups of drugs that have become most useful today. It presents a concept of the sympathomimetic stimulation of the blood vessel and the modus operandi of such drugs as guanethidine and methyldopa, which reduce the availability of norepinephrine to the neuroeffector site as compared with phenoxybenzamine, which appears to block the ability of catecholamines to stimulate the blood vessel.

Ganglionic blocking agents

It can be seen from Table 1 that the ganglionic blocking agents such as hexamethonium, mecamylamine (Inversine), and pentolinium (Ansolysen) are quite potent antihypertensive agents (4, 5). However, as will be obvious in Table 2, their side effects are a limiting factor. These agents block the ganglia to the parasympathetic as well as to the sympathetic nervous system. The side effects resulting from the parasympathetic blockade become quite prohibitive, especially those caused by inhibition of the motor activities related to motility of the gastrointestinal tract, salivation, and focusing of the eyes. The antihypertensive response to the ganglionic blocking agents indicates that these agents are as potent as any drugs that are currently available and used with any regularity. Furthermore, tolerance to mecamylamine does not usually develop, and the antihypertensive effectiveness of this drug, which is completely absorbed from the gastrointestinal tract, is enhanced by the concurrent administration of diuretics. Unfortunately, gastrointestinal inhibition, even to the point of severe ileus, limits the value of this drug. Despite its potency as an antihypertensive agent, the side effects have led to its replacement by drugs which limit their activity to inhibition of the sympathetic nervous system.

Diuretics

Diuretics such as chlorothiazide are all about equally effective in doses of equivalent strength; when the various diuretics are compared, using the previously described criteria, the response rate is about 40−50% (Table 4). There seems to be no advantage of one diuretic over the other, and therefore chlorothiazide can be used as a prototype for comparison with other agents. When the diuretic is given in conjunction with rauwolfia, ganglionic blocking agents, methyldopa (Aldomet), or guanethidine (Ismelin)—whether used singly or in any of various combinations—it enhances the antihypertensive response to these sympathetic depressant drugs and therefore makes it possible to use smaller doses of them. This, in turn, reduces the incidence and severity of side effects. The diuretic, given concurrently, also reduces the incidence of tolerance that develops to the sympatholytic agent.

When guanethidine is given in combination with a diuretic, the limiting factor is the side effects rather than inability to obtain antihypertensive responsiveness with increased dosage. Variability of blood pressure response may limit the degree of dose titration that can be attempted. If the blood pressure is reduced too low during the day, excessive hypotension and syncope may occur, especially in the morning causing the patient to refuse medication. One advantage of guanethidine is that the entire dosage can be given in the morning, thus eliminating the need for giving divided doses throughout the day.

Side Effects

The incidence of side effects, using three drug programs as examples, is summarized in Table 2. Column 1 shows the percentage of patients experiencing various side effects while taking rauwolfia and chlorothiazide with the ganglionic blocking agent pentolinium; column 2 gives the same information concerning side effects related to guanethidine given with the diuretic chlorothiazide. It is quite obvious that the greatest progress that has been made since the days when drugs such as pentolinium and mecamylamine (i.e., ganglionic blocking agents) were the cornerstones of therapy has been in the area of reduction of side effects. As noted previously, the ganglionic blocking agents block the parasympathetic as well as the sympathetic nervous system. Contrariwise, blockade with guanethidine given alone or in combination with a diuretic is limited to the sympathetic component of the autonomic nervous system, as is apparently achieved with methyldopa also (Fig. 1). Therefore the incidence and severity of side effects is sharply reduced when guanethidine and chlorothiazide are given in combination,

Table 2. Side Effects with Various Antihypertensive Drugs and Drug Regimens (% of Number Treated)

Side effect	*Rauwolfia and chlorothiazide and pentolinium: 75 patients treated (%)*	*Guanethidine and chlorothiazide: 30 patients treated (%)*	*Alpha methyldopa: 38 patients treated (%)*
Nasal congestion	48	4	--
Constipation	36	--	--
Diarrhea	--	12	--
Weakness	32	40	8
Dizziness	32	12	--
Syncope	12	4	--
Increased appetite	20	--	--
Weight gain	12	--	--
Nausea and vomiting	4	--	--
Blurred vision	40	4	--
Impotence[a]	50	16	--
Failure of ejaculation[a]	--	36	--
Drowsiness	8	8	37[b]
Dry mouth	28	--	--
Anorexia	8	8	--
Photophobia	12	12	--
Urinary retention	4	--	--
Drug fever	--	--	8

a % of male patients only

b Temporary drowsiness; disappears with continued administration as compared to the ganglionic blocking agent, and this is true at equivalent antihypertensive doses. Methyldopa, although limited in potency as compared to guanethidine, is relatively free of side effects (Table 2).

Improvement of Symptoms

In Table 3 the improvement of symptoms related to hypertension is summarized. There appears to be very little difference related to the drug regimen in the relief of those symptoms. The important thing is the degree of blood pressure control obtained, and this would appear to be the principal determinant of symptomatic relief of the symptoms directly related to blood pressure elevation. This is in contrast to the incidence of side effects, which are directly related to the particular drug being administered. We can conclude from this observation that the important parameter in the treatment of hypertension is blood pressure reduction. If that can be achieved, then the symptoms related to blood pressure elevation are relieved.

Summary of Observations on Blood Pressure Response

The results of using some drugs that have been evaluated over the past 20 years for their effectiveness in controlling the blood pressure of patients with essential hypertension have been summarized. The following conclusions can be drawn:

1. The ganglionic blocking agents are potent antihypertensive medications and are about as potent as any agent available today for the reduction of blood pressure. The effectiveness of these agents is markedly enhanced by the addition of diuretic agents. The limiting factor in the use of these drugs is the high incidence of side effects attributable primarily to the parasympathetic blockade.

Table 3. Symptomatic Improvement with Various
Antihypertensive Drug Regimens (% of Number Treated)

Regimen	Angina	Heart failure	Headache	Retino-pathy
Rauwolfia and hexamethonium	77	81	72	76
Rauwolfia and pentolinium	77	65	78	59
Rauwolfia and mecamylamine	82	81	71	60
Rauwolfia and chlorothiazide and mecamylamine	73	96	80	82
Rauwolfia and chlorothiazide and pentolinium	67	91	77	75
Guanethidine and chlorothiazide	40	75	62	75

2. Drugs which are limited in their activity to depression of the sympathetic nervous system without involving the parasympathetic nervous system have allowed the therapist to reduce the blood pressure in hypertensive patients with a much lower incidence of side effects compared to those encountered with the ganglionic blocking agents. This characteristic has permitted significant improvement of treatment programs based on the current antihypertensive armamentarium.

3. Use of multiple drugs that depress the sympathetic nervous system, given in combination with diuretic agents, has increased the antihypertensive effectiveness of the therapeutic program and at the same time reduced the incidence of side effects. This in turn makes the successful treatment of hypertension an attainable goal.

4. The greatest achievement over the past eight years has been the availability of drugs and drug programs which are as effective as earlier drugs in reducing the blood pressure and which at the same time have a lesser incidence of side effects.

DISCUSSION

The results of studies on blood pressure response to diuretic drugs (which increase excretion of salt and water) and to drugs that decrease transmission of impulses over the sympathetic nervous system, given alone and in combination, indicate that effective modes of therapy are available for the treatment of hypertension. Although the ganglionic blocking agents used 15 or more years ago were quite potent antihypertensive agents, the incidence of side effects prohibits their use by the clinician who is not completely knowledgeable concerning the clinical pharmacology of these drugs. Recent advances have made available drugs whose pharmacodynamic effects are primarily limited to the sympathetic nervous system, permitting sharp reduction in the incidence of side effects.

Who Should Be Treated?

When should hypertension be treated? Many formulas have been devised over the years, but most specialists working actively in this field have concluded that the primary parameter is the degree of fixed diastolic blood pressure elevation. Therefore, for purposes of therapeutic simplicity, it would appear that the main factor to consider when deciding whether or not antihypertensive drug therapy is indicated, is the severity of diastolic hypertension. Obviously, the existence of vascular complications increases the urgency of the need for antihypertensive therapy. Equally obvious, however, is the fact that early therapy is preferable, before vascular damage has occurred, especially to large vessels supplying critical tissue beds.

Table 4. Comparison of Blood Pressure Response in Patients with Hypertension Given Various Oral Diuretics (% of Number Treated)

Drug (diuretic)	Dose/Day (mg)	No. of patients	Normotensive[a]		Significant response[b]	
			Supine (%)	Upright (%)	Supine (%)	Upright (%)
Chlorothiazide	1,000	50	18	24	36	46
Hydrochlorothiazide	100	54	20	22	39	39
Flumethiazide	1,000	17	12	47	41	53
Chlorthalidone	100–200	30	17	27	40	40
Quinethazone	100–200	29	17	24	41	41
Ethacrynic acid	150–400	15	7	20	53	53

[a] Normotensive: arterial pressure reduced to 140/90 mm Hg or less

[b] Significant response: mean arterial blood pressure reduced more than 20 mm Hg

Table 5. When Should Hypertension Be Treated?

1. Diastolic pressure above 105 mm Hg – age under 65 years

2. Diastolic pressure above 90 mm HG – men under 45 years, women under 35 years

3. Diastolic pressure above 90 mm HG – Negroes of any age, either sex

Referring to Table 5, the blood pressure should be evaluated carefully during a control period, and this then becomes the baseline blood pressure. On the basis of these observations, certain conclusions can be reached. In accordance with the observations of the Veterans Administration Cooperative Study Group (8), a diastolic pressure above 105 mm Hg is a definite indication for antihypertensive therapy. Pressures between 90 and 105 mm Hg are borderline hypertension. For patients in this category, most of the specialists working in the field have concluded that antihypertensive drug therapy is indicated, but the data supporting these conclusions are not absolutely incontrovertible. Therefore, for those patients who are especially prone to progressive vascular disease, it is my opinion that antihypertensive therapy should be implemented when the blood pressure elevation is in this range—particularly in Negroes, men of either the black or white race less than 45 years of age, or women less than 35 years of age. Naturally it is taken for granted that any surgically correctible causes of blood pressure elevation have been ruled out and that the patient has, in fact, bona fide essential hypertension.

Results of Therapy

The important parameter for measuring effectiveness of treatment of hypertension is the degree of blood pressure reduction, irrespective of the therapeutic program employed. When the blood pressure is well controlled, vascular deterioration is arrested and the prognosis is sharply improved. Figure 2 summarizes the mortality among patients with malignant hypertension, i.e., severe diastolic blood pressure elevation with papilledema, comparing effectively treated patients with those who received no antihypertensive drugs. In the group of untreated patients, the mortality at the end of five years was 100%, whereas in the group of treated patients the mortality was 25% (9). It was of interest, as recorded previously, that during the first two years most of those patients who died succumbed to progressive renal failure, whereas after the second year those treated patients who died succumbed to major vascular catastrophes associated with atherosclerotic disease, not from small vessel disease such as that seen in the patients with renal failure.

The results of treatment and five-year followup are summarized in Table 6. It is obvious that those whose hypertension prior to antihypertensive therapy was more severe did less well than those with milder hypertension, whether treated or untreated. However, for all grades of severity, when comparing comparable patients, the treated patients had a much improved outlook.

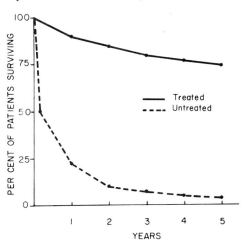

Fig. 2. Comparison of the mortality rate over a period of five years for treated and untreated patients with malignant hypertension. It can be seen that the mortality has been reduced by 75% in the group of patients receiving treatment. (Only patients on effective therapeutic programs were included in this study—e.g., diuretic plus ganglionic blocking agents, ganglionic blocking agents plus rauwolfia, or guanethidine plus methyldopa and a diuretic.) (Reprinted from Moyer, J. H., and Flynn, J. (9), by permission of J. B. Lippincott Co.)

278   J. H. Moyer

Table 6. Results of Treatment in 301 Patients[a]
(% of Total Number)

Pretreatment diastolic blood pressure (mm Hg)	Death in less than five years	
	Treated (%)	Untreated (%)
100 to 120	7	15
120 to 140	13	38
More than 140	19	59

[a] Only patients receiving effective drug therapy such as diuretics with ganglionic blocking agents or guanethidine and methyldopa, or ganglionic blocking agents with rauwolfia, or similar combinations were included in this study.

Planning the Therapeutic Program

In Figure 3 an attempt has been made to fit the various drugs into an overall comprehensive approach to the treatment of hypertension. The diuretics are the basis of all therapeutic programs. For more mildly hypertensive patients, methyldopa (Aldomet) or reserpine can be added to the diuretic. Generally speaking, those patients who need and accept a tranquilizer will do very well with a combination of diuretic and reserpine in this group with milder disease. However, executives and professional people do not tolerate rauwolfia very well; these people do better on a therapeutic program of methyldopa and the diuretic. One advantage of reserpine is that it can be used in a fixed dosage, whereas methyldopa has to be administered in a sequential dose titration, starting with 250 mg and increasing in 250 mg increments until the blood pressure is adequately regulated in the standing position.

Usually it has been my practice not to give methyldopa in doses exceeding 1500 mg per day (6 tablets). If the blood pressure response to the diuretic plus methyldopa (or diuretic plus reserpine) is not adequate in this group, then adjunctive medications may be added as indicated in columns 3, 4, and 5 of Figure 3. Hydralazine must be given by a dose titration procedure, usually starting with 10 to 12.5 mg per *dose*, three or four times a day as a rule—i.e., with each meal and at bedtime. If the response is not adequate, then the dose can be increased to 25 mg three or four times a day.

Hydralazine has a relatively short duration of action. Therefore, in treating those patients whose blood pressure tends to peak at some regular time during the day, the pressure can be controlled by the administration of hydralazine each day about two hours before the peak period, which allows for more even control of the blood pressure.

REGIMENS FOR THE MANAGEMENT OF UNCOMPLICATED HYPERTENSION

Severity Diastolic Blood Pressure (mm. Hg)	Mild (90 - 120)		Moderately Severe (121 - 140)	Severe (more than 140)
	Alternative #1	Alternative #2		
Initial Therapy	Diuretic	Diuretic	Diuretic	Diuretic plus Guanethidine
Supplemental Therapy - A	Reserpine	Methyldopa	Guanethidine	Methyldopa
Supplemental Therapy - B	Hydralazine	Hydralazine	Methyldopa	Hydralazine
Supplemental Therapy - C	Propranolol	Propranolol	Hydralazine plus Propranolol	Propranolol
Remarks	When Tranquilizer Indicated	—	—	Ganglionic Blockade If Necessary

Fig. 3. In this regimen schedule, "hydralazine plus propranolol" as indicated for moderately severe hypertension (Supplemental Therapy–C) does not necessarily mean that these must always be given together; for all degrees of hypertension, propranolol may be used to offset the cardiac effects of hydralazine and is occasionally beneficial when used with the other antihypertensive agents indicated, if tachycardia is a problem.

Propranolol is administered in a dose of 10 mg four times a day, increasing it in 10-mg increments at each dose until a total of 40 mg per dose has been reached. Doses in excess of this amount produce side effects which outweigh the therapeutic benefit of the propranolol. This drug has its effect primarily on the adrenergic receptors in the heart and therefore reduces tachycardia and blood pressure elevation related to a theoretical increase in cardiac output.

For patients with more severe disease, guanethidine (Ismelin) must usually be added to the therapeutic program, starting with a dose of 12.5 mg each morning and increasing it in 12.5-mg increments until adequate reduction in pressure is obtained. Although doses as high as 400 mg per day can be employed, the maximum daily dose usually does not exceed 150 mg. The side effects become quite significant when doses in excess of this amount are used, thus making it difficult to keep the patient on the drug. When a dose of 150 mg per day has been reached, it is usually best to maintain this dose along with a diuretic and add methyldopa in a sequential dose titration pretty much as indicated above. Other adjunctive drugs can be used as outlined under Alternative 1 (Fig. 3) and with essentially the same reasoning.

CONCLUSIONS

1. Effective antihypertensive drugs for reduction of blood pressure have been available for 20 years. More recently available drugs, although not more potent, have substantially fewer and less severe side effects and are therefore more practical to use as therapeutic agents.

2. When patients treated effectively for five years or more are compared with untreated patients, mortality is seen to be greatly reduced, irrespective of the therapeutic program employed. This is true of patients who previously had malignant hypertension as well as those with nonmalignant hypertension, who had diastolic blood pressure elevation of various grades of severity.

3. The effectiveness of any therapeutic program is determined by the degree of *sustained* blood pressure reduction that can be achieved. Long-term treatment can be undertaken successfully only if distressing side effects can be kept to a minimum and the development of tolerance avoided. This requires the careful working out of a program specifically adapted to the individual needs of the patient, both as to drugs employed and the dosage of each drug.

REFERENCES

1. Mills, L. C., and Moyer, J. H. 1952. The treatment of hypertension with orally and parenterally administered purified extracts of veratrum viride and a comparison with ganglionic (hexamethonium) and adrenergic blocking agents. A.M.A. Arch. Internal Med. 90:587.
2. Moyer, J. H. 1953. Hydralazine (Apresoline)–Pharmacological observations and clinical results in the treatment of hypertension. A.M.A. Arch. Internal Med. 91:419.
3. Miller, S. I., Ford, R. V., and Moyer, J. H. 1953. Dibenzyline–Results of therapy in patients with hypertension and a comparison with hexamethonium, 1-hydrazinophthalazine (Apresoline) and semi-purified extracts of veratrum. New Engl. J. Med. 248:576.
4. Moyer, J. H., Snyder, H. B., Johnson, I., Mills, L. C., and Miller, S. I. 1953. Results with oral hexamethonium alone and in combination with 1-hydrazinophthalazine (Apresoline) in the treatment of hypertension. Amer. J. Med. Sci. 225:379.
5. Moyer, J. H., and Brest, A. N. 1961. Drug therapy of hypertension: V. Observations on the results with ganglion blocking agents given in combination with rauwolfia and chlorothiazide. A.M.A. Arch. Internal Med. 108:231.
6. Brest, A. N., Novack, P., Kasparian, H., and Moyer, J. H. 1962. Guanethidine. Dis. Chest 42:359.
7. Brest, A. N., Onesti, G., Heider, C., Seller, R. H., and Moyer, J. H. 1964. Comparative effectiveness of pargyline as an antihypertensive agent. Amer. Heart J. 68:621.
8. Veterans Administration Cooperative Study Group on Antihypertensive Agents: Effects of treatment on morbidity in hypertension: Results in patients with diastolic blood pressures averaging 90 through 114 mm. Hg. 1970. J.A.M.A. 213:1143.
9. Moyer, J. H., and Flynn, J. 1971. Role of arterial hypertension in coronary atherosclerosis. Pages 137–145 in H. I. Russek and B. L. Zohman, eds. Coronary heart disease. Lippincott, Philadelphia.

A NEW PERSPECTIVE: THE RENIN-ALDOSTERONE SYSTEM IN ANALYSIS AND TREATMENT OF HYPERTENSIVE PATIENTS

JOHN H. LARAGH

The renin-angiotensin-aldosterone system is now understood to play a vital role in regulation of electrolyte and blood pressure homeostasis. In the past twelve years, it has been shown that a derangement of the hormonal system is critically involved in the pathogenesis of malignant hypertension (1−3) and possibly in renovascular hypertension (4) as well as in the pressor consequences of primary aldosteronism and of oral contraceptive usage (5,6). However, these conditions represent the more egregious hypertensive states in which abnormalities of renin-aldosterone are the more easily demonstrated, and altogether these disturbances comprise only a small portion of the large hypertensive population.

The role of the renin-angiotensin-aldosterone axis in the pathogenesis and natural history of so-called essential hypertension remains unsettled. The investigations to date, while not altogether in agreement, have most often reported normal aldosterone excretion in these patients. However, certain abnormal features have been described such as a failure of normal suppression of aldosterone with sodium loading (7) or a failure of aldosterone to increase normally with sodium deprivation (8). On the other hand, more convincing abnormalities in plasma renin activity have been reported so that while this measurement is normal in the majority of these patients, in significant fractions it may be either subnormal (8−15) or abnormally increased (9,10).

Two new approaches led my group to believe that more subtle associations might be exposed between renin and aldosterone and the etiology and natural history of that large group of patients now necessarily classified under the cognomen of essential hypertension. One was the availability of sensitive isotope dilution and radioimmunoassay methods permitting coincident and reliable quantitative measurements of the various components of the system; the other was the broader application of an approach to the definition of normalcy which relates a normal value to a dynamic index of salt balance.

Accordingly, in this chapter, I would like to first consider the methodology that we have employed and its validation. The second part will consider the application of these criteria to the study of more than 200 patients who presented with essential hypertension. In these studies we have also related plasma renin activity to aldosterone excretion values, first to determine whether the dynamic relationships between the two hormones were similar to those of the normal control subjects. Second, it was hoped that deviations in these relationships might permit the perception of abnormal subpopulations in the patient group. Finally, we have looked at various clinical correlates to see whether deviations in natural history of the disease might be meaningfully related to demonstrable abnormalities in hormonal patterns. This could mean that "profiling" of hypertensive patients with respect to renin and aldosterone patterns could have broad application not only to understanding but also for forecasting prognosis and for determining when and how to treat these patients.

ANALYTICAL METHODS

We are now extremely pleased with our analytical methods which have been many years in development. Plasma renin activity is measured by a sensitive and specific radioimmunoassay procedure which quantitates the angiotensin I produced during incubation. This method is reproducible to ± 12% (SD), permits processing of many samples, and is highly sensitive (16). The procedure is inherently simpler than most others since EDTA, which is added in collection of blood, performs three functions; anticoagulation, angiotensinase inhibition, and converting enzyme blockade. These latter two effects are exploited by incubating at the pH optimum of 5.7 for renin. At the same time this provides the greatest possible sensitivity and precision, features especially important in studying low-renin patients. Moreover, since our method involves no extractions there is no chance for losses to occur during analysis.

Commercial kits are now available which attempt to simplify plasma renin activity measurements. These kits have some value for learning purposes. But if the procedure is to become routine we recommend the purchase of a large and therefore uniform source of antibody and the separate purchase of freshly prepared iodinated angiotensin I; the latter should be purified by use of the fourth column described by Gocke et al. (18).

Aldosterone excretion ratio is also measured by double isotope dilution (17) and more recently, by radioimmunoassay (19). Metabolism ward procedures and analytic methods for measuring plasma and urine electrolytes, and blood urea nitrogen have also been described previously (20).

CRITERIA FOR NORMAL VALUES

Our first approach to the problem of establishing normal values was the development of a nomogram for both renin activity and aldosterone secretion as related to sodium excretion over a wide range of physiological variation. Such a nomogram permits more precise definition of normalcy than does the traditional bracketed range approach, because each value of a hypertensive patient can be related to similar values obtained from normal subjects at precisely the same rate of sodium excretion.

Normal values were defined by submitting normal volunteers to the same dietary regimens utilized in the hypertensive patients. Some of the normal volunteers were studied while housed on the metabolic ward, others were not hospitalized but received a constant dietary regimen in the metabolic kitchen, and a third group was on unrestricted diets. As seen in Figure 1, irrespective of the dietary control, a close relationship exists between the rate of sodium excretion and both plasma renin activity and aldosterone excretion. Particularly in the case of aldosterone excretion, there appears to be no difference in the values obtained whether or not dietary intake is rigidly controlled. In the case of plasma renin activity, occasional values appear inappropriately high in patients not under dietary control. However, no subjects eating random diets exhibited inappropriately low values. Therefore, under most situations the 24-hour urinary

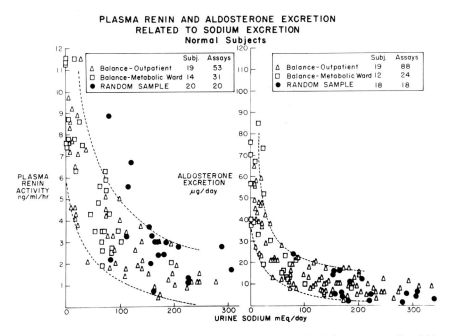

Fig. 1. Relation of both noon plasma renin activity and of the corresponding 24-hr urinary excretion of aldosterone to the concurrent daily rate of sodium excretion. For these normal subjects, the data describe a similar dynamic hyperbolic relationship between each hormone and sodium excretion. Of note is the fact that subjects studied on random diets outside of the hospital exhibited similar relationships, a finding which validates the use of this nomogram in studying out-patients of subjects not receiving constant diets.

sodium excretion rate can be used as an indicator in determining normalcy of the hormonal activity, even when dietary intake is not rigidly controlled.

Certain theoretical considerations also support the validity of relating these hormonal activities to the 24-hour rate of sodium excretion. Since the kidney is the major route through which sodium is normally eliminated, the daily rate of sodium excretion obviously reflects the extent to which the kidney is being directed to either retain or release sodium. The hormonal activity is thus linked to the target organ response rather than to changes in the homeostatic function which probably is subserved, i.e., sodium balance.

One might think it most appropriate to relate changes in hormonal activity to changes in overall balance, since changes in the latter probably initiate the hormonal responses and sodium balance is probably the homeostatic function which the system is designed to regulate. In fact, however, this approach is not only more laborious, but the errors inherent in measurement and calculation of balance make it a relatively insensitive index as compared with measurement of daily urinary sodium excretion. In fact, when balance is measured there is a lag of as much as three days between changes in balance and the final adjustment of the renin-aldosterone system (19).

Also, it is more meaningful to relate changes in renin and aldosterone activity to sodium output rather than to the dietary intake, since serial daily studies have revealed that changes in renin and aldosterone activity closely follow changes in sodium excretion rate even before equilibrium is achieved (18). From a technical standpoint too, sodium output from day to day is more readily monitorable than is dietary intake. This approach has the additional advantage of being applicable to the study of out-patients on random diets.

The nomographic index presented in Figure 1 clearly shows the continuum of the interrelationships. The need for a continuous index of this sort is underlined by the hyperbolic shape of the curve. Thus, a small change in sodium excretion at a high level of hormone activity involves a greater hormone response than a similar change at other levels. This phenomenon might be completely overlooked in the bracketed ranges in traditional usage. In this way, it has been possible to classify our patients more accurately into low, normal, and high renin groups over a wide range of salt balance.

In Figure 1, the renin values appear to inscribe a broader normal range than aldosterone. This is partially, at least, an illusion because if the scale on the ordinate is either reduced for renin or stretched out for aldosterone, the curves become similar. Even then, however, renin values have a slightly greater spread, perhaps because they reflect only one point in time, whereas the aldosterone measurement is an integrated reflection of the day's secretion.

These results suggest certain guidelines which should be observed in the classification of patients with essential hypertension. Thus it is apparent that the high renin patients may not be detected if they are studied when on a low salt diet. Also, in patients studied when the urinary sodium excretion is above 150 mEq/day, it may be difficult to identify those with subnormal plasma renin activity. If only one point on the curve is available for classification of a patient, the sample should probably be collected when the urinary sodium excretion is between 40 and 100 mEq/day. To accomplish this we have developed a simple dietary instruction sheet which the patient uses for about a week before the 24-hour urine collection is made.

RESULTS

Patterns of Plasma Renin Activity, Aldosterone and Sodium Excretion in Uncomplicated Essential Hypertension

Table 1 presents a breakdown of the frequency of abnormalities occurring in an unselected population of patients with benign essential hypertension. All patients had diastolic blood pressures greater than 95 mm Hg determined on three separate occasions.

A total of 146 patients were admitted to the metabolic ward and evaluated on the fifth day of a fixed dietary regimen. Most were studied on two or more different levels of constant sodium intake. Renin activity was measured in samples collected at noon, after the patients were ambulatory for about four hours (1). The excretion of the acid labile conjugate of aldosterone was estimated in a 24-hour urine specimen collected on the same day (17,18). Another 73 patients were studied in the outpatient department. Antihypertensive and diuretic drugs were withdrawn for at least three weeks prior to a study and a normal diet was prescribed. Known causes of hypertension were excluded by a workup which included intravenous pyelography and, often, renal angiography. Patients with malignant hypertension, congestive heart failure, or evidence of parenchymal renal disease were also excluded.

Table 1. Hormonal Patterns and Their Frequency in Essential Hypertension

Renin		Aldosterone	
Low	27%	Low	5–8%
		Normal	13–21%
		High	1–2%
Normal	57%	Low	2–6%
		Normal	36–54%
		High	3–6%
High	16%	Low	–
		Normal	8–12%
		High	6–9%

At first, the results of the outpatients were separated from those of the inpatients. However, the distribution of abnormalities was quite similar in both groups. This fact, together with the previously mentioned studies indicating that the results obtained in normal subjects maintained either on controlled regimens or random diets did not differ, permitted pooling of the data.

Classification of Patients

In classifying patients into low, normal, or high renin categories, two problems should be recognized. First, one must consider that the renin status of the patients might vary with time. This has not yet been observed in preliminary longitudinal studies of patients re-evaluated at intervals of one to three years. Second, it is possible that the renin status might change with sodium intake so that it would be normal at one level and abnormal at another. In fact, a minor fraction (about 10%) of the patients do exhibit this latter phenomenon, but even in these, classification was usually not difficult since one or two of the values were clearly normal or abnormal with the inconsistent result located in a borderline area.

Since abnormal categories were defined by purely quantitative differences, one cannot necessarily presume the existence of three qualitatively different homogeneous groups. Indeed, it is possible that the hypertensive patients could, in fact, represent more or less than three different populations, with or without some overlap in the borderline zones. However, one large but continuous and homogeneous population seems quite unlikely since large group deviations from the normal range appear both on the high and the low side. Thus, using this approach, we have found that 57% of the hypertensive population exhibited normal plasma renin activity, 27% were low, and 16% were abnormally high (Table 1). A problem arises in attempting to classify these patients further according to their corresponding aldosterone measurements since, unlike plasma renin activity, aldosterone excretion rates are more apt to move from an abnormal category to a normal category or vice versa depending on the particular state of sodium balance as indicated by the urinary sodium excretion. For this reason, ranges are given for the frequency of abnormalities in aldosterone excretion as shown on the right hand side of Table 1. These ranges reflect the two extremes of variation. The minimum value in each instance is an estimate developed from the application of "strict" criteria. "Strict" criteria mean that the patient consistently exhibited a particular hormonal pattern regardless of sodium excretion. The higher value in each case is an estimate of the frequency distribution based on "loose" criteria. Using "loose" criteria, all patients were included in a particular category who exhibited the hormonal pattern either consistently or inconsistently.

The tendency for some low-renin patients to be inconsistent in maintaining a given normal or abnormal category with respect to their aldosterone secretion is

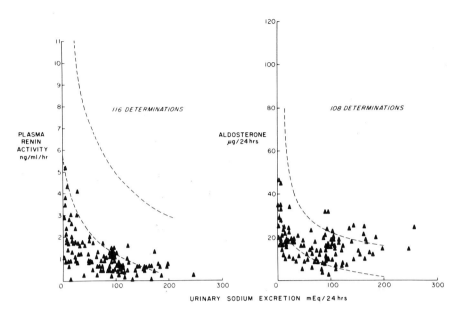

Fig. 2. Low-renin essential hypertension, 59 patients. Noon plasma renin activity and the corresponding daily aldosterone excretion in relation to the concurrent daily rate of sodium excretion. This subgroup of essential hypertension is the one which seems to have a better prognosis. These patients are relatively protected from the development of heart attacks or strokes.

illustrated in Figure 2, where renin and aldosterone data for all patients of the "low-renin" type are plotted against urinary excretion. In this particular group, aldosterone excretion appears normal or high when sodium excretion is greater than 90 mEq/day. However, in the same patients aldosterone excretion is often below normal when the urinary sodium excretion falls below 40 mEq/day. In other words, the aldosterone excretion response to changes in sodium excretion may differ from normal so that the hormone can appear to be relatively unresponsive to both extremes of sodium balance. These unresponsive characteristics of the aldosterone secretory response have been noted by others during sodium loading (7) and sodium deprivation (8). However, in the present study our two- or three-point analyses of individuals indicate that those in this low-renin group are not homogeneous in their secretory responses. Thus, the majority of patients exhibited normal percentage changes in renin in relation to sodium balance. However, three different types of aldosterone response were noted: 1) a normal response, 2) a blunted change in percentage, and 3) a virtual absence of response. The fixed behavior or autonomy of adrenal cortex in the latter group might suggest primary or pseudo-primary (hyperplasia) aldosteronism. However, in primary aldosteronism high aldosterone excretion is associated with hypokalemia and removal of the adrenal adenoma usually cures the hypertension. In contrast, the low renin essential hypertensive patients usually exhibit normal aldosterone excretion rates. However, in certain respects, this group resembles patients with pseudo-primary aldosteronism who are also usually normokalemic (21,22).

Interrelationships Between Renin Activity, Aldosterone Excretion, and Sodium Excretion in Normal and Hypertensive Subjects

Figure 3 attempts to depict the interaction of the three interdependent variables: plasma renin activity, aldosterone excretion, and urinary sodium excretion. The circles represent the values derived from 42 normal volunteers. The squares are values from 36 patients with high renin essential hypertension, and the triangles represent values from 59 patients with low renin essential hypertension. It is possible that this method of classification may uncover additional or dimensionally different abnormal groups since three variables determine the final position. In fact, in the low renin group of our initial analysis, four patients who were difficult to classify could be definitely separated into an abnormal zone by the application of this analysis. This was

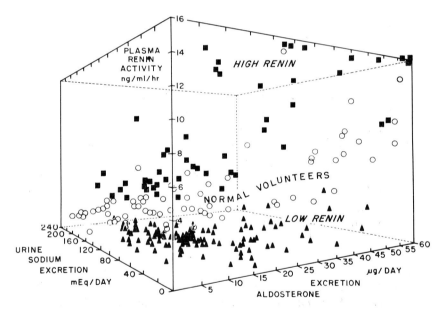

Fig. 3. Three dimensional plot of the relationship between concurrent measurements of plasma renin activity, aldosterone excretion, and urinary sodium excretion. The *open circles* are normal subjects. The *triangles* are patients with low-renin hypertension and the *squares* are high-renin patients. The plot, by introducing the strength of the third variable (aldosterone), may aid in classifying patients with borderline renin abnormalities.

attributable to the strength of the aldosterone value in determining the final position. This analysis is difficult to visualize on paper and practical application requires construction of a three dimensional model or a computer analysis for introduction of other variables such as blood pressure and the state of potassium balance.

Clinical Correlates of Renin Subgroups

An analysis of the clinical features and natural history of these patients with essential hypertension indicates that the biochemical deviations have meaningful clinical correlates. The evidence supporting this is based on both a retrospective and prospective follow-up of 219 patients studied over the last five years.

The mean ages of patients with low renin (46) and high renin (43) hypertension did not differ significantly but those with normal renin activity were significantly younger (37.5 years). There were, however, no differences in the known duration of hypertension between any of the groups, with the average being seven years.

There was a significantly greater incidence of black patients of 42% in the low renin group as compared to only 24% in the normal renin group and 11% in the high renin categories. These results tend to confirm the impression that low renin hypertension is relatively more common in blacks (11,12).

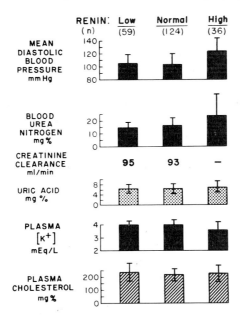

Fig. 4. Mean diastolic blood pressures and clinical biochemical features of the three renin subtypes of essential hypertension.

Figure 4 presents relevant clinical data for the three subgroups. Of note are the findings that both the mean diastolic pressure and blood urea nitrogen were significantly higher, while the plasma potassium was significantly lower in the high renin patients as compared to the other two groups. All other routine indicators showed no significant differences including plasma uric acid, plasma cholesterol, and fasting blood sugars (not shown). It is of some interest to note that there were no significant differences between the degree of diastolic hypertension or the blood urea nitrogen-plasma potassium or plasma cholesterol levels in the normal and low renin groups. However, perhaps as one might expect, the more severe hypertension with a tendency to azotemia and hypo-kalemia in the high renin group was also accompanied by a greater incidence of grade II and III retinopathy and of proteinuria.

Cardiovascular Complications in the Three Subgroups

Left ventricular hypertrophy as defined by electrocardiographic and roentgeno-graphic criteria occurred with fairly equal frequency in the three renin sub-groups, with the incidences ranging from 15–22%. However, a most striking difference emerges from this analysis. A complete absence of the occurrence of heart attack or stroke among the patients with low renin essential hypertension was recorded. In contrast, these complications occurred with a frequency of 11–14% in the normal and high renin groups respectively. The complete absence of either strokes or heart attacks in low renin essential hypertension is highly significant; statistical analysis of the results indicates that the highest possible incidence of such events in a low renin hypertensive population at large would be 4.9% (5% confidence limits).

In Figure 5 all the measurements are presented of plasma renin activity in 19 patients of the study who suffered either a stroke or heart attack or both at some time before or after the measurement was made. It can be seen that all of the values fall into the normal range or high range. The one value in the suppressed renin area is that from a patient who, on another occasion, had a clearly normal value for plasma renin activity of 1.8 ng/ml/hr when the urinary sodium excretion was 163 mEq/day. Both of these values are depicted as open circles. Thus, this one patient did not conform consistently to the pattern of low renin hypertension since the other value was well within the normal limits.

The high incidence of blacks in the low renin hypertension group perhaps seems to present a paradox. That low renin essential hypertension previously, and in the present studies, has been found to be relatively common in black populations (11,12) seems difficult to reconcile with the high incidence of malignant and severe hypertension in blacks. Also, strokes and heart attacks are certainly well recognized complications of hypertensive disease in black popula-tions. The answer to this seeming paradox may lie in the fact that hypertension as such is much more common in the black population. Indeed, in a recent

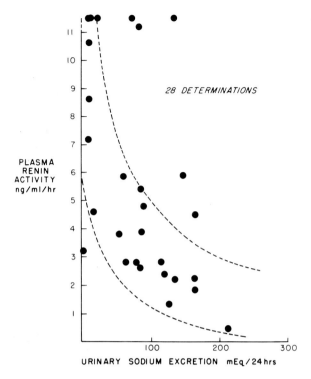

Fig. 5. Plasma renin activity of 19 hypertensive patients who, either before or after the measurement, suffered a documented myocardial infarction or stroke or both. See text for explanation of symbols. Note that all of such patients exhibited either a normal or an elevated plasma renin activity. Accordingly, to date, no low-renin patients have been observed to develop these cardiovascular complications.

report (23) the black population in the inner city of Washington, D.C. had an approximately 50% incidence of hypertension. The low incidence of blacks (11%) observed in the high renin group of the present study may simply be caused by the fact that patients with malignant hypertension have been excluded from the study, and it is conceivable that black patients with high renin essential hypertension are more prone to develop malignant hypertension.

Renin as a Risk Factor

In some previous studies of renin and aldosterone in essential hypertension, the values were not always related to an index of sodium balance. No matter how precise the method of measurement, the physiological meaning of such measurements remains uncertain.

The data presented here describe and provide validation for an analysis of variations in the activity of two hormones, renin and aldosterone. The approach is based on the fact that both hormones fluctuate continuously according to the daily rate of salt excretion by the kidneys, and aldosterone is used as an indicator of balance. This procedure is simpler, more reliable than complete balance studies, and can be applied to the evaluation of outpatients on random diets.

Using nomograms of hormonal behavior, it has been possible to define more precisely various subgroups of patients with essential hypertension in which renin or aldosterone is abnormally low or high. Moreover, these renin subgroups have been shown to have clinical relevance. Accordingly, this approach appears useful for identifying qualitative differences among patients designated as essential hypertensives.

In patients with essential hypertension, abnormalities in plasma renin are more consistent at all levels of sodium excretion than are abnormalities in aldosterone excretion. That is to say, patients with defects in renin activity demonstrate their defect at various levels of sodium excretion so that in general the slope of their response, while not always parallel to the norm, is shifted below or above normal. In particular, some patients with low renin essential hypertension exhibit normal aldosterone excretion at intermediate levels of sodium excretion but move out of the normal zone, at either the high or low extremes. Thus, the aldosterone secretory behavior of this group is variably unresponsive, or viewed in another way, the endocrine response of some has quite a different slope from the normal.

It was found that the normal renin patients exhibit an entirely normal aldosterone secretory response. Accordingly, it may prove appropriate to retain the term "essential hypertension" only for this normal renin, normal aldosterone group in which no abnormalities are yet identifiable.

Perhaps the strongest validation for the approaches used herein has been the associated survey of the clinical features and natural history of 219 patients with essential hypertension (10). Of particular note is the observation that no heart attacks or strokes have yet been observed in 59 patients with low renin essential hypertension. This finding, if it can be confirmed in prospective studies and with larger numbers, could have important implications for understanding pathogenesis and planning therapeutic strategy.

These observations may also go a long way in explaining the fact that certain hypertensive patients tolerate remarkably high blood pressures for prolonged periods of time. Moreover, it should be pointed out that the benign nature of low renin essential hypertension is similar to the usually benign nature of primary aldosteronism (1–3), another condition in which renin is similarly suppressed (6,21,24).

In contrast to the low renin group, hypertensive patients with normal or high renin exhibited a significant incidence of cardiovascular complications. These findings are in keeping with vasculotoxic effects of renin which have already been implicated as a mechanism of severe vasculitis in human malignant hypertension, a situation in which renin and aldosterone are both markedly increased (2,3). In malignant hypertension, it is likely that a vicious cycle develops, characterized by inappropriate release of excesses of renin into the circulation as a result of renal damage. Renin then induces more angiotensin, more aldosterone, and more hypertension, leading in turn to more renal damage. The system cannot be compensated because the target organ, the kidney, cannot respond appropriately to the hormonal signals. The idea that these two hormones together, present in excess, are involved in the vasculitis of this syndrome is supported by animal experiments in which simultaneous excesses of renin and aldosterone induce vasculitis (25). Altogether such observations raise the possibility that renin, in milder excess, with or without aldosterone participation, might play a role in more slowly developing vascular damage of hypertensive disease. In this context, further studies may also be needed to determine whether renin abnormalities are similarly related to vascular disease, heart attacks, and strokes in the normotensive population.

Renin Measurements and Therapeutic Strategy

These studies in defining nonhomogeneity of patients traditionally classified as essentially hypertensive at the same time indicate that the patients classified into different renin subgroups may have quite a different prognosis. These results indicate that, given two equally hypertensive individuals the one with a normal or high plasma renin ought to be treated sooner and more vigorously than the one with a low plasma renin level.

Thus, when measured under appropriate circumstances plasma renin levels can be used as a risk factor, useful for deciding when and how intensively antihypertensive drug therapy should be applied. However, in using renin measurements as a determinant of prognosis, a realistic approach is required. It already appears that renin measurements are probably a more relevant and more meaningful guide than traditional risk factors (i.e., tobacco, hyperlipidemia, obesity). At the same time a low plasma renin level does not per se confer immortality on a hypertensive patient. Our data simply indicate that such patients are at much less risk for heart attack and stroke than are similar normal and high renin patients. Therefore it still behooves the conscientious physician to evaluate the total clinical problem in planning treatment and to consider all other risk factors as they apply to the individual patient.

Such hormonal profiling may not only be useful in forecasting prognosis and for deciding when to treat, but it may also have great value in planning how to apply antihypertensive drug therapy. Thus recent reports (26) indicate that all of the various antihypertensive drugs have different and specific effects on the renin system. It therefore seems possible and likely that in the application of these drugs, the selection of agents that can correct the renin abnormalities might produce a more specific blood pressure response and a better prognosis. This promising approach could develop new criteria for more rational drug therapy, specifically "tailored" to correct the abnormal biochemical profiles.

In this vein, a recent study (27) indicates that those patients with low renin essential hypertension respond best to volume depletion therapy with either a sulfonamide diuretic (chlorthalidone 100 mg o.d.) or an aldosterone blocker (spironolactone 50 mg b.i.d.). Either of these agents given alone is sufficient to normalize the blood pressure in more than half of these low renin patients, with another sizeable fraction being greatly improved.

On the other hand, patients with high renin forms of hypertension (malignant hypertension, renovascular and renal hypertension, high renin essential hypertension) have been found to respond uniquely to propranolol (28). Moreover, the effectiveness of this agent was shown to be directly related to the degree of elevation of control plasma renin levels and to the degree to which renin secretion was reduced by the drug.

Thus antihypertensive drugs of this type can be used to both identify and treat renin-dependent forms of hypertensive disease. Propranolol is also effective in some patients with normal renin essential hypertension. In contrast, however, the drug is quite ineffective and may be contraindicated in low renin essential hypertension since its negative inotropic action on the heart is not accompanied by a pressure drop so that heart failure can be induced.

For those residual hypertensive patients requiring combination drug therapies, more work is required to define the effects of these regimens—for example, blood pressure responses in relation to the renin system. However, the future is bright. Indeed, hormonal profiling promises to provide a basis for simplified individualized and more rational treatment programs for the vast majority of hypertensive patients.

REFERENCES CITED

1. Laragh, J. H., Ulick, S., Januszewicz, W., Deming, Q. B., Kelly, W. G., and Lieberman, S. 1960. Aldosterone secretion and primary and malignant hypertension. J. Clin. Invest. 39:1091.
2. Laragh, J. H., Angers, M., Kelly, W. G., and Lieberman, S. 1960. Hypotensive agents and pressor substances. The effect of epinephrine, norepinephrine, angiotensin II and others on the secretory rate of aldosterone in man. J.A.M.A. 174:234.
3. Laragh, J. H. 1960. The role of aldosterone in man: evidence for regulation of electrolyte balance and arterial pressure by renal-adrenal system which may be involved in malignant hypertension. J.A.M.A. 174:293.
4. Dustan, H. P., Tarazi, R. C., and Frohlich, E. D. 1970. Functional correlates of plasma renin activity in hypertensive patients. Circulation 41:555.
5. Newton, M. A., Sealey, J. E., Ledingham, J. G. G., and Laragh, J. H. 1968. High blood pressure and oral contraceptives. Changes in plasma renin and renin substrate and in aldosterone excretion. Amer. J. Obstet. Gynec. 101:1037.
6. Laragh, J. H., Cannon, P. J., and Ames, R. P. 1963. Aldosterone secretion and various forms of hypertensive cascular disease. Ann. Internal Med. 59:117.

7. Luetscher, J. A., Weinberger, M. H., Dowdy, A. J., Nokes, G. W., Balikian, H., Brodie, A., and Willoughby, S. 1969. Effects of sodium loading, sodium depletion and posture on plasma aldosterone concentration and renin activity in hypertensive patients. J. Clin. Endocr. 29:1310.

8. Weinberger, M. H., Dowdy, A. J., Nokes, G. W., and Luetscher, J. A. 1968. Plasma renin activity and aldosterone secretion in hypertensive patients during high and low sodium intake and administration of diuretic. J. Clin. Endocr. 28:359.

9. Ledingham, J. G. G., Bull, M. B., and Laragh, J. H. 1967. The meaning of aldosterone in hypertensive disease. Circ. Res. 20 and 21 (Suppl. II):177.

10. Brunner, H. R., Laragh, J. H., Buhler, F. R., and Baer, L. 1972. Essential hypertension: renin and aldosterone, heart attack and stroke. New Engl. J. Med. 286:441.

11. Helmer, O. M. 1964. Renin activity in blood from patients with hypertension. Canad. Med. Assoc. J. 90:221.

12. Creditor, M. C., and Loschky, U. K. 1967. Plasma renin activity in hypertension. Amer. J. Med. 43:371.

13. Jose, A., Crout, J. R., and Kaplan, N. M. 1970. Suppressed plasma renin activity in essential hypertension: roles of plasma volume, blood pressure, and sympathetic nervous system. Ann. Internal Med. 72:9.

14. Fishman, L. M., Kuchel, O., Liddle, G. W., Michelakis, A. M., Gordon, R. D., and Chick, W. T. 1968. Incidence of primary aldosteronism in uncomplicated "essential" hypertension. J.A.M.A. 205:497.

15. Kaneko, Y., Ikeda, T., Takeda, T., Inoue, G., Tagawa, H., and Ueda, H. 1968. Renin release in patients with benign essential hypertension. Circulation 38:353.

16. Sealey, J. E., Gerten-Banes, J., and Laragh, J. H. 1972. The renin system: variations in man measured by radioimmunoassay or bioassay. Kidney International 1:240.

17. Laragh, J. H., Sealey, J. E., and Sommer, S. C. 1966. Patterns of adrenal secretion and urinary excretion of aldosterone and plasma renin activity in normal and hypertensive subjects. Circ. Res. 19 (Suppl. I):158.

18. Gocke, D. J., Gerten, J., Sherwood, L. M., and Laragh, J. H. 1969. Physiological and pathological variations of plasma angiotensin II in man. Circ. Res. 24, 25 (Suppl. I): 131.

19. Sealey, J. E., Buhler, F. R., Laragh, J. H., Manning, E. L., and Brunner, H. R. 1972. Aldosterone excretion: physiologic variations in man measured by radioimmunoassay or double isotope dilution. Circ. Res. 31:367.

20. Heinemann, H. O., Demartini, F. E., and Laragh, J. H. 1959. The effect of chlorothiazide on renal excretion of electrolytes and free water. Amer. J. Med. 26:853.

21. Baer, L., Sommers, S. C., Krakoff, L. R., Newton, M. A., and Laragh, J. H. 1970. Pseudo-primary aldosteronism: an entity distinct from true primary aldosteronism. Circ. Res. 26, 27 (Suppl. I):203.

22. Baer, L., Brunner, H. R., Buhler, F. R., and Laragh, J. H. 1972. Pseudo-primary aldosteronism, a variant of low-renin essential hypertension. In J. Genest and E. Koiw, eds. Hypertension 1972, p. 459. Springer, Berlin, New York.

23. Finnerty, F. A. 1971. Hypertension is different in blacks. J.A.M.A. 216:1634.

24. Conn, J. W. 1964. Plasma renin activity in primary aldosteronism. Importance in differential diagnosis and in research of essential hypertension. J.A.M.A. 190:134.

25. Masson, G. M. C., Mikasa, A., and Yasuda, H. 1962. Experimental vascular disease elicited by aldosterone and renin. Endocrinology 71:505.

26. Laragh, J. H., Baer, L., Brunner, H. R., Buhler, F. R., Sealey, J. E., and Vaughan, E. D., Jr. 1972. Renin, angiotensin and aldosterone system in pathogenesis and management of hypertensive vascular disease. Amer. J. Med. 52:633.

27. Vaughan, E. D., Jr., Buhler, F. R., Gavras, I., Brunner, H. R., Baer, L., and Laragh, J. H. 1972. Spirolactone compared to diuretic therapy in analysis and treatment of normal and low renin hypertensions. Circulation 66 (Suppl. II):83.

28. Buhler, F. R., Laragh, J. H., Baer, L., Vaughan, E. D., Jr., and Brunner, H. R. 1972. Propranolol inhibition of renin secretion: a specific approach to diagnosis and treatment of renin-dependent hypertensive diseases. N. Engl. J. Med. 287:1209.

Disorders of Cardiac Rhythm

PROGRESS IN THE PREVENTION OF
SUDDEN CARDIAC DEATH

PETER L. FROMMER

To discuss the prevention of sudden cardiac death, we must first define it. Then, after considering the population involved, premonitory symptoms, pathology and pathophysiology, we can discuss possible prophylactic therapy and the delivery of this therapy.

DEFINITION

For the purposes of this discussion, I propose a very broad definition of sudden cardiac death as death attributable to a primary cardiac cause or mechanism occurring within 24 hours of the onset of acute symptoms in a person who has symptomatically mild cardiac disease or who is thought to be free of it. This is a rather all-encompassing definition. For most analyses, it becomes important to identify specific subsets of this group.

The 24-hour upper limit may be very useful for some epidemiologic purposes, but if one is interested in pathophysiology, one probably wants to look differently at the group dying almost instantly from the group dying 12–24 hours after the onset of symptoms. Similarly, if one is considering very early therapy and emergency care systems, the differentiation may become important between instantaneous therapy and delays of five minutes, 15 minutes, one hour, and longer.

A rather simple and pragmatic time frame that is often used is equating sudden death with death before hospitalization, generally limiting it to deaths occurring within 24 hours of the onset of symptoms.

Implicit in any of these definitions involving time is the assumption that the onset of acute illness can be defined precisely. Often, this is not the case. Consider, for example, the man who had chest discomfort, nausea, and weakness for five minutes, then felt completely well and resumed his normal activities for two hours, only to drop dead within a minute after complaining of renewed chest pain. Did he die within one minute after the onset of acute illness, or did he die two hours after the onset? There is obviously a need for defining what constitutes "the acute illness."

"Unexpectedness" is implicit to some physicians in the definition of sudden cardiac death; to others it is explicit. Unfortunately, unexpectedness is very difficult to define. Is it an increased risk for death by a factor of five, or ten, or what? Was it unexpected by the patient, his physician, his wife? Because of this vagueness and potential confusion, "unexpectedness" is excluded from the definition.

The basis for attributing a sudden death to a primary cardiac cause or mechanism and the certainty of this conclusion warrant consideration. Data from medical examiners show that, in adults, sudden death is caused by cardiac factors in an overwhelming proportion of instances unless there are clinical circumstances suggesting a different etiology. Indeed, the more one narrows the time limit from 24 hours to shorter periods, the higher the cardiac incidence. It exceeds 90% for deaths occurring within one hour in persons for whom reasonable history of the immediate events is available. In medical examiners' series other causes for sudden medical deaths include fatty liver, stroke, pneumonia, pulmonary embolism, gastrointestinal bleeding, and drugs. Of sudden cardiac deaths in adults, more than 90% are associated with and apparently caused by arteriosclerotic heart disease. Although they account for only a small fraction of the sudden cardiac deaths, the list of other causes is long and interesting, and contains some pathophysiologically important subsets—for example, aortic stenosis, hereditary and infectious cardiomyopathies, other forms of cardiomyopathy, rheumatic heart disease, cor pulmonale, cyanotic heart disease, and the toxic manifestations of therapeutic drugs.

The certainty of the diagnosis warrants consideration. Is there autopsy evidence of an acute cardiac process? Is there an autopsy showing chronic arteriosclerotic heart disease with no acute process but with no other cause for death? Is there no autopsy, but convincing laboratory or electrocardiographic evidence of an acute cardiac process? Is it the best clinical diagnosis based on a good history? Or is it simply a wastebasket diagnosis?

THE POPULATION INVOLVED

Emphasis is placed on these varied definitions, implications, and criteria to call attention to their variety and to their importance in any discussion of sudden cardiac death. Other highly important factors which will influence the observations include sex, age, to a lesser extent race, and, perhaps most importantly, the selection of cases—how, by whom, and for what reason? By medical examiners looking only at unexplained death? By a death certificate analysis? Or by a total look at all deaths in a defined demographic base?

What are the characteristics of the population with sudden cardiac death? About 60% of deaths caused by ischemic heart disease occur before hospitalization. With this definition, there are about 400,000 sudden cardiac deaths annually in the United States. Half of these victims, even in the age group below 65 years, have a definite history of arteriosclerotic heart disease—generally, a previous myocardial infarction, sometimes only angina pectoris—and about 40% have hypertension. There is some overlap between these groups, but the important point is that even in the group below age 65, less than 25% of sudden cardiac deaths are in persons free of overt cardiovascular disease.

The risk factors for sudden cardiac death are basically the same as those for arteriosclerotic heart disease and myocardial infarction: hypertension, smoking, lipid disorders, and so forth. However, since the majority of sudden cardiac death patients have previously known heart disease and very often myocardial infarction, the most important risk factor is a history of myocardial infarction and its severity, particularly with respect to the residual impairment of cardiac function. Thus, such factors as residual S-T segment abnormalities, cardiomegaly, heart failure, and frequent premature ventricular contractions, particularly those occurring early in the cardiac cycle with the "R on T" phenomenon, become important. (However, it is to be emphasized that premature ventricular contractions in the absence of symptoms or findings of heart disease carry very little, if any, additional risk for sudden cardiac death—certainly not for sudden cardiac death in the near future.)

PREMONITORY SYMPTOMS

The presence of antecedent potentially premonitory signs varies according to how hard one inquires and how one interprets his findings. About 25% or even more of the victims have seen a physician in the two weeks before their death, but it now seems that these are largely routine visits for known cardiac disease or for totally unrelated problems. On questioning the family, one can often get a retrospective history, with all its pitfalls, which quite often indicates new or increased symptoms in the days immediately prior to sudden cardiac death. Often this may be a new chest discomfort, sometimes increase in an anginal pattern, often just a vague chest discomfort, or particularly breathlessness for no apparent reason. And then there are the usual symptoms referred to the musculoskeletal system or the gastrointestinal tract. Overwhelming fatigue or emotional changes such as depression seem to occur in a quarter of patients in the experience of some investigators.

Although on questioning family and acquaintances, a substantial majority of victims seem to have had the development or exacerbation of one or more of the above symptoms, we do not know the other side of the coin, *i.e.*, what fraction of patients with such symptoms go on to sudden cardiac death or myocardial infarction, and what fraction do not.

PATHOLOGY AND PATHOPHYSIOLOGY

Even in patients less than 65 years of age, advanced multivessel coronary arteriosclerosis is a frequent finding at autopsy. Old myocardial infarction is found in about 40–50% of patients, and an additional 20–25% have small fibrotic scars less than 1 cm in size. In about 15% of victims, substantial narrowing is restricted to only one of the major coronary arteries. In medical examiner series of sudden cardiac death in patients less than 65 years old, there is even a small percentage of victims who do not have substantial coronary artery disease, who have no other cardiac disease or other finding with autopsy and toxicologic study, and yet in whom the clinical circumstances strongly suggest a cardiac mechanism for death.

The autopsy confirmation of a cardiac basis for a sudden death is confounded by several factors. From autopsies on traumatic and other obviously noncardiac deaths, it is evident that coronary artery disease has a high prevalence in the adult population; accordingly, finding only chronic coronary artery disease without acute obstruction or evidence of acute myocardial damage is not conclusive evidence, and one would like to have a complete and otherwise negative autopsy as well as a strong clinical history for the acute terminal event. There is some argument about the frequency of acute coronary obstruction, but it seems to be present in about 40% of sudden cardiac deaths, with occlusion caused by thrombosis in half of these and plaque rupture in a comparable or slightly greater fraction. Another confounding factor is that when myocardium is deprived of its arterial supply, histologic changes become visible on light microscopy only after 6–12 hours, and the person must remain alive during those hours; if death occurs before this time, the presence of infarcting myocardium can be detected only by special staining techniques which depend on enzyme depletion or altered intracellular electrolyte concentrations, or by electron microscopy. Finally, as discussed subsequently, there is now sound clinical evidence that death can be caused by rhythm disturbances without associated acute infarction, and autopsy findings in these circumstances cannot be expected to reveal acute changes.

In about 10% of medical examiner cases, findings at autopsy indicate the onset of myocardial damage at a time which clearly antedates symptoms which the patient has related to his family. Some of this may be attributable to a failure to communicate, but in a substantial number of cases sudden cardiac death can be the consequence of an initially silent, recent myocardial infarction.

The most important findings about the pathophysiology of sudden cardiac death are coming from emergency ambulance or rescue systems which are equipped and staffed for cardiac resuscitation. In persons who have collapsed and are found to have a fatal rhythm disturbance, *i.e.*, ventricular fibrillation or cardiac standstill, ventricular fibrillation is found almost universally if the patient is seen within four minutes, whereas ventricular standstill is found with increasing frequency with later arrival. This tells us nothing about the events or rhythms leading up to this rhythm, but it does suggest that the fatal rhythm is generally ventricular fibrillation and that standstill is a sequela.

More importantly, emergency ventricular defibrillation has resulted in a survival rate of approximately 15%. Survivors are defined as persons defibrillated, hospitalized, and discharged alive. In these patients, a full 50% fail to evolve electrocardiographic, enzymatic, or other evidence of acute myocardial infarction. The vast majority are known to have arteriosclerotic heart disease based on a prior history of myocardial infarction or angina pectoris, or the subsequent findings at coronary angiography. However, the important point is that at least in this group, sudden cardiac death would not have been caused by very early death following myocardial infarction. On the contrary, it would have been death caused by a rhythm disturbance—ventricular fibrillation—in association with otherwise apparently stable coronary heart disease.

The trigger mechanism which converts chronic coronary artery disease into acute myocardial infarction or sudden cardiac death is controversial and undoubtedly attributable to multiple factors. The circumstances surrounding specific cases may point to possible mechanisms, for example, physical stress (or the vagotonia following abrupt cessation of physical stress), transient hypertension, emotional stress, autonomic disorder, and so forth. However, in a substantial proportion of cases—probably a majority—it is difficult to implicate any of these mechanisms from the limited history available. Regardless of the trigger mechanism, ventricular fibrillation seems to be a common, final pathway for the vast majority of sudden cardiac deaths; a few sudden deaths are caused by very rapid heart failure and a very few by standstill, cardiac rupture, or other causes.

PROPHYLACTIC AND EARLY THERAPY

If ventricular fibrillation plays such an important role in sudden cardiac death, and if patients at high risk for sudden cardiac death can be recognized, what is the role of chronic prophylactic antiarrhythmic agents? Unfortunately, drugs which have been most effective in suppressing ventricular irritability in the coronary care unit are not suitable for chronic, oral administration. Furthermore, the orally effective agents which seem most effective in suppressing ventricular irritability are found to have side-effects with substantial frequency. It is also important to remember that while these drugs clearly have been shown to reduce ventricular irritability, there are no studies to show an associated reduction in mortality from such therapy. (Most carefully designed studies have been content to show a decrease in ventricular irritability.) It must also be remembered that even a ten-fold enhanced risk for sudden cardiac death does not carry with it any imminent danger of this catastrophe, and protracted periods of therapy would have to be used. However, it is likely that the high-risk patient is intermittently at periods of much higher risk; if these points in time could be recognized, antiarrhythmic therapy could be focused appropriately. Similarly, if there were a better insight into what may trigger fatal arrhythmias or the pathophysiologic antecedents thereto, we might have other methods of therapeutic intervention, possibly agents which diminish the workload of the heart, or drugs which diminish the potential for ventricular fibrillation by myocardial catechol depletion or by diminishing automatic stimuli which cause irritability, or surgical revascularization by aortocoronary vein grafting. It must be emphasized that the clinical indications and reasonable goals of such procedures are far from settled. Their potential for preventing sudden cardiac death is a hypothesis, and their use would be dictated primarily by other goals, or, in the case of new drug regimens, in carefully designed clinical trials.

The possible advantages and disadvantages of early prophylactic therapy of the patient with suspected myocardial infarction by intramuscular atropine or lidocaine administration were discussed previously in this volume by Dr. Epstein. Suffice it to say that presently these are important topics for clinical research under conditions in which the patient can be observed carefully and treated appropriately. Neither is a proved prophylactic method.

Emergency medical care systems are receiving considerable attention, and justifiably so. No one would argue that they can represent a complete or even ideal solution to the problem of sudden cardiac death. After all, 50% of sudden cardiac deaths occur "instantly" or unwitnessed. The systems pose logistic and cost problems in areas of low or very high population density, and in large measure they are focused on the end result of a disease process rather than on its prophylaxis. However, good emergency care systems can make a difference, to a limited extent by resuscitation and reversal of ventricular fibrillation, but to a substantially greater extent by preventing complications of myocardial infarction and perhaps by reducing the extent of myocardial involvement through promoting the early entry of the patient into the medical care system.

Emergency cardiac rescue systems have been most successful in communities in which they are incorporated into an excellent overall emergency medical care system. Indeed, we need a general and marked upgrading of our total emergency medical care systems, which must be as capable of handling cardiovascular emergencies as they are of treating traumatic emergencies. We have learned that appropriately trained paramedical personnel can give excellent emergency cardiovascular therapy, not only by external cardiac massage, but by defibrillation, electrocardiographic monitoring, and administration of medications intramuscularly and intravenously. Such systems have depended on excellent and continued training. They utilize radiotelemetry links with physicians, both for oral communications and for transmission of electrocardiograms; however, skilled and experienced personnel can perform these maneuvers effectively even if these communication links are lost.

However, ambulances and their staffs are only one element of any emergency medical care system. Nowhere is the old adage about the chain and its weakest link more true than in emergency care. Patients must be informed about the indications for seeking medical help. Steps must be taken to overcome the great reluctance people have in seeking such help. They must have ready access to the system. The system must respond promptly. Only then can it begin to deliver care. And the ambulance is not the last link in the emergency care system. The patient must be brought to a facility where he can be handled promptly and effectively, and often this means a prompt admission to the coronary care facility.

Having discussed a number of the facets of the problem of sudden cardiac death, it might be best to conclude by emphasizing that the best prevention for sudden cardiac death applicable to the general population is to take the steps for preventing or minimizing arteriosclerosis. Much of what has been said is particularly relevant to those who already have clinically manifest coronary heart disease. This is the group most easily identified as being at greater risk; this is the group which is probably the most receptive to advice; and this group certainly deserves our efforts and attention. However, we should not forget that the fundamental solution would be preventing or minimizing arteriosclerosis. We do not yet know all the answers, but there is a body of information from which we can advise the smoker, the hypertensive, the person with lipoprotein disorders, and those with sedentary habits. Let us make preventive cardiology an integral part of medical practice.

THE ROLE OF HIS BUNDLE RECORDINGS IN
THE DELINEATION OF RHYTHM DISTURBANCES

DEMETRIOS KIMBIRIS, LEONARD S. DREIFUS,
and MICHAEL R. KATZ

The electrophysiologic basis for the interpretation of cardiac arrhythmias has been greatly accelerated by the development of ultramicroelectrode and His bundle recording techniques. While the recognition of cardiac dysrhythmias preceded both the electrocardiogram and electrophysiology studies (1–4) it has been only within the past decade that rather precise information has become available for both the identification of cardiac dysrhythmias and the electrophysiologic basis for the action of antidysrhythmic drugs. At the outset, we would like to indicate the great contributions of Wenckebach, Lewis, Mobitz, Winterberg, Scherf, Katz, Pick, Langendorf, Hoffman, and many others who have contributed so much to the understanding of cardiac dysrhythmias. Although electrogram recordings from the atrioventricular (A-V) transmission system were made several years ago (5, 6), it was not until 1969 that Scherlag and coworkers (7) developed a very useful technique to obtain transvenous recordings of the intracardiac events including atrial, His bundle, and ventricular electrograms. Atrial electrograms had been obtained by transvenous cardiac electrodes in man by Hellerstein (8) and later by Dreifus and Najmi (9) utilizing a high resistance circuit to prevent intracardiac hazards with polyethylene catheters filled with saline solution, which could be floated into the right atrium for the recording of intraatrial events. These techniques, along with esophageal electrodes, aided the identification of independent activation of atria and ventricles and helped to identify accurately electrical wave forms in living man. It is the purpose of this chapter to describe the advantages and pitfalls of intracardiac electrocardiography.

The techniques for the recording of His bundle, left and right bundle electrograms have been extensively described previously (7). We recommend that an additional atrial electrogram always be recorded from the upper right atrium.

LOCALIZATION OF A-V CONDUCTION DELAY

The deflection of the atrial electrogram recorded with a bipolar electrode catheter from the upper right atrium close to the S-A node, corresponds to the beginning of the P wave of the surface electrocardiogram. The atrial deflection (A) of the His bundle electrogram corresponds to atrial activity from an area adjacent to the A-V node. For practical purposes, therefore, the P-A interval can be regarded as the intraatrial conduction time. The A-H interval represents the A-V nodal conduction time, and the H-V interval represents the His bundle to the beginning of the ventricular depolarization conduction time, which for the most part is conduction through the left and right bundle branches. The normal values for the different intervals of the A-V conduction are: P-A, 30–50 msec; A-H, 60–120 msec; and H-V interval, 35–55 msec.

PROLONGED P-R INTERVAL

Prolongation of the P-R interval or the A-V conduction can occur individually within the atria, the A-V node, the His bundle, left or right bundle branch, the Purkinje system or, as usually is the case, coexists in one or more levels. Intraatrial delay can occur in acquired or congenital atrial disease or during atrial pacing. A-V nodal delay may be caused by organic, chronic, or acute disease (acute posterior wall myocardial infarction), increased vagal tone (carotid sinus

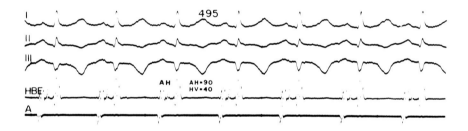

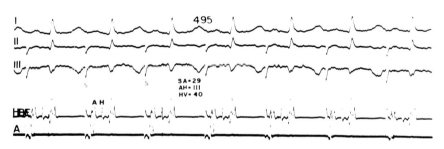

Fig. 1. Upper strips: Leads 1, 2, 3, simultaneously recorded HBE and right atrial electrogram (*A*). Sinus rhythm is present with a cycle length of 495 msec (A-H = 90 msec, HV = 40 msec). *Lower strips:* Right atrial pacing with a cycle length of 495 msec, identical to sinus rate but A-H interval now increased to 111 msec and HV = 40 msec. Inhomogeneous input to A-V node may be responsible for increase of A-H interval with pacing.

pressure), various drugs, or atrial pacing. Delay in the His bundle, left or right bundle branches, and the Purkinje system is always attributable to organic heart disease. Figure 1 shows two simultaneous His bundle recordings, right atrial electrograms with surface electrocardiogram leads from the same patient at comparable heart rates during sinus tachycardia (upper strips) and during right atrial pacing (lower strips). The stimulus to A interval (P-A or S-A) became prolonged, as did the A-H interval. If the pacing rate is increased, first degree A-V block will develop. Hence, first degree A-V block can easily be explained on the basis of an inhomogenous input into the A-V node or anatomical disruptions which fragment the wave front as it enters the head of the A-V node. This may cause subsequent delay between the atria and His bundle (10–12).

It has been shown that in most patients with left bundle branch system block and in a large majority of those with right bundle branch system block and left

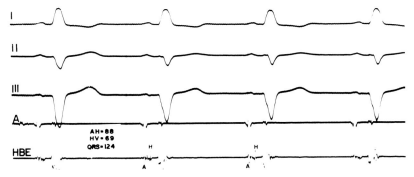

Fig. 2. Simultaneous recording of a surface ECG leads 1, 2, 3, with atrial (*A*) and His bundle electrogram (*HBE*) in a patient with LBBB. The H-V interval is prolonged to 69 msec.

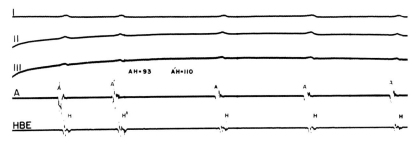

Fig. 3. Recording as in Figure 2 from the same patient. After manipulation of a catheter into the right ventricle, prolonged ventricular asystole is seen. Regular, as well as premature atrial P waves are seen in the surface ECG leads. In the HBE an H deflexion is seen following each A wave of the atrial electrogram. A-H interval = 93 msec. The atrial premature wave A'_1 to H'_1 interval is prolonged to 110 msec. No QRS complexes are seen.

anterior division block, the H-V interval may be prolonged (13). The extent of the His Purkinje conduction delay rarely exceeds 80–90 msec, and hence the P-R interval rarely becomes increased. P-R intervals greater than 280–300 msec are most often engendered by A-V conduction delay above the His bundle. His bundle electrocardiography has contributed significantly to the understanding of conduction within the A-V transmission system and has predicted the clinical significance of these conduction disorders and requirements for intracardiac pacemakers. One fact must be emphasized, that in the presence of a left bundle branch system block, His bundle electrocardiography or cardiac catheterization must be accompanied by a backup system to immediately pace the ventricles, in case the catheter should strike the right bundle branch system and produce complete A-V block and asystole (Figs. 2 and 3).

ATRIOVENTRICULAR BLOCK

Within recent years an abundance of information has become available concerning the anatomy, pathology, electrophysiology, and clinical significance of disturbances of the A-V conduction. Wenckebach (3), in his original paper in 1899, described the progressive prolongation of the a-c interval (interval between atrial and ventricular contractions) until one ventricular contraction dropped out. Following a pause, the a-c interval was shortest, which suggested improved conductivity. Impairment of conductivity was judged from the increment of the a-c interval and was most marked in the second conducted beat and much less in subsequent beats. This resulted in quickening of the radial pulse. However, the increment of the a-c interval was often again greater immediately before the dropped beat, in the presence of higher conduction ratios, resulting in a slowing of the pulse. When Mobitz (14) for the first time classified incomplete A-V conduction disturbances in 1924, he termed the above variety Type 1, which subsequently became known by the name "Wenckebach periodicity." In contrast, Mobitz (15) called a block Type 2, when a ventricular complex blocked out without any change in the P-R interval of the electrocardiogram in the immediately preceding beats. He also mentioned that in the Type 2 variety, often many successive ventricular beats dropped out causing prolonged asystole, despite preceding periods of 1:1 conduction with a normal P-R interval. Hence it must be reemphasized that the original classification of the two types of partial heart block was based entirely on variations or consistency of the A-V conduction time.

However, microelectrode studies in which precise mapping of the A-V conduction delay was identified (16–20) demonstrated the precise site of block. More recent studies using His bundle electrocardiography made it abundantly apparent that from the clinical standpoint it was the location of the block that largely determined the significance (21–23). Therefore the variation or consistency of the P-R interval essentially made very little difference. In a more recent study by Haiat et al. (21), as well as earlier studies by Lenégre (24–26) and Scanlon et al. (27), the clinical significance of Type 1 versus Type 2 block was readily apparent. In general, A-V block associated with a narrow QRS complex (less than 120 msec) usually indicates block within the A-V node, while block occurring in the presence of a QRS complex greater than 120 msec suggests a more peripheral block, usually within the fascicles of the Purkinje system (10). Invariably, clinical symptoms are associated with Type 2 block with wide QRS complexes, but variations in the location of both types of A-V conduction are readily apparent both from electrocardiographic as well as His bundle studies (Figs. 2 and 3).

Several pertinent facts have emerged from His bundle recordings made in the presence of A-V block. Narula et al. (23) have pointed out the significance of intranodal block associated with Wenckeback periodicity in the face of an acute posterior myocardial infarction. Block occurs invariably above the His bundle in these cases (Fig. 4). However, these investigators have shown that block of Wenckebach variety can occur within the fascicles of the bundle branch systems. This has been demonstrated with microelectrode studies between close myocardial fibers (10).

Confusion of the classification and significance of A-V block occurs, when one talks exclusively of the progressive or sudden increase of the P-R interval before the dropped beat (10–20). These criteria can be applied only in the presence of a regular supraventricular rhythm and second degree A-V block associated with conduction ratios greater than 2:1 (10). Furthermore, instances of atrial fibrillation associated with higher grades of A-V block cannot be considered in this classification. His bundle electrocardiography has added im-

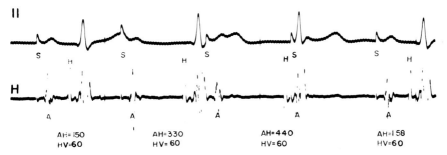

Fig. 4. Simultaneous recording of lead 2 surface ECG and His bundle electrogram (*HBE*) during right atrial pacing. Typical Wenckebach phenomenon is seen. The stimulus (*S*) or A to H interval is progressively prolonged, H-V interval is stable, and the fourth A is not followed by H or QRS (block above the His bundle).

measurable information to the differentiation of the site of block in the presence of these confusing conduction disturbances (28). However, the requirement for the insertion of a permanent cardiac pacemaker is predicated on the development of symptomatology related to neurologic manifestations, congestive heart failure, or alternating bradycardia-tachycardia syndromes, which are disturbing to the patient. Lenégre (24–26) has insisted that symptomatology must exist before pacemakers are inserted.

An acute myocardial infarction, associated with wide QRS complexes, offers a guarded prognosis and the prophylactic insertion of a temporary transvenous pacemaker may be indicated. Hence, His bundle recordings, either in the presence of chronic A-V block or acute myocardial infarction, may be of very little value to the clinician in ascertaining whether pacemakers should be inserted. Thus the clinical evaluation of the patient is preeminent in this decision.

The introduction of intracardiac electrocardiography has enhanced the diagnosis of very complex cardiac arrhythmias and has allowed for more precise differentiation of supraventricular from ventricular arrhythmias. Atrial and/or ventricular pacing may be necessary to stress the A-V transmission system and induce or terminate specific cardiac arrhythmias (29–32). Computer logic for the introduction of intracardiac pacing impulses has added greatly to the understanding of both experimental and clinical electrographic dysrhythmias.

Atrial Arrhythmias

Although many atrial arrhythmias arise within the atrial myocardium and are secondary to degenerative or inflammatory disease, other rhythms such as atrial flutter and atrial fibrillation may result from sinus node default. Within recent years, the tachycardia-bradycardia syndromes have been well identified and appropriately studied by intracardiac electrocardiography (33). Other studies using rapid atrial stimulation have elicited apparent or latent sinus node disease. Following over-drive of the atria or sinus pacemaker, the return cycle of the sinus pacemaker should not exceed 1.5 sec. However, in patients with sinus node disease, subsidiary pacemaker disease usually exists, as well. Consequently, long periods of asystole may be observed in the electrocardiogram (34, 35). The riddle of paroxysmal supraventricular tachycardia has now been solved by intraatrial and His bundle electrograms. There is no doubt that repetitive atrial tachycardias mature from a single atrial premature systole entering the A-V node during a specific portion of the relative refractory period or secondary to prolongation of the A-V interval, allowing a U-turn back to the atria in a reciprocal fashion (29). Whether the delay of A-V transmission is engendered by the premature systole or is caused by delayed A-V transmission, the reciprocating mechanism (Fig. 5) is clear (29, 36–38). The precise plotting of this pathway within the A-V transmission system was first described by Watanabe and Dreifus in 1965 and may be the cause of both repetitive atrial tachycardias, as well as apparent Mobitz Type 2 A-V conduction disorders (16, 17). It also becomes quite clear that paroxysmal nodal and atrial tachycardia are probably similar and that it is only a matter of definition as to the degree of delay within the upper portions of the A-V node or lower portions that discerns between these two rhythms. It is interesting that these mechanisms respond to properly timed atrial or ventricular premature depolarization (39, 40) as seen in Figure 6. These rhythms are now treated by permanent pacemaker implantations and particularly by the use of bifocal atrial synchronous or sequential pacing. On the other hand, the paroxysmal supraventricular tachycardias and those caused by

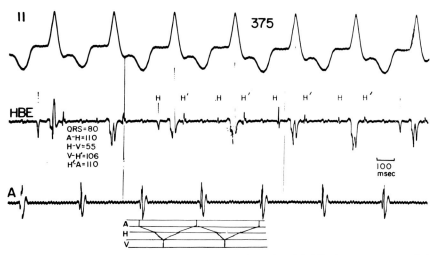

Fig. 5. Lead 2 surface ECG, His bundle (*HBE*) and atrial (*A*) electrogram recorded during reciprocal supraventricular tachycardia. H' follows the QRS complexes, and suggests a U-turn within the A-V junction.

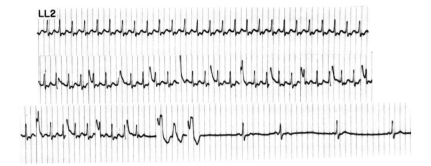

Fig. 6. Lead 2 ECG during supraventricular tachycardia, associated with Wolf-Parkinson-White syndrome and right ventricular stimulation terminated the tachycardia.

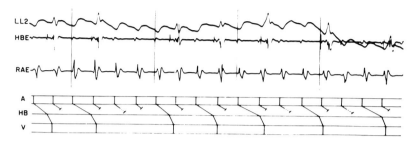

Fig. 7. Simultaneous recordings of the standard lead 2 (*LL2*), His bundle electrogram (*HBE*), and right atrial electrogram (*RAE*) in a patient with atrial flutter and varying conduction ratios. The ladder diagram shows periods of 2:1, 4:1, and 3:1 A-V conduction. Note that every QRS complex is preceded by a His deflection with essentially identical H-Q interval, but no His potential is seen following a right atrial excitation that is not conducted to the ventricles. Some of the oblique lines representing concealed conduction are dotted as the depths of penetration cannot be judged from the His bundle recording.

ectopic atrial mechanisms, can often be distinguished by noting the mode of onset or termination in the His bundle electrograms.

Quite often, the identification of atrial flutter and fibrillation cannot be made by surface electrocardiograms. However, intraatrial electrograms have frequently documented the presence of these arrhythmias and have directed more specific and pertinent therapy. A combination of His bundle electrograms and intraatrial electrograms have aided considerably in the understanding of the various conduction ratios associated with atrial flutter (41). However, in most clinical cases of atrial flutter, it cannot be readily determined whether those impulses penetrating deeper into the A-V junction did partially invade the His bundle or were blocked within the NH region of the A-V node. A His bundle electrogram shown in Figure 7 failed to reveal such information. However, in some instances, multiple levels of concealment with decrement in the excitation wave front can be observed as shown in Figure 8. Hopefully, other His bundle recordings will

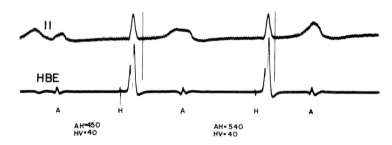

Fig. 8. Simultaneous lead 2 ECG and His bundle recording (*HBE*) from a patient with heart block of the Wenckebach type. Decremental excitation of the His bundle is seen in the second and fourth H deflection.

give us more information as to the depth of penetration both in atrial flutter and fibrillation (41). In a previous study, location of the His bundle deflections varied in position relative to QRS inscription (42). Even in the presence of spontaneous atrial fibrillation without evidence of A-V conduction block, His bundle deflections have been recorded before, superimposed and beyond the QRS inscription.

Ventricular Arrhythmias

In spite of sophisticated recording techniques, the differentiation between supraventricular and ventricular tachycardias remains one of the most difficult exercises in clinical electrocardiography. Although A-V dissociation may be easily identified, the precise site of impulse formation is still elusive. His bundle electrograms, however, have contributed significantly to the actual site of impulse formation and along with the reasoning developed by the concept of fascicular blocks, the actual ventricle and region of that ventricle can be almost definitely identified.

Impulses which arise above the N region of the A-V node usually show a rather normal A-H interval. On the other hand, impulses which arise below the N region often show a short H-V interval, with the atrial impulse being inscribed in a dependent manner relative to the degree of retrograde conduction delay through the N region of the A-V node. Hence, the relative degree of conduction delay from the site of impulse formation within the NH or His region to the ventricle versus the retrograde delay determines the position of the atrial complex relative to the QRS (43). On the other hand, impulses arising within the fascicles of the A-V node usually show either a very short H-V time or the His bundle electrogram may be embraced with the QRS complex or follow the QRS, if conduction delay from the site of impulse formation retrograde through the fascicles is extraordinarily prolonged (44). Furthermore, aberrancy of junctional beats can be ruled out by observing a short His-Q interval, usually less than 35 msec. However, decremental conduction and delay towards the His bundle catheter cannot be completely ruled out (42).

REFRACTORY PERIOD OF THE A-V TRANSMISSION SYSTEM

The electrophysiologic behavior of A-V transmission has been identified by the use of the extra stimulus method (45) for the determination of A-V nodal and subjunctional refractoriness (46). Refractoriness, as usually defined, is related to the ability for an impulse to propagate from a site of electrically induced impulse formation so that it may be recorded on the surface electrogram. Hence, refractoriness in an electrophysiologic sense has been based on the plotting of strength interval curves which always require conduction from the stimulating

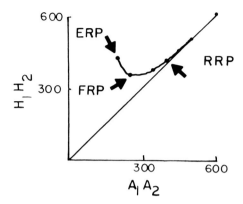

Fig. 9. Plot of A_1-A_2 interval against H_1-H_2 responses. As the A_1-A_2 interval is shortened from 600 msec to 500 msec there is an equal decrease in the H_1-H_2 interval and the plot lies along the line of identity. With further shortening of the A_1-A_2 interval there is at first a smaller decremental shortening of the H_1-H_2 interval (Relative Refractory Period) and the curve leaves the line of identity. This is engendered by an increase in A_2-H_2 conduction time. The functional refractory period is reached at the point of the shortest H_1-H_2 interval for a corresponding A_1-A_2 interval. This occurs as seen in Figure 10. A_1-A_2 interval is decreased by 50 msec from 450 to 400 msec. The increase of the A_2-H_2 interval is 10 msec; hence, H_1-H_2 is 420 msec or a reduction of only 30 msec. The H_1-H_2 interval represents the shortest interval that A-V conduction can occur. Any further reduction of the A_1-A_2 interval either increases the H_1-H_2 interval or engenders A-V block (Effective Refractory Period).

site. On the other hand, refractoriness, as it relates to the A-V transmission system, is quite complex. One must first realize that the refractoriness of each individual fiber type must be considered. Generally speaking, fibers in the proximal portion of the A-V transmission system have a shorter refractory period than do those more distal (19). Furthermore, one still must consider that it is the interrelationship of conduction within the various zones of the A-V transmission system that finally affects total A-V conduction or the P-R interval (18, 41). Severe delay in the more proximal regions of the A-V node may permit further recovery in the tissues below a site of delay; thus conduction may totally improve through the entire A-V transmission system, rather than show further deterioration (41).

A-V nodal refractoriness or more specifically, responsiveness in humans, may be defined during sinus rhythm or atrial pacing with His bundle and atrial electrograms (43). After every eighth to tenth atrial depolarization (A_1), a premature atrial stimulus (A_2) is introduced and the His bundle depolarization, which is the A-V nodal output, marked H_1 and H_2 respectively, is recorded (Figs. 9 and 10). The extra atrial stimulus is introduced progressively more premature-ly and the A_1-A_2 interval becomes progressively shorter. As is shown in Figures 9 and 10 the A_1-A_2, and the H_1-H_2 intervals closely parallel each other along a

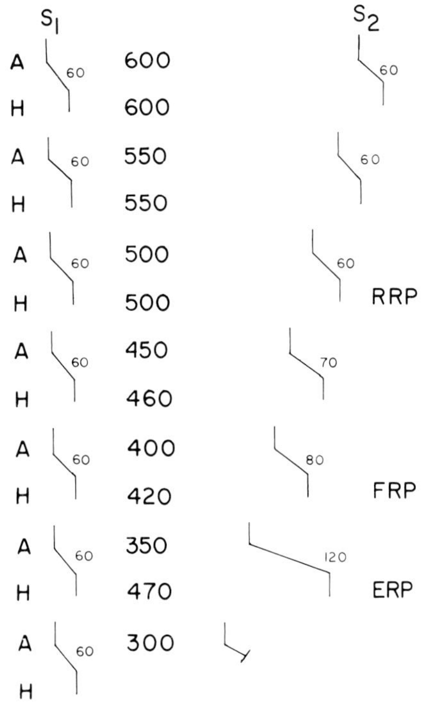

S₁ S₂

A	60	600	60
H		600	
A	60	550	60
H		550	
A	60	500	60
H		500	RRP
A	60	450	70
H		460	
A	60	400	80
H		420	FRP
A	60	350	120
H		470	ERP
A	60	300	
H			

Fig. 10. Determination of refractory periods of the A-V transmission system (*see text*).

line of identity, until the latter interval shortens less than the corresponding A_1–A_2 interval. This is described as the point of relative refractoriness. Continued shortening of the A_1–A_2 interval produces a progressively shorter H_1–H_2 interval until a point is reached at which further shortening of the A_1–A_2 interval is associated with a sharp increase in the H_1–H_2 interval. The shortest H_1–H_2 interval is then defined as the functional refractory period of the A-V junction as it is the shortest interval in which an impulse can reach the ventricles. The shortest A_1–A_2 interval in which A_2 can propagate to the His bundle is defined as effective refractory period. Beyond that point, further shortening of this interval will result in block (Fig. 10). Perhaps a better designation of this phenomenon would be the A-V responsiveness.

A-V CONDUCTION IN THE PRESENCE OF A-V BYPASS FIBERS

Considerable information has been obtained by precise mapping of the atria and ventricles in the presence of Wolff-Parkinson-White syndrome and related A-V conduction abnormalities associated with a short P-R interval. Intraventricular conduction time may be properly assessed by His bundle and ventricular excitation mapping techniques (47). Furthermore, the actual refractory period of both the A-V node and bypass fibers can be accurately determined by pacing and intracardiac electrocardiography (48). Thus decisions as to precise therapy have been determined by these techniques. In the presence of bypass fiber tracts of the Kent variety, the presence of fusion has been easily established by His bundle recordings. During normal sinus rhythm, conduction occurs through both the normal pathway and the Kent bundle. During premature atrial stimulation

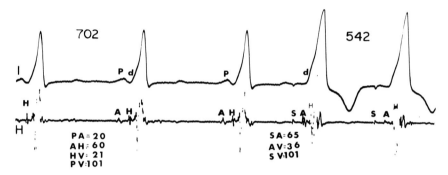

Fig. 11. Lead 2 simultaneously recorded with His bundle electrogram (*H*). The first 3 beats (cycle length 702 msec) are inscribed as fusion complexes and a delta wave is seen. PA = 30 msec, A-H = 60 msec, and H-V = 21 msec. Total A-V conduction is 101 msec. With right atrial pacing, the QRS is increased to 150 msec. The stimulus (*S*) to A interval (*PA*) is now prolonged to 65 msec and the A-V interval is shortened to 25 msec. The H deflection is inscribed within the QRS complex.

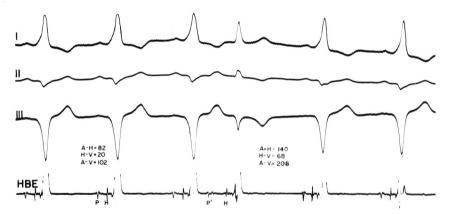

Fig. 12. Determination of the refractory period of the accessory fibers by the extra stimulus method. The shortest A_1-A_2 interval which could conduct via the accessory pathways was greater than 352 msec. At 352 msec block occurred in the accessory fibers and all conduction was through the A-V node with normalization of the QRS complexes.

the normal conduction through the A-V node and His bundle is normally delayed and therefore the stimulus (S) to H interval is prolonged. The conduction through the Kent bundle is not subject to any delay and the S-V interval remains foreshortened and unchanged. Therefore, pre-excitation occurs as before, but because of the delay of the normal pathway conduction, more ventricular mass is pre-excited and the QRS appears more wide and deformed. The His bundle deflexion moves into and at times beyond the QRS complex (Fig. 11). However, very early premature systoles or rapid atrial stimulation may produce block in the Kent bundle and normal intraventricular conduction can then ensue (Fig. 12).

In the presence of James bundle (syndrome with short P-R interval and normal QRS), the A-H interval is not increased by premature atrial stimulation. The A-V transmission occurs through the posterior fiber tracts which insert into an area below the N region of the A-V node and hence, conduction to the ventricles proceeds without eliciting the usual intranodal delay (47). A delta wave is not observed in these cases. In the presence of Mahaim fibers, the extra stimulus atrial premature method will show increase in the A-H interval with decrease or no change in the H-V intervals, depending on whether or not pre-excitation exists. A delta wave or early pre-excitation of the ventricles may still take place via paraspecific fibers which cause delay in the QRS complex and stimulate a delta wave. When both Mahaim fibers and James fibers exist, the situation becomes a little more complex. The surface electrocardiogram may show short P-R interval and wide and distorted QRS complexes similar to those seen with Kent bundle pre-excitation. With the extra atrial stimulus method, the A-H or H-V intervals will not change since the A-V node is bypassed.

EPILOGUE

The introduction of His bundle recordings has offered much in the identification and confirmation of complex cardiac arrhythmias. We now understand better how reciprocal tachycardias are initiated and terminated as well as the relative importance of studying the various conduction times within the layers of the A-V transmission system. With the introduction of hemiblocks to the analysis of electrocardiography, His bundle recordings contributed to the understanding of premature systoles and the differentiation of supraventricular from ventricular beats. What remains to be attained, however, is the ability to identify precisely conduction towards the atria, ventricle, or His bundle catheter and relate these timing events to the actual electrophysiologic events in that particular situation. One can imagine that delay towards the His bundle recording site may exceed either retrograde or forward conduction in some instances, and therefore the inscription of atrial, His, and ventricular electrograms may be misleading as to the site of impulse formation or direction. As brush microelectrode techniques to identify A-V transmission are developed by Van Capelle (13), a greater correlation will be achieved between clinical scalar electrocardiography, His bundle electrograms, and what is actually the electrophysiologic mechanism.

REFERENCES CITED

1. Adams, R. 1827. Dublin Hospital Rep. 4:353.
2. Stokes, W. 1846. Dublin Quart. J. Med. Sci. 2:73.
3. Wenckebach, K. F. 1899. Zur Analyse des unregelmassigen Pulses. Z. Klin. Med. 37:475.
4. Hay, J. 1906. Bradycardia and cardiac arrhythmia produced by depression of certain functions of the heart. Lancet 1:139.
5. Giraud, G., Puech, P., and Latour, H. 1960. The physiological electrical activity of Tawara's node and of His' bundle in man. Endocavitary electrocardiographic registration. Bull. Acad. Nat. Med. (Par.) 144:363.
6. Watson, H., Emslie-Smith, D., and Lowe, K. G. 1967. The intracardiac electrogram of human atrioventricular conducting tissue. Amer. Heart J. 74:66.
7. Scherlag, B. J., Lau, S. H., Helfant, R. H., et al. 1969. Catheter technique for recording His bundle activity in man. Circulation 39:13.
8. Hellerstein, H. K., Pritchard, W. H., and Lewis, R. L. 1949. Recording of intracavitary potentials through a single lumen, saline filled cardiac catheter. Proc. Soc. Exp. Biol. Med. 71:58.
9. Dreifus, L. S., and Najmi, M. 1965. The right atrial electrogram. A bedside procedure for the diagnosis of cardiac arrhythmias. Dis. Chest 48:6.
10. Dreifus, L. S., Watanabe, Y., Haiat, R., and Kimbiris, D. 1971. Atrioventricular block. Amer. J. Cardiol. 28:371.
11. Truex, R. C. 1966. Anatomical consideration of the atrioventricular junction. Pages 333–340 in L. S. Dreifus and W. Likoff, eds. Mechanism and therapy of cardiac arrhythmias. New York, Grune & Stratton.
12. Janse, M. J. 1969. Influence of the direction of the atrial wave front on A-V nodal transmission in isolated hearts of rabbits. Circ. Res. 25:439.
13. Van Capelle, F. J. L., Janse, M. J., Varghese, P. J., Freud, G. E., Mater, C., and Durrer, D. 1972. Spread of excitation in the atrioventricular node of isolated rabbit hearts studied by multiple microelectrode recordings. Circ. Res. 31:602.
14. Mobitz, W. 1924. Über die unvollständige Störung der Erregungsüberleitung zwischen Vorhof and Kammer des menschlichen Herzens. Z. Ges. Exp. Med. 41:180.
15. Mobitz, W. 1928. Über den partiellen Herzblock. Z. Klin. Med. 107:449.
16. Watanabe, Y., and Dreifus, L. S. 1965. Inhomogeneous conduction in the A-V node. A model for re-entry. Amer. Heart J. 70:505.
17. Watanabe, Y., and Dreifus, L. S. 1967. Second degree atrioventricular block. Cardiov. Res. 1:150.
18. Watanabe, Y., and Dreifus, L. S. 1968. Sites of impulse formation within the atrioventricular junction of the rabbit. Circ. Res. 22:717.
19. Watanabe, Y., and Dreifus, L. S. 1968. Newer concepts in the genesis of cardiac arrhythmias. Amer. Heart J. 76:114.
20. Dreifus, L. S., and Watanabe, Y. 1971. Localization and significance of atrioventricular block. Amer. Heart J. 82:435.
21. Haiat, R., Dreifus, L. S., and Watanabe, Y. 1969. Fate of A-V block: An electrocardiographic study. Pages 73–97 in J. Han, ed. Symposium on cardiac arrhythmias. Charles C Thomas, Springfield, Ill.
22. Narula, O. S., Scherlag, B. J., Javier, R. P., et al. 1970. Analysis of the A-V conduction defect in complete heart block utilizing His bundle electrograms. Circulation 41:437.
23. Narula, O. S., Sherlag, B. J., Samet, P., et al. 1971. Atrioventricular block localization and classification by His bundle recordings. Amer. J. Med. 50:146.

24. Lenégre, J., and Morear, P. 1963. Le block auriculo-ventriculaires chroniques. Etude anatomique, clinique et histologique. Arch. Mal. Coeur. 56:867.
25. Lenégre, J. 1964. Etiology and pathology of bilateral bundle branch block in relation to complete heart block. Progr. Cardiov. Dis. 6:409.
26. Lenégre, J. 1965. Les lesions due système de His-Tawara dans les blocs auriculo-ventriculaires d'un haut degré. Cardiologia 46:261.
27. Scanlon, P. J., Pryor, R., and Blount, G., Jr. 1970. Right bundle branch block associated with left superior or inferior intraventricular block: associated with acute myocardial infarction. Circulation 42:1135.
28. Narula, O. S., and Samet, P.: Analysis of right bundle branch block (RBBB) and left axis deviation (LAD) by His bundle recordings [abstract]. Circulation 44(Suppl. 3):1, 53.
29. Goldreyer, B. N., and Bigger, J. T., Jr. 1969. Spontaneous and induced reentrant tachycardia. Ann. Internal Med. 70:87.
30. Haft, J. I., Lau, S. H., Stein, E., et al. 1968. Atrial fibrillation produced by atrial stimulation. Circulation 37:70.
31. Cohen, H. E., Meltzer, L. E., Lattimer, G., et al. 1971. Treatment of refractory supraventricular arrhythmias with induced permanent atrial fibrillation. Amer. J. Cardiol. 28:472.
32. Barold, S. S., and Linhart, J. W. 1970. Recent advances in the treatment of ectopic tachycardias by electrical pacing. Amer. J. Cardiol. 25:698.
33. Goel, B. G., and Han, J. 1970. Atrial ectopic activity associated with sinus bradycardia. Circulation 42:853.
34. Lange, G. 1965. Actions of driving stimulus from intrinsic and extrinsic sources on in situ cardiac pacemaker tissues. Circ. Res. 17:499.
35. Narula, O. S., Samet, P., and Javier, R. P. 1972. Significance of the sinus node recovery time. Circulation 45:140.
36. Bigger, J. T., Jr., and Goldreyer, B. N. 1972. The mechanism of supraventricular tachycardia. Circulation 45:673.
37. Goldreyer, B. N., and Bigger, J. T., Jr. 1971. Site of reentry in paroxysmal supraventricular tachycardia in man. Circulation 43:15.
38. Han, J. 1970. The mechanism of paroxysmal atrial tachycardia. Sustained reciprocation. Amer. J. Cardiol. 26:329.
39. Lister, J. W., Cohen, L. S., Bernstein, W. H., et al. 1968. Treatment of supraventricular tachycardias by rapid atrial stimulation. Circulation 38:1044.
40. Hunt, N. C., Cobb, F. R., Waxman, M. B., et al. 1968. Conversion of supraventricular tachycardias with atrial stimulation. Evidence for reentry mechanisms. Circulation 38:1060.
41. Watanabe, Y., and Dreifus, L. S. 1972. Levels of concealment in second degree A-V block. Amer. Heart J. 84:330.
42. Kimbiris, D., Dreifus, L. S., and Watanabe, Y. 1971. The nature of A-V transmission in the presence of atrial fibrillation [abstract]. Circulation 44(Suppl. 2):62.
43. Goldreyer, B. N. 1972. Intracardiac electrocardiography in the analysis and understanding of cardiac arrhythmias. Ann. Internal Med. 77:117.
44. Massumi, R. A., De Maria, A., McFarland, J., Amsterdam, E. A., and Mason, D. T. 1972. Fascicular rhythms in myocardial infarction: Diagnostic significance [abstract]. Circulation 46(Suppl. 2):89
45. Hoffman, B. F., Moore, E. N., Stuckey, J. H., et al. 1963. Functional properties of the atrioventricular conduction system. Circ. Res. 13:308.
46. Damato, A. N., Lau, S. H., Patton, R. D., et al. 1969. Study of atrioventricular conduction in man using premature atrial stimulation and His bundle recordings. Circulation 40:61.
47. Befeler, B., Castellanos, A., Jr., Castillo, C. A., and Myerberg, R. J. 1972. Arrival of excitation at the right ventricular apex in WPW type A with and without right bundle branch block [abstract]. Circulation 46(Suppl. 2):117.
48. Wellens, H. J., and Durrer, D. 1972. Effects of digitalis in Wolff-Parkinson-White syndrome [abstract]. Circulation 46(Suppl. 2):114.

IDENTIFICATION AND TREATMENT OF FASCICULAR BLOCKS IN CLINICAL SETTINGS

JOHN E. BATCHELDER and CHARLES FISCH

In recent years the concept of fascicular blocks has generated considerable interest both as an electrocardiographic and clinical concept. The first description of experimentally induced bundle branch block appeared in 1910 when Eppinger and Rothberger (1) produced complete heart block by sectioning the bundle of His or both bundle branches. They commented at that time that by severing the posterior division, they were able to produce an "unusual" ECG. In 1921, Wilson and Herrmann (2) published an ECG which demonstrated right bundle branch block (RBBB) and left anterior hemiblock (LAH) and stated that this was produced by "cutting the anterior division of the left bundle." The first clinical case suggesting fascicular conduction disturbance was reported by Wilson (3) in 1934. He published three cases of RBBB with an rS pattern in leads II and III and suggested that this was caused by block in the right bundle and the anterior division of the left bundle. In 1950, Rosenbaum (4), one of the leading proponents and contributors to the concept of fascicular blocks, described a patient with an acute myocardial infarction and RBBB with intermittent LAH and left posterior hemiblock (LPH). In 1964, Lepeschkin (5) suggested that in the presence of slow idioventricular rhythm a wide QRS complex was strong evidence of the presence of bilateral bundle branch block, while a QRS complex of normal duration supported block above the bifurcation of the bundle of His. In 1968 Watt and associates (6) demonstrated the existence of RBBB and LAH and LPH in the dog and baboon hearts. In 1969 Watt and Pruitt (7) demonstrated, by cutting the posterior division of the left bundle branch, reversal of the Rs pattern in leads II, III, and AVF to a qR pattern in these leads, while the QRS duration was increased by only 0.01 second.

The first clinical cases of simultaneous impairment of conduction in all three fascicles were reported by Rosenbaum and associates in 1969. They described four cases of RBBB and LAH progressing to RBBB and LPH with a prolongation of the PR interval (8). Three of the four cases also demonstrated a high degree of atrioventricular block.

Supported in part by the Herman C. Krannert Fund, USPHS Grants HL-06308, HL-05636 and HL-05749, the American Heart Association, the Indiana Heart Association, and the AMA Committee for Research on Tobacco and Health.

The above described experimental and clinical observations have led to the general acceptance of the concept of a trifascicular conduction system. Some investigators, however, feel the approach is rather simplistic and that further anatomical, electrophysiological, and clinical studies are needed.

The purpose of this chapter is to describe the current state of knowledge of trifascicular conduction, but by no means do we suggest that the final word regarding this interesting concept has been written.

ANATOMY

The anatomy of the specialized conduction system has been studied by a number of investigators (4,9,10). The results indicate that the bundle of His measures approximately 1–2 cm by 0.8–1.2 mm and can be divided into two portions. The penetrating portion extends from the atrioventricular (A-V) node to the origin of the left bundle. The branching portion begins where the fibers of the posterior division of the left bundle leave the bundle of His and ends at the origin of the right bundle and the anterior division of the left bundle. The initial part of the penetrating portion lies protected within the central fibrous body, but when it leaves this protective environment it lies relatively close to the mitral and tricuspid valves. The distal end of the branching portion of the bundle of His lies in the area of the noncoronary and right aortic cusps and also in the area of the insertion of the septal leaflet of the tricuspid valve on the membranous septum. Since the posterior division of the left bundle leaves the bundle of His first, there is a short segment of the bundle of His which contains only the fibers of the right bundle and of the anterior division of the left bundle. The right bundle is a long, thin structure measuring about 45–50 mm by 1–2 mm. The initial portion of the right bundle lies near both the aortic and tricuspid valves while the remainder of the right bundle courses along the ventricular septum, then travels subendocardially to the base of the anterior papillary muscle of the right ventricle. The left bundle is a much thicker structure and leaves the bundle of His at a right angle. The narrowest portion of the main left bundle is at its origin. The left bundle courses through the membranous septum and where this portion of the septum is thin, it lies close to the noncoronary and right coronary aortic cusps. The posterior fibers divide early and therefore escape a close relationship to the membranous septum and the aortic valve. The anterior division of the left bundle measures about 25 mm by 3 mm and initially runs with the right bundle in the vicinity of the tricuspid and aortic valves, coursing closer to the aortic valve than does the right bundle. The remainder of the left anterior division courses down the left septal surface and terminates at the anterior papillary muscle of the left ventricle. The posterior division is exposed to the left ventricular inflow while the anterior division is influenced by the turbulent left ventricular outflow.

The initial portion of the right bundle is supplied by the right coronary artery while the second portion is supplied by the left anterior descending artery (4,10). The main left bundle has a dual blood supply, receiving branches from both the right coronary artery and the left anterior descending artery. The anterior division of the left bundle has only a single source of blood, that from the left anterior descending coronary artery, while the posterior division receives blood from both the anterior and posterior descending coronary arteries. This difference in blood supply is probably one of the reasons why block of the posterior division of the left bundle is infrequent. Not only does the posterior division separate early from the left bundle and run a short course in the path of the nonturbulent in-flow tract of the left ventricle, but it also has a dual blood supply. Therefore, to be involved by ischemic heart disease, the coronary artery disease must, as a rule, be extensive. On the other hand, the anterior division of the left bundle is much more vulnerable and more often affected by coronary artery disease. A recent paper (11) reports the development of transient LPH during exercise testing in four patients. It is interesting to note that in one patient the disease was confined to the right coronary artery. The authors suggested, and this has been supported by others (10,12), that some patients have a single blood supply to the posterior division of the left bundle and in these cases the vulnerability of the posterior division is increased.

PATHOLOGY

Lenegre (13) describes two types of pathological processes involving the conduction system. The first is a slowly progressive change which he defined as a "primary sclero-degenerative" process usually involving the right bundle, progressing to bilateral bundle branch block, and finally resulting in complete heart block. The QRS is, as a rule, wide and the ventricular rate relatively slow. In his series only 25% of the patients had evidence of ischemic heart disease. This process, commonly referred to as Lenegre's disease, implies a primary degenerative process of the conduction system. The second type of pathological process was that caused by ischemic heart disease.

Lev (10) described sclerosis of the left side of the cardiac skeleton resulting in A-V block. This process is manifest by age-dependent progressive fibrosis and by calcification of the mitral annulus, the central fibrous body, the base of the aorta, and a portion of the muscular ventricular septum. It usually becomes apparent at the age of about 40 years with damage of the A-V node, bundle of His, or the proximal segments of the bundle branches. Lev felt that this was perhaps the most common cause of permanent complete A-V block (10). This disorder is now known as Lev's disease.

As indicated earlier, the specialized conduction system lies in close proximity to the mitral and tricuspid valves, the noncoronary cusps of the aortic valve, and the membranous septum. It is thus reasonable to assume that surgical procedures in these areas may result in various degrees of damage to the conduction system. Thus, LAH has been reported with mitral valvulotomy, surgical correction of both discrete subvalvular aortic stenosis and idiopathic hypertrophic subaortic stenosis (IHSS), as well as with aortic valve surgery (14). Fascicular blocks have also been reported in 14 patients following tricuspid valve replacement (15). Five of the 14 developed RBBB and LAH and three had RBBB alone.

An incidence of 8.2% of RBBB and LAH has been observed in 291 patients after complete repair of tetralogy of Fallot (16). Of interest was the fact that this group of patients had an increased morbidity and mortality when compared to patients without complicating RBBB and LAH. Of the patients with RBBB and LAH 41% developed complete A-V block as compared to only 4% of patients without intraventricular conduction defects. The patients with fascicular block also demonstrated a significant incidence of ventricular arrhythmias and sudden death. The authors suggest that this group of patients might benefit from prophylactic pacemaker insertion. In another study dealing with a similar group of patients, a 7% incidence of RBBB and LAH was reported (17).

Conduction abnormalities have been reported in association with congenital heart disease (14). Approximately 15% of patients with ventricular septal defect have LAH. Endocardial cushion defects are also frequently associated with LAH. Fascicular conduction defects are occasionally seen with corrected transposition. In the cyanotic group of congenital disorders LAH has been reported in patients with tricuspid atresia and a single ventricle. Intraventricular conduction abnormalities only rarely accompany isolated right ventricular hypoplasia and cor biloculare (14).

It appears that the most common cause of RBBB and LAH is coronary artery disease (13,18–21). In a large series of patients with RBBB and LAH, disease of the coronary arteries was the underlying cause in 36% (21). In other series (13,19) the incidence ranged from 50 to 80% (13,19,20). Hypertension and aortic valve disease are also not uncommonly associated with RBBB and LAH (13,18–21). In a significant number of patients, however, the etiology remains obscure. The incidence of patients in whom this occurs varies from 10.7% to 30% from series to series (4,13,19–21). Some of the patients without an obvious etiology may have RBBB and LAH secondary to "subclinical" coronary artery disease, but a significant incidence is probably attributable to Lev's or Lenegre's disease.

Coronary artery disease is also the most common cause of RBBB and LPH. An incidence as high as 41% has been reported (21). Whatever the etiology, the pathologic process is usually diffuse before the posterior division becomes involved. It has been said that the posterior division is involved more easily by disease originating in the vicinity or at the site of the posterior division because of the otherwise "protective environment" (4). Thus, one of the most common causes of LPH remains Lenegre's disease.

ELECTROCARDIOGRAPHIC DIAGNOSIS

The electrocardiographic diagnosis of LAH is fairly straightforward while the diagnosis of LPH is plagued with a number of unresolved problems. The criteria for LAH include a QRS axis of $-45°$ to $-60°$, a Q in leads I and AVL, a small R and moderate S wave in leads II and III. The S wave in lead III must be larger than in lead II. In pure LAH, the QRS complex is never wider than 0.10 second (4) (Figs. 1,2). The point of disagreement regarding the above criteria is the range of left axis deviation. Left ventricular hypertrophy and variations in the anatomical position of the heart (horizontal and/or counterclockwise rotation) may be associated with a prominent left axis deviation. If $-30°$ is accepted as the lower limit for LAH, the incidence of false positive diagnosis of LAH is increased. At the same time a lower limit of $-60°$, while reducing the number of false positive diagnoses, increases false negative diagnoses. For this reason, $-45°$ has been suggested as the lower range of axis deviation acceptable for the diagnosis of LAH (4). Other obvious causes of abnormal left axis deviation such as inferior myocardial infarction, pulmonary emphysema, Wolff-Parkinson-White syndrome, and hyperkalemia should be excluded before the diagnosis of LAH is made (22). The Q in lead I may be lost as a result of an anterior infarction (23). The QRS in V_1, V_2, and V_3 in patients with LAH may suggest an anteroseptal myocardial infarction (4,24). If the Q wave is secondary to the LAH, recording from one interspace higher will increase the magnitude of the Q wave, while a tracing obtained one interspace lower will disclose a small R wave. LAH may

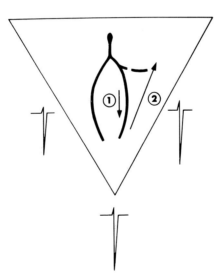

Fig. 1. Diagrammatic presentation of LAH with leads II, III, and AVF projected on the Einthoven triangle.

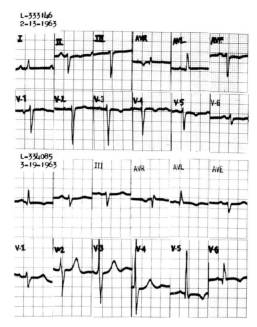

Fig. 2. Two examples of LAH.

also simulate a lateral infarction with a Q wave in AVL and, furthermore, when LAH is associated with RBBB the R/S ratio in the lateral precordium is decreased and this may be mistaken for a lateral myocardial infarction. The opposite may also be true, namely, that LAH may mask an anterior infarction by changing a QS complex to an rS complex if the electrodes are applied in a position lower than normal. LAH can also mask an inferior infarct by producing an initial small R wave in II, III, and AVF.

The fact that an ECG diagnosis of LPH is much more difficult than that of LAH was emphasized by Watt and Pruitt (7). They also stressed the importance of serial ECG tracings in the diagnosis of LPH. The following are the most widely accepted criteria (18) for the diagnosis of LPH: 1) a QRS axis of about $+120°$ with a prominent S in lead I; 2) a Q in lead III; 3) a relatively tall R in leads II and III; 4) the absence of other causes for similar QRS patterns such as a vertical position or pulmonary disease; and 5) the presence of clinical evidence of left ventricular disease (Figs. 3,4,5). Thus, it is obvious that LPH is not a specific ECG abnormality and its presence must be supported by clinical findings. LPH can simulate an anterior infarction with a small Q wave recorded in leads V_1, V_2, and V_3 if the tracing is recorded from sites slightly lower than the conventional position (4). On the other hand, by placing the precordial leads somewhat higher than normal, LPH can mask an anterior infarction by generating an initial small R wave.

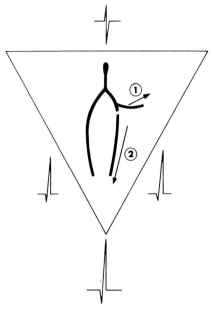

Fig. 3. Diagrammatic presentation of LPH with leads II, III, and AVF projected on the Einthoven triangle.

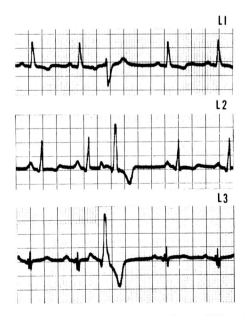

Fig. 4. Atrial premature complex with aberrancy due to LPH and RBBB (V leads not shown).

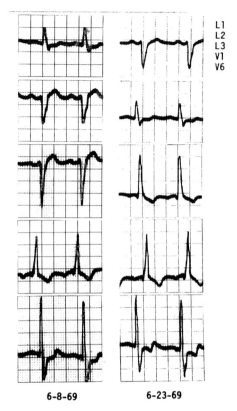

6-8-69   6-23-69

Fig. 5. Right bundle branch block with LAH on June 8, 1969 and LPH on June 23, 1969.

FASCICULAR BLOCK

Incidence

The most common form of fascicular block is LAH. An incidence of 4.58% among 1,658 consecutive patients was reported. In the same series, the incidence of RBBB and LBBB was 3.19% and 1.02% respectively (4). In our own study of 1,000 consecutive hospital patients the overall incidence of LAH was 4.7% and in a nonhospital population of 700 individuals over the age of 65 years, the incidence was 11%. In a large epidemiologic survey the overall incidence of LAH was 5.3% while the incidence of isolated LAH was 2.24% (25). In our study, 3.9% of the hospital patients had isolated LAH, while the incidence of this abnormality in the 65 years and older age group was 7.6%. Ostrander (25) found no increase in mortality with isolated LAH. In large series an incidence of about

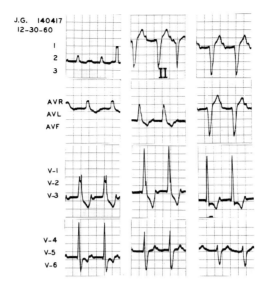

J.G. 140417
12-30-60

Fig. 6. Right bundle branch block with LAH and prolonged P-R interval (trifascicular block?).

1% of combined RBBB and LAH has been reported (4,18,26). In our own group of patients the incidence was 0.6% (Fig. 6). LAH usually precedes the appearance of RBBB (26).

Because of its rarity, little data are available on the incidence of LPH. In a large autopsy series only four patients were found who satisfied the ECG criteria for RBBB and LPH (27). Rosenbaum has been able to accumulate 29 cases of RBBB and LPH (4). In our series of 1,000 consecutive patients, none demonstrated unequivocal LPH. A number of reasons have been suggested to explain the low incidence of LPH and have been outlined above. These are related not only to difficulties in the ECG interpretation but also to the favorable anatomical relationships of the posterior division of the left bundle branch to the surrounding structures.

Fascicular Blocks and Atrioventricular Block

Several authors have reported on the incidence of A-V conduction defects following RBBB and LAH (4,18,21,26,28). The incidence varies from 7.7% to 13.6% (18,21,26,28) (Fig. 7). On the other hand, chronic high degree of A-V block is preceded by RBBB and LAH in 40 to 59% of the cases. The incidence of A-V block caused by fascicular block is derived from the studies of the surface ECG, which has its limitations. For example, Narula and Samet (29) reported

332 J. E. Batchelder and C. Fisch

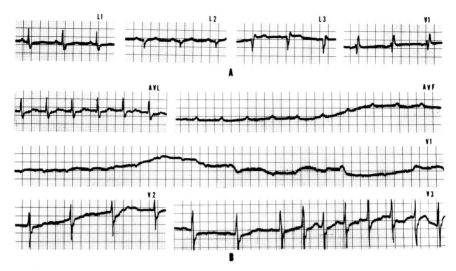

Fig. 7. Right bundle branch block with LAH (*A*) followed by transient complete A-V block and ventricular standstill. The P-R interval in *A* is within normal limits.

that 72% of the patients with RBBB and LAH had increased H-V times implying that these patients might actually have conduction delay in all three fascicles. Some 22% of these patients had second degree or third degree A-V block. At the same time, 62% in this subgroup with episodes of high degree of A-V block and prolonged H-V time, had *normal* P-R intervals during normal sinoventricular conduction. In the same study, the authors reported that 100% of the patients with RBBB and LPH had increased H-V times. In another series, dealing with similar patients, an incidence of 62% of complete heart block was reported (4). Stokes-Adams attacks were seen in 59% of the patients with A-V block.

The problem of treatment, or more specifically the place of pacing in acute myocardial infarction complicated by intraventricular conduction defect, remains unsettled. Of 480 patients with acute infarction, 4.8% had RBBB and LAH (30) (Fig. 8). One is never sure, however, whether the block antedated the infarction or developed following the infarction. The mortality of patients with acute myocardial infarction complicated by RBBB and LAH is high (31). Roos and Dunning (32) reported a 70% mortality for patients with RBBB and LAH and a 100% mortality in patients with RBBB and LPH.

A 71% incidence of complete heart block has been reported in patients with bilateral bundle branch block and a 13% incidence with isolated right or left bundle branch block (33). The mortality in patients who progressed to complete heart block was high. Of the 31 patients treated prophylactically with pacemakers because of a sudden development of bundle branch block, nine devel-

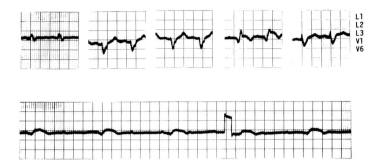

Fig. 8. Acute anterior myocardial infarction complicated by RBBB and LAH, progressing to complete heart block.

oped complete heart block and eight of these nine died. A high incidence of arrhythmias was also observed during pacemaker insertion (33).

The incidence of complete heart block in acute infarction varies from 3.4 to 5.9% from series to series (34−36). Lenegre (13) emphasized that patients with anterior infarcts tend to develop permanent A-V block with wide QRS complexes, while in those with inferior infarcts the heart block is often transient and the QRS complexes are narrow. The mortality is usually much higher with the former type of infarction and A-V block. Friedberg, Cohen, and Donoso (34) reported a series of nine patients with an inferior infarct complicated by complete heart block and a narrow QRS. Two of the nine died. In their series, eight patients had an anterior infarct with complete heart block and a wide QRS complex; of these, seven died. In another study (35), a mortality of 40% was reported in patients with inferior myocardial infarction with complete heart block and a 75% mortality was seen in patients with anterior myocardial infarction and complete A-V block. The high mortality is most likely attributable to associated severe myocardial infarction frequently complicated by shock and heart failure, and is not primarily caused by the heart block. Most authors (33−36) agree that complete heart block in the presence of acute infarction is still an indication for temporary pacing, although convincing data as to its effectiveness in acute myocardial infarction are lacking.

REFERENCES CITED

1. Eppinger, H., and Rothberger, J. 1910. Ueber die Falgen der Durchschneidung der Tawareschen Schenkel des Reizleitungssystems. Z. Klin. Med. 70:1.
2. Wilson, F. N., and Herrmann, G. R. 1921. An experimental study of IBBB and of the refractory period of the heart of the dog. Heart 8:229.
3. Wilson, F. N. 1934. Electrocardiogram of an unusual type in right bundle branch block. Amer. Heart J. 9:472.

4. Rosenbaum, M. B., Elizari, M. V., and Lazzari, J. O. 1970. The hemiblocks. Tampa Tracings, Oldsman, Florida.
5. Lepeschkin, E. 1964. The electrocardiographic diagnosis of bilateral bundle branch block in relation to heart block. Prog. Cardiov. Dis. 6:445.
6. Watt, T. B., Freud, G. E., Durrer, D., and Pruitt, R. D. 1968. Left anterior arborization block combined with right bundle branch block in canine and primate hearts: an electrocardiographic study. Circ. Res. 22:57.
7. Watt, T. B., and Pruitt, R. D. 1969. Left posterior fascicular block in canine and primate hearts. An electrocardiographic study. Circulation 40:677.
8. Rosenbaum, M. B., Elizari, M. V., Lazzari, J. O., Nau, G. T., Levi, R. J., and Halpun, M. S. 1969. Intraventricular trifascicular blocks. The syndrome of right bundle branch block with intermittent left anterior and posterior hemiblock. Amer. Heart J. 79:306.
9. Hudson, R. E. B. 1949. Surgical pathology of the conducting system of the heart. Amer. Heart J. 38:604.
10. Lev, M. 1964. Anatomic basis for atrioventricular block. Amer. J. Med. 37:742.
11. Bobba, P., Salerno, J. A., and Casari, A. 1972. Transient left posterior hemiblock. Circulation 46:931.
12. Frink, R. J., and James, T. N. 1972. The normal blood supply to the His bundle and proximal bundle branches. Amer. J. Cardiol. 29:263.
13. Lenegre, J. 1964. Etiology and pathology of bilateral bundle branch block in relation to complete heart block. Prog. Cardiov. Dis. 6:409.
14. Pryor, R., and Blount, S. G., Jr. 1966. The clinical significance of true left axis deviation. Amer. Heart J. 72:391.
15. Aravindokshon, V., Elizari, M. V., and Rosenbaum, M. B. 1970. Right bundle branch block and left anterior fascicular block following tricuspid valve replacement. Circulation 42:895.
16. Wolff, G. S., Rowland, T. W., and Ellison, R. C. 1972. Surgically induced right bundle branch block with left anterior hemiblock. Circulation 46:587.
17. Chesler, E., Beck, W., and Schrire, V. 1972. Left anterior hemiblock and right bundle branch block before and after surgical repair of tetralogy of Fallot. Amer. Heart J. 84:45.
18. Lasser, R. P., Haft, J. I., and Friedberg, C. K. 1968. Relationship of right bundle branch block and marked left axis deviation to complete heart block and syncope. Circulation 37:429.
19. Byahatti, V., DePasquale, N. P., and Crampton, R. S. 1970. Indirect graphic studies in bilateral bundle branch block. Chest 58:223.
20. Entman, M. L., Estes, E. H., Jr., and Hackel, D. B. 1967. The pathologic basis of the electrocardiographic pattern of parietal block. Amer. Heart J. 74:202.
21. Scanlon, P. J., Pryor, R., and Blount, S. G., Jr. 1970. Right bundle branch block associated with left superior or inferior intraventricular block. Circulation 42:1123.
22. Castellanos, A., Jr., Maytin, O., Arcebol, A. G., and Lemberg, L. 1969. Alternating and co-existing block in the divisions of the left bundle branch. Dis. Chest 50:103.
23. Castellanos, A., Jr., and Lemberg, L. 1971. Diagnosis of isolated and combined block in the bundle branches and the divisions of the left branch. Circulation 43:971.
24. McHenry, P. L., Phillips, J. F., Fisch, C., and Corya, B. R. 1971. Right precordial qrS pattern due to left anterior hemiblock. Amer. Heart J. 81:498.
25. Ostrander, L. D. 1971. Left axis deviation: prevalence, associated conditions, and prognosis. Ann. Internal Med. 75:23.
26. Watt, T. B., and Pruitt, R. 1969. Character, cause and consequence of combined left axis deviation and right bundle branch block in human electrocardiograms. Amer. Heart J. 77:460.
27. Strickland, A. W., Horan, L. G., and Flowers, N. C. 1972. Gross anatomy associated with patterns called left posterior hemiblock. Circulation 46:2/6.
28. Rothfield, E. L., Zucker, I. R., Tiu, R., and Parsonnet, V. 1969. The electrocardiographic syndrome of superior axis and right bundle branch block. Dis. Chest 55:306.

29. Narula, O. S., and Samet, P. 1971. Right bundle branch block with normal, left or right axis deviation. Amer. J. Med. 51:432.
30. Scheinman, M., and Brenman, B. 1972. Clinical and anatomic implications of intraventricular conduction blocks in acute myocardial infarction. Circulation 46:753.
31. Scanlon, P. J., Pryor, R., and Blount, S. G., Jr. 1970. Right bundle branch block associated with left superior or inferior intraventricular block. Circulation 42:1135.
32. Roos, J. C., and Dunning, A. J. 1970. Right bundle branch block and left axis deviation in acute myocardial infarction. Brit. Heart J. 32:847.
33. Godman, M. J., Lassero, B. W., and Julian, D. G. 1970. Complete bundle branch block complicating acute myocardial infarction. New Engl. J. Med. 282:237.
34. Friedberg, C. K., Cohen, H., and Donoso, E. 1968. Advanced heart block as a complication of acute myocardial infarction. Role of pacemaker therapy. Prog. Cardiov. Dis. 10:466.
35. McNally, E. M., and Benchimol, A. 1968. Medical and physiological considerations in the use of artificial cardiac pacing. Amer. Heart J. 75:380.
36. Schlerger, J., Iraj, I., and Edson, J. N. 1970. Cardiac pacing in acute myocardial infarction complicated by complete heart block. Amer. Heart J. 80:116.

GUIDELINES FOR THE USE OF DRUGS, CARDIOVERSION, PACING, AND PACEMAKERS IN CARDIAC ARRHYTHMIAS

LEONARD S. DREIFUS, IRANY M. de AZEVEDO, and MICHAEL R. KATZ

It was stated wisely by the late Charles Wolferth that "in the management of serious arrhythmias any fool can push a button, but it takes a wise and mature clinician to properly outline the course and management of patients with serious cardiac arrhythmias." Fortunately, the clinician has at his fingertips a wide variety of both pharmacologic agents and electronic methods to reestablish sinus rhythm and prevent subsequent cardiac arrhythmias. It is the purpose of this discussion to set forth several guidelines which may offer an approach to the management of patients with serious and disturbing cardiac dysrhythmias.

VENTRICULAR TACHYCARDIA AND FIBRILLATION

The most serious of all cardiac dysrhythmias is recurrent ventricular tachycardia, or ventricular fibrillation. Although it appears profoundly presumptuous to discuss the management of recurrent ventricular tachycardia in the coronary care setting, I feel it is necessary to restate many of the problems encountered when ordinary therapy fails. Precordial shock is always utilized in the face of ventricular fibrillation and is the initial approach with sustained ventricular tachycardia and hypotension or shock. Most importantly, a pharmacologic program must be organized to protect the patient from recurrent ventricular arrhythmias. The use of a 50–100 mg bolus of lidocaine, followed by an intravenous drip of 1–4 mg/min, is mandatory. If lidocaine alone fails to inhibit the reemergence of these arrhythmias, procainamide in a bolus of 100–200 mg must be administered, followed by an intravenous drip of procainamide of 1–4 mg/min along with the lidocaine. Often a compromise can be reached between 2 mg of lidocaine and 2 mg of procainamide used in conjunction with each other. If the use of these two agents alone or in combination cannot prevent the recurrence of these serious arrhythmias, it is possible to add Inderal, 1–2 mg, every 30 min in a slow, intravenous drip.

Therapeutic failure after use of these agents invariably identifies a very serious problem. Other antiarrhythmic agents, for so-called intractable situations, are still experimental or sometimes hazardous. Bretylium tosylate,

300–600 mg, can be attempted either intravenously or intramuscularly. It is important to withhold other antiarrhythmic agents at the time bretylium is administered (1). The side-effects of bretylium often outweigh its usefulness, and marked hypotension may prevent further use. Disopyramide phosphate has shown important antiarrhythmic effects when other agents, such as procainamide, lidocaine, and propranolol, have failed to control the ventricular arrhythmia. Disopyramide phosphate can be administered orally in a dose of 100–200 mg every six hours (2). The use of diphenylhydantoin has been less than satisfactory in the ventricular arrhythmias, but a dose of 300–500 mg intravenously can be attempted.

Intractable ventricular arrhythmias often can be controlled by fixed-rate cardiac pacing in conjunction with antiarrhythmic agents. If atrioventricular (A-V) block is not present, passage of a transvenous pacemaker into the right atrium with overdrive pacing utilizing rates from 90–120/min is effective in controlling the reemergence of the ventricular arrhythmias. It is wise to continue antiarrhythmic agents, although in smaller doses, if pacing is successful. If there is a question of A-V block, ventricular overdrive pacing is selected. More recently, the use of a bifocal pacemaker with atrial and ventricular sequential activation has proved successful in the most intractable of the recurrent ventricular arrhythmias. Preservation of atrial contribution to ventricular filling will increase coronary flow and cardiac output.

Most importantly, all possible mechanisms for the initiation and continuation of intractable ventricular arrhythmias should be identified. Acid-base imbalance or electrolyte imbalance, particularly hypokalemia, must be corrected, or else any therapeutic approach to the control of ventricular arrhythmias will be inadequate (3, 4).

ATRIAL FIBRILLATION AND ATRIAL FLUTTER

Many techniques and programs have matured over the past decade in the management of paroxysmal atrial flutter and atrial fibrillation. We have passed from the most conservative management with digitalis alone to programs using precordial shock at the onset of each issue of atrial flutter or fibrillation (5).

It would appear now that the use of precordial shock is reserved for those cases of atrial flutter and atrial fibrillation which are associated with hypotension and which appear intractable to antiarrhythmic drug therapy (6). Hence, there would be no hesitation to use dc shock in a patient who is showing rapid deterioration or a shock-like state. Thereafter, maintenance of sinus rhythm must be managed with precise antiarrhythmic drug therapy.

Elective precordial shock is reserved for those patients who require reestablishment of sinus rhythm and who have not been converted with other pharmacologic agents. Elective precordial shock is rarely utilized, since very potent antiarrhythmic drugs can be used alone or in combination for conversion to sinus rhythm (6). In most instances, however, antiarrhythmic drugs must be utilized to maintain sinus rhythm after conversion.

The use of digitalis in the presence of paroxysmal atrial flutter, atrial fibrillation, and atrial tachycardia may be summarized as follows. Initially, digitalis is administered either orally as 0.5 mg of digoxin or intravenously as 0.4 mg of Cedilanid or 0.25 mg of digoxin. Following the initial dose of digitalis and the achievement of a maximum cholinergic response, propranolol, 0.5–1 mg, is administered intravenously. The sequence of drug administration may be repeated at the end of 30 min–one hour, two hours, and three hours if necessary (Figs. 1 and 2). Invariably, after the first or second doses of combined therapy, an adequate ventricular rate is achieved, and only oral maintenance therapy of Inderal, 5–10 mg, four times daily, and digoxin, 0.25 mg daily, is necessary (7, 8).

Conversion of atrial flutter or atrial fibrillation to sinus rhythm can be achieved as follows. After adequate digitilization has been achieved, quinidine, 0.2–0.3 g, can be administered every two hours for five doses. If there is failure to achieve sinus rhythm within that period of time, quinidine is increased to 0.4 g every two hours for five doses plus propranolol, 10 mg every six hours on the

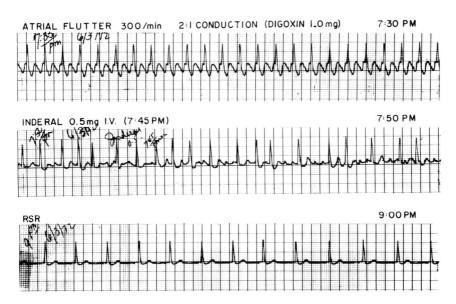

Fig. 1. Lead 1. Upper strip shows an atrial flutter with 2:1 A-V conduction. Digoxin, 1.0 mg, was given prior to 7:30 p.m. without slowing of the ventricular rate. Middle strip, 0.5 mg of propranolol was given intravenously at 7:45 p.m. and the ventricular rate slowed by 7:50 p.m. Lower strip, sinus rhythm was reestablished without further drug therapy at 9:00 p.m.

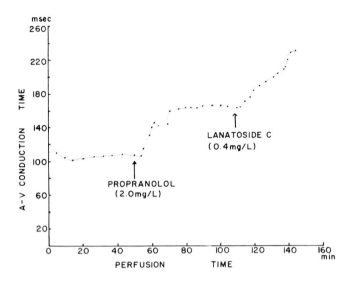

Fig. 2. Effect of combined propranolol and lanatoside C on A-V conduction. Enhancement of A-V conduction delay by combined therapy most likely accounts for marked slowing of ventricular rate in the presence of atrial flutter, as seen in Figure 1.

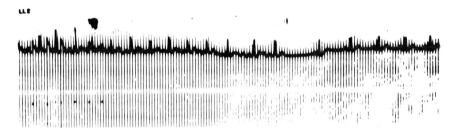

Fig. 3. Lead 2, conversion of atrial flutter to sinus rhythm with right atrial pacing. Note pacing artifacts at lower left-hand portion of the strip. Multiple conversions can be performed by this method.

next day. Failure to convert at this dosage may invite increasing side-effects. Evidences of congestive heart failure or pulmonary disease are contraindications to the use of propranolol. Precordial shock may be the method of choice under these circumstances.

Reentry mechanisms producing atrial flutter and atrial tachycardia can be terminated by right atrial pacing and can offer an alternative method of therapy when precordial shock is not possible, such as in the setting of an acute myocardial infarction (Fig. 3) (9).

Some comment should be directed to identify the mechanism of repetitive tachycardias. It now is possible to locate the point of reciprocation. The U-turn can be in the atria or upper regions of the A-V junction or below the bundle of His (10). For those mechanisms which are known to be reciprocating above the bundle of His, the use of propranolol with or without digitalis appears most efficient. Rhythms reciprocating below the bundle of His often respond to antiarrhythmic drugs, such as propranolol, procainamide, or lidocaine. The use of electrocardiography of the bundle of His to identify these mechanisms properly is mandatory in many intractable cases where drug therapy has failed.

TACHYCARDIA-BRADYCARDIA SYNDROMES

Sinus node default can be responsible for the appearance of rapid supraventricular mechanisms. Although the sick sinus syndrome has been known for many years, its precise management was not appreciated until the development of cardiac pacing. Rapid supraventricular mechanisms alternate with a very slow bradycardia. Bradycardia permits diastolic depolarization and slow conduction. Hence, the atria are vulnerable for subsequent issues of rapid supraventricular rhythms (Fig. 4). The use of antiarrhythmic drugs, such as quinidine, propranolol, and digitalis, may further aggravate the bradycardia by depressing sinus node rhythmicity. These patients respond dramatically to cardiac pacing. The introduction of bifocal pacing for this mechanism has been extremely gratifying. Antiarrhythmic drugs may be necessary for a short period after bifocal pacemaker implantation, but after three or four months the requirement for antiarrhythmic drugs usually diminishes. Ventricular pacing alone often will prevent the onset of supraventricular tachycardia and will guarantee the preservation of an adequate ventricular rate.

A-V HEART BLOCK

While cardiac pacemaking has prolonged and improved the quality of life for patients with chronic A-V heart block, certain guidelines must be expressed in the selection and management of patients who do have or will develop high

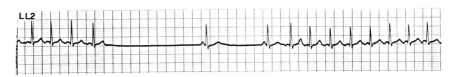

Fig. 4. Lead 3, a rapid supraventricular rhythm is seen at the left- and right-hand portions of the strip. Sinus arrest with two junctional escape beats is seen in the middle of the strip. Failure of the sinus mechanism with periods of tachycardia requires cardiac pacing.

grades of A-V block. Lenégre distinctly stated that the requirement for cardiac pacing in the face of A-V heart block was the appearance of either cardiovascular or neurologic symptoms (11). Extensive investigation has attempted to identify the precise site of A-V transmission block (11–17). Most patients with block above the bundle of His do not require pacing, since they do not have symptoms of either congestive heart failure or syncope (12, 14). No hard and fast rule can be made as to who will or will not require cardiac pacing. Patients with intraventricular conduction block usually demonstrate Mobitz 2 variety of A-V block, and in most instances these patients have symptoms of syncope or congestive heart failure (12, 14). Cardiac pacing is absolutely indicated in these individuals. While rate itself cannot be used generally as a guideline for cardiac pacing, it seems apparent that rates below 40/min frequently are associated with inadequate cardiac output, fatigue, syncope, and the emergence of ectopic ventricular beating. Hence, cardiac pacemakers are inserted most often for Mobitz type 2 block or block below the bundle of His. Much attention has been directed to the prediction of who will develop heart block when two or more fascicles of the A-V transmission system are blocked. The concepts of hemiblock

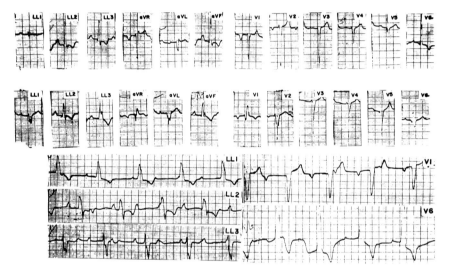

Fig. 5. Upper strip, 12 lead ECG. A right axis of +90 is present. Q waves are present in 2, 3, and aVF, and a Q wave pattern is present in V_4-V_5. Posterior hemiblock is present with anterioseptal infarction. Second strip: the QRS is now widened to 0.14 sec and deep slurred S wave in 1, aVL, and V_6, an RSR' is present in V_1. An extreme right-axis deviation is present in right bundle branch block; in addition, left-posterior hemiblock is present. Ventricular demand pacing should have been instituted in the presence of RBBB plus posterior hemiblock, because high-grade block (*lower strip*) appeared within a few hours, followed by cardiac arrest.

by Rosenbaum et al. (18) and the clinical course of fascicular block have established a new basis for the identification and management of these conduction disorders.

In the presence of an acute myocardial infarction, the development of bifascicular block is hazardous, and temporary transvenous pacing is indicated. Some clinics have even selected the use of temporary demand transvenous pacing in patients developing either right or left bundle branch system block and have not reserved this method of therapy only for bifascicular or trifascicular blocks. This question still seems unsettled, and no great division of opinion would exist if prophylactic temporary pacing were instituted in these individuals (Fig. 5).

Antiarrhythmic drug therapy, such as the use of isoproterenol and atropine, has been largely abandoned, except for a temporary holding measure during the organization of temporary transvenous pacing. Long-term use of pharmacologic agents to enhance either sinus rhythmicity or A-V conduction has largely failed. Most attempts to lower or raise potassium levels, or the administration of steroids, have met with complete or inadequate control of the mechanisms.

WOLFF-PARKINSON-WHITE (WPW) TACHYCARDIA

As more information has emerged concerning the anomalous pathways associated with the Wolff-Parkinson-White syndrome, many intractable arrhythmias associated with this syndrome have been treated successfully by cardiac pacing. Cardiac pacing is valuable in those patients who require surgical interruption of either the preexcitation bypass or A-V conduction system for control of the cardiac arrhythmia (19) or in those patients in whom a properly timed premature stimulus either in the atria or ventricle will interrupt the reciprocating tachycardia and terminate the rhythm (20). The implantation of either a radio frequency pacemaker or a magnetically activated demand pacemaker can be effective in the termination of repetitive tachycardia associated with a WPW syndrome. Adequate study of the refractory periods of both the normal and bypass conduction fibers should be performed before pacemakers are inserted and in patients with recurrent WPW intractable to usual antiarrhythmic therapy (21). Precordial shock still remains the treatment of choice in WPW tachycardia not responding to antiarrhythmic therapy.

REFERENCES CITED

1. Watanabe, Y., de Azevedo, I. M., and Dreifus, L. S. 1972. Electrophysiologic antagonism of quinidine and bretylium tosylate. Circulation 11-40 (Suppl).
2. Dreifus, L. S., Filip, Z., Sexton, D. M., and Watanabe, Y. 1973. Electrophysiological and clinical effects of a new anti-arrhythmic agent: Disopyramide phosphate. Amer. J. Cardiol. 31:129.

3. Watanabe, Y., and Dreifus, L. S. 1967. Interactions of quinidine and potassium on atrioventricular transmission. Circ. Res. 20:434.
4. Watanabe, Y. 1965. Antagonism and synergism of potassium and anti-arrhythmic agents. Pages 86–103 in E. Bajusz, ed. Electrolytes and cardiovascular diseases. S. Karger, Basel.
5. Lown, B., Perlroth, M. G., Kaldbly, S., and Tadaaki, A. 1963. Cardioversion of atrial fibrillation. New Engl. J. Med. 269:325.
6. Dreifus, L. A. 1970. Use of D.C. shock in the treatment of cardiac arrhythmias. Mod. Treat. 7:188.
7. Pamintuan, J. C., Dreifus, L. S., and Watanabe, Y. 1970. Comparative mechanisms of anti-arrhythmic agents. Amer. J. Cardiol. 26:512.
8. Dreifus, L. S. 1972. Clinical correlates of the electrophysiological action of digitalis in the heart. Semin. Drug Treat. 2:179.
9. Dreifus, L. S. 1971. Indication for cardiac pacing. Page 140 in L. E. Meltzer and J. J. Kitchell, eds. Current concepts of cardiac pacing and cardioversion. Charles Press, Inc., Philadelphia.
10. Mandel, W. J., Kermaier, A. J., Blum, R. L., and Hayakawa, H. 1972. Critical prolongation of A-V conduction time as the inciting mechanism in reentrant tachycardia. J. Electrocardiol. 5:39.
11. Lenégre, J., and Moreau, P. Le bloc aureculo-ventricularis chronique-étude anatomique, clinique et histologique. Arch. Mal. Coeur 56:867.
12. Haiat, R., Dreifus, L. S., and Watanabe, Y. 1972. Fate of A-V block, an electrocardiographic study. Page 76 in J. Han, ed. Cardiac arrhythmias. Charles C Thomas, Springfield, Ill.
13. Watanabe, Y., and Dreifus, L. S. 1967. Second degree atrioventricular block. Cardiov. Res. 1:150.
14. Dreifus, L. S., and Watanabe, Y. 1971. Atrioventricular block. Amer. J. Cardiol. 28:374.
15. Watanabe, Y., and Dreifus, L. S. 1972. Levels of concealment in second degree and advanced second degree A-V block. Amer. Heart J. 84:330.
16. Damato, A. N., Larr, S. H., and Berkowitz, W. D. 1970. Second degree A-V block. Amer. J. Cardiol. 25:91.
17. Rosen, K. M., Loeb, H. S., and Chuquinina, R. 1970. Site of block in acute myocardial infarction. Circulation 42:925.
18. Rosenbaum, M. B., Elizari, M. V., Lazzari, J., Nair, G. J., Halpern, M. S., and Levi, R. J. 1972. The differential manifestations of hemiblocks, bilateral bundle branch block and trifascicular blocks. Page 145 in R. C. Schlaub and J. W. Hurst, eds. Advances in electrocardiography. Grune and Stratton, New York.
19. Dreifus, L. S., Nichols, H., Morse, D., Watanabe, Y., and Truex, R. 1968. Control of recurrent tachycardia of Wolff-Parkinson-White syndrome by surgical ligation of the A-V bundle. Circulation 36:1030.
20. Durrer, D., Shoo, J., Schulenburg, R. M., and Wellens, J. J. 1967. The role of premature beats in the initiation and the termination of supraventricular tachycardia in the Wolff-Parkinson-White syndrome. Circulation 36:644.
21. Castillo, C. A., and Castellanos, A., Jr. 1970. His bundle recordings in patients with reciprocating tachycardias and Wolff-Parkinson-White syndrome. Circulation 42:271.

Progress in Cardiac Disease
of Infectious Etiology

THE CHANGING SCENE IN RHEUMATIC FEVER

GEORGE C. GRIFFITH

Rheumatic fever is defined as a systemic poststreptococcal nonsuppurative inflammatory disease with protean manifestations of varying severity and duration (1).

In the past, rheumatic fever has been known as acute arthritis, acute inflammatory rheumatism, and by various other designations all of which have directed special attention to the joint inflammation and very little attention to the systemic manifestations.

In 1866, Ludwig Aschoff described the granulomatous lesions associated with the pathologic changes in the myocardium. In 1877, such clinicians as Sibson (2) called attention to the heart involvement in association with the arthritis occurring in a family group. Sir James Mackenzie (3) described the changes in the pulse, in the heart rate and rhythm, in the myocardium, in the heart valves, and the seriousness of an associated pneumonia. He attributed the infection to an organism called *Diplococcus rheumaticus.*

Osler (4) defined rheumatic fever as an acute infection dependent upon an unknown infective agent, and he described its clinical manifestations of arthritis, myocarditis, and a marked tendency to inflammation of the endocardium and the heart valves. F. Griffith, of London, first associated the onset of rheumatic fever with beta-hemolytic streptococcal infection of the nasopharynx, as described in his article published in 1934 (5). In 1931, Paul Dudley White (6) defined rheumatic fever as a systemic disease with a streptococcal antecedent, and he stated that of all heart disease cases under the age of 20, 93% were rheumatic in type.

In 1964, J. Willis Hurst (7) described the manifestations of rheumatic fever following the T. Ducket Jones criteria and definitely linked it to an invasion of the nasopharynx by the Group A beta-hemolytic streptococcus. He emphasized that the diagnosis should be confirmed by the sedimentation rate, the C-reactive protein level, and the elevated titers of an antibody to one or more streptococcal antigens, such as antistreptolysin-O, antistreptokinase, antihyaluronidase, and/or anti-DPNase. The titers continue to be elevated from months to years after the streptococcus invasion.

The concept of a systemic poststreptococcus nonsuppurative inflammatory disease caused by a hypersensitive faulty antibody-antigen reaction is universally accepted.

INCIDENCE

The incidence of rheumatic fever has been on the decline since the turn of the century. In its annual summary for the years 1969 through 1971, the Center for Disease Control reports (8) show a steady decline in the incidence of rheumatic fever, from 10,470 cases in 1961 to 2,793 cases in 1971. Conversely, the incidence of streptococcal sore throat and scarlet fever has increased from 338,410 cases in 1961 to 433,405 cases in 1970. Thus, we note a steady yearly decline in rheumatic fever and a yearly increase in the cases of streptococcal sore throat and scarlet fever. These facts are contrary to our concept that streptococcal control reduces the incidence of rheumatic fever.

In a study conducted in Navy training camps in the 1940's, the incidence of streptococcal infection was 5%, and of those so infected 5% developed rheumatic fever with carditis (1).

Admission data from the House of the Good Samaritan, by B. F. Massell (9), show that over a period of 40 years the incidence of rheumatic fever changed very little until the last 5 years, when a decrease of 11.9% occurred.

In 1947, the incidence of acute rheumatic fever was 2% of all school children, with the highest rate occurring in the northeastern and Rocky Mountain states. The study of 17,366 Denver school children, completed in 1965 by Morton, Huhn, and Litchy (10), showed a definite change in the incidence and the clinical picture, illustrated by 1.7 cases per 1,000 among the 10-year-old children, increasing to 3.1 per 1,000 at the age of 15. The socio-economic status showed less than one-half this incidence and a less florid clinical picture in the higher status group.

Sievers and Hall (11) showed a marked decrease in the incidence of firm rheumatic fever since 1930 in Great Britain: from 2.5 cases per 10,000 to a low of 0.7 per 10,000. Studies in other western countries have shown a similar reduction in incidence, in mortality, and in acute manifestations. In a study carried out in 1968 in a large city in southern Iran (12), 10,676 school children between the ages of 6 and 17 were examined, and this study revealed an incidence of 3.5 per 1,000. A study involving 33,361 subjects, conducted in a town in northern India from mid-1966 to 1969 (13), revealed an incidence of 3.3 per 1,000 population. The worldwide incidence of rheumatic fever (Table 1) varies from continent to continent and nation to nation, as shown in the statistical study published in 1972 by the British Medical Association (14). Few clear-cut patterns can be determined, except for the low incidence in Sweden, Norway, Scotland, Denmark, and Yugoslavia.

In Los Angeles County there has been a gradual downward trend in the incidence of rheumatic fever (15). With a population of 7,300,000, an average of 100 cases of acute rheumatic fever are reported each year in Los Angeles County. In Childrens Hospital of Los Angeles, there have been only 47 cases of

Table 1. Rheumatic Fever Death Rate per
Million Population for 1966 (14)

Continent	Country	% Rheumatic fever (male & female)
America	Argentina	12.6
	Canada	2.2
	Chile	20.4
	Colombia	32.0
	Mexico	15.4
	United States of America	5.2
Asia	China (Taiwan)	45.7
	Japan	17.3
	Philippines	28.9
Europe	Austria	2.9
	Belgium	8.8
	Czechoslovakia	12.1
	Denmark	1.5
	Finland	4.1
	France	5.0
	Germany (Federal Republic)	5.8
	Greece	5.7
	Hungary	2.6
	Ireland	6.3
	Netherlands	2.3
	Norway	0.6
	Poland	48.2
	Portugal	7.4
	Sweden	0.4
	Switzerland	2.2
	United Kingdon (England, Wales,	3.2
	N. Ireland,	17.1
	Scotland)	0.8
	Yugoslavia	1.8
Oceania	Australia	2.3
	New Zealand	7.7

acute rheumatic fever in 58,548 admissions of patients under the age of 16 years. Further evidence of the decreasing incidence is shown in the records of the Hospital of the Good Samaritan in Los Angeles, where admissions for valvular surgery for the years 1968 to 1972 total one-third of the number admitted from 1960 to 1964.

Scarlet fever and rheumatic fever occurred in less severe forms even before the 1945 antibiotic age. Therefore, it is believed that the falling incidence and lessened severity of rheumatic fever are attributable to a change in the virulence of the streptococcus and an improvement in the host resistance.

It is estimated that in the United States, 27 million people have organic heart disease, of which the estimated number of rheumatic heart disease cases is 1,670,000—or about 1 in every 26 cases of organic heart disease. However, this represents a marked decrease when compared to the 7 of every 10 patients in the New England survey reported in 1931 by Paul Dudley White (6).

CLINICAL PICTURE

Fulminating acute rheumatic fever, with the classical features of fever, sweating, carditis, and migrating arthritis has become an infrequent entity. The cyclic and monocyclic types are likewise uncommon. The frequency of the subclinical type probably will never be known, and undoubtedly accounts for the small number of patients with rheumatic valvular disease encountered in the 1960's.

Fever may be absent, moderate, or severe. When fever is present it usually subsides in 8 to 10 days. A fever of $102°$ to $104°F$ is seldom seen. The hot, dry skin, alternating with profuse, hot sweating, the dry mouth, and the restlessness occur infrequently. Migrating polyarthralgia in the larger joints has replaced the red, hot, swollen, painful joint manifestations. Arthritis may be totally absent.

Carditis is the most important diagnostic criterion, and should be searched for with diligence. Tachycardia out of proportion to the fever, a pericardial friction rub, apical systolic murmur, and aortic diastolic murmur are diagnostic findings. Rapid dilation of the heart in all of its chambers seldom occurs at this point in time, so congestive failure is very rarely seen. A prolonged P-R interval following a streptococcus throat infection may be the only diagnostic sign of carditis, and this is infrequent.

Chorea is an almost unknown entity, occurring in very few poststreptococcal infections. Erythema marginatum is rare, but is seen in the same frequency as carditis. Epistaxis, subcutaneous nodules, and erythema nodosum are very rarely seen. Pneumonitis, which formerly occurred in 11% of patients with rheumatic fever, is rarely found.

With the marked decrease in the severity of the disease, the Jones criteria for diagnosis cannot be fully depended upon. Throat culture, sedimentation rate, C-reactive protein, and antistreptolysin-O titers yielding positive findings are more dependable diagnostic criteria in the mild or the subclinical rheumatic fever syndromes.

TREATMENT

Beginning with the use of sulfa drugs in the form of sulfadiazine, followed by the use of penicillin and the broad spectrum antibiotics, the treatment of the Group A hemolytic streptococcal infection of the nasopharynx has become specific. Therapy must be initiated early and continued until the throat culture is negative. The efficacy of such treatment is illustrated by an educational program for physicians and parents undertaken in Orange County, California, where there have been no reported cases of rheumatic fever in the past 10 years. In this program, every sore throat is cultured, the treatment started, and altered only when the report from the Public Health Department is returned (it takes about 12 hours). Antibiotics are discontinued only when the throat cultures of both the patient and the members of the patient's family are negative.

Treatment for the rheumatic fever itself is clearly defined. Acetyl-salicylic acid in dosage sufficient to produce a blood level of 30 mm/100 ml is easily maintained when the aspirin is given with food and plenty of water. If a diagnosis of carditis is made, then cortisone is prescribed, and continued until the active rheumatic state has passed.

Many studies have shown that ACTH or cortisone are not superior to aspirin in the prevention of permanent cardiac damage. Prednisone is the preferred form, and is used when aspirin is not tolerated, or fails to give prompt relief.

REASONS FOR THE CHANGING PICTURE

All of the available evidence suggests that the severity of rheumatic fever and carditis has diminished gradually since 1900, but at an accelerated rate of diminution since the antibiotic age began in 1946 (16).

With prompt treatment of the streptococcal infection and continuation of treatment until it is fully eradicated, and with the use of adequate doses of aspirin and prednisone, the disease has become less severe and the acute manifestations of carditis have lessened. In rheumatic fever cases, long-term prophylaxis with antibiotics or sulfonamide has resulted in fewer recurrent attacks.

There is a belief that an altered virulence of the streptococcus, together with the improvement in the socio-economic conditions in the western world may have, of themselves, changed the picture for the better. The future of rheumatic fever and rheumatic heart disease is uncertain because of subclinical rheumatic carditis. The reduction in the presence of florid rheumatic fever and classical carditis has resulted in an overall diminishing incidence of the disease.

With increased vigilance and prompt treatment of the Group A streptococcus infections, there is good reason to believe that the favorable trend will continue.

REFERENCES CITED

1. Griffith, G. C. 1947. Rheumatic fever: Its recognition and treatment. J.A.M.A. 133: 974–981.
2. Sibson, F. 1877. Vol. 4, p. 526 *in* J. R. Reynolds, ed. A system of medicine. Macmillan, London.

3. Mackenzie, J. 1913. Diseases of the heart, p. 283. Oxford Medical Publications, London.
4. Osler, W., and McCrae, T. 1921. Principles and practice of medicine, 10th ed., p. 358. Appleton, New York.
5. Griffith, F. 1934. Serological classification of streptococcus pyogenes. J. Hygiene 34:542–584.
6. White, P. D. 1931. Heart disease, pp. 822–841. Macmillan, New York.
7. Hurst, J. W., and Logue, R. B. 1966. The heart, pp. 519–610. McGraw-Hill, New York.
8. U.S. Department of Health, Education, and Welfare: Morbidity and mortality: Annual supplement, 1969, 1970, 1971. 18 (No. 54):5–10 (Sept) 1970; 19 (No. 53):4–10 (Aug) 1971; 20 (No. 53):4–10 (June) 1972.
9. Massell, B. F., Amezcua, F., and Pelargonio, S. 1964. Evolving picture of rheumatic fever: Data from 40 years at the House of the Good Samaritan. J.A.M.A. 188:287–294.
10. Morton, W. E., Huhn, L. A., and Litchy, J. A.: Rheumatic heart disease epidemiology: observations in 17,366 Denver school children. J.A.M.A. 199:879–884.
11. Sievers, J., and Hall, P. 1971. Incidence of acute rheumatic fever. Brit. Heart J. 33:833–836.
12. Joorabchi, B., Tahernia, A. C., et al. 1971. Epidemiology of rheumatic heart disease in Iran. J. Trop. Med. Hygiene 74:203–205.
13. Berry, J. N. 1972. Prevalence survey for chronic rheumatic heart disease and rheumatic fever in northern India. Brit. Heart J. 34:143–149.
14. Wood, P. H. N., and Benn, R. T. 1972. Statistical Index published by the British Medical Association. Ann. Rheumatic Dis. 31:73.
15. California State Department of Public Health. 1960. A manual for the control of communicable diseases, p. 316.
16. Besterman, E. 1970. The changing face of acute rheumatic fever. Brit. Heart J. 32:579–582.

THE CHANGING SCENE IN BACTERIAL ENDOCARDITIS

GEORGE C. GRIFFITH and SOL BERNSTEIN

Bacterial endocarditis is now designated as infective endocarditis, an old term used in the 1800's and early 1900's by such early cardiologists as Sir James Mackenzie (1). The designation "infective endocarditis" is now in common usage, and was defended by Humphries, Weinberg, and Roberts in a symposium presented at the American Heart Association Scientific Clinical Session in November of 1972, in Dallas, Texas.

The Oslerian classification of bacterial endocarditis into the acute and sub-acute types is obsolete, except when used in reference to the seriousness of the clinical symptoms. No longer can the term "bacterial" be used because many other infective organisms are recognized, such as *Fungi, Bacteroides, Haemophilus influenzae, Pseudomonas, Klebsiella, Serratia, Aerobacter, Candida,* and others.

INCIDENCE AND CHANGING FLORA

In 1913, Mackenzie (1) stated that the incidence of bacterial endocarditis was unknown. He reported 40 cases of infective endocarditis, all caused by bacteria. In 1931, White reported on a series of 45 cases, all caused by common bacteria (2). He called attention to reports of other isolated cases attributable to the meningococcus, typhoid bacillus, plague bacillus, and *Brucella.* The infection agents in these two series are very similar (Table 1).

In 1965, Uwaydah and Weinberg (3) reviewed the cases of bacterial endo-carditis at the Massachusetts General Hospital from 1944 to 1964. The infective agents were studied in a total of 328 cases during two periods: from 1944 to June, 1958; and from July, 1958 to June, 1964. Their findings are reported in Table 2. From their study we note very little difference in the proportionate number of cases: 228 in 14 years to 100 in 6 years. The flora showed a decrease in the incidence of *Streptococcus viridans* and very little change in the incidence of *Staphylococcus aureus.*

A great difference in the incidence and flora is seen in separate studies we carried out in two Los Angeles hospitals (Table 3): a 10-year (1961–1971) study in a private hospital (Hospital of the Good Samaritan) without a walk-in emergency admitting service; and a one-year (July 1, 1971 to June 30, 1972) study in the Los Angeles County-University of Southern California Medical

Table 1. Causative Organisms of Bacterial Endocarditis
in Two Pre-Antibiotic Periods, 1913 and 1931

Infective agent	Mackenzie, 1913: 40 cases (1)	White, 1931: report of Thayer's cases (2)
Streptococcus	26	114
Pneumococcus	5	28
Gonococcus	2	22
Bacillus influenza	5	8
Staphylococcus aureus	0	26
Staphylococcus albus	1	1
Unclassified	1	0

Center, which has a 24-hour emergency service. In the private hospital, the incidence of bacterial endocarditis was 1 in 3,750 cases; in the general hospital the incidence was much greater, 1 in 1,609 cases.

The infecting organisms differ greatly. In the private hospital the infective organism was bacterial; in the general hospital there was a wide variety of infecting organisms.

There was also a difference in the type of patient treated. In the private hospital most infective endocarditis occurred in the older age group with established heart disease. Of the 36 cases, 7 followed implantation of a valvular prosthesis. In the general hospital, 35 cases occurred in young addicts who were either "skin poppers" or "mainline pushers." Patients with established heart disease accounted for 28 cases. Of the 35 addicts, 7 died from lesions on both the right and left sides of the heart; 3 of the addicts had tricuspid disease in association with left-sided valvular disease, mainly of the aortic valve. Of the 14 patients who died in the nonaddict group, 2 had aortic, mitral, and tricuspid involvement; and all died from embolism and congestive failure. The addicts with tricuspid involvement showed more pulmonary complications.

These findings are confirmed in the recent report by Roberts (4). Weinberg (4) reported similar findings in a study of infective endocarditis found in patients at Massachusetts General Hospital. He made special reference to prosthetic valve endocarditis occurring early and late, with most of the organisms being of the gram-positive type. It was observed that the gram-positive organisms adhered to valvular structures, while gram-negative organisms frequently attached to the free wall endocardium.

Skin popper: a narcotics addict who uses the needle to inject a drug under the skin—not into a vein. Mainline pusher: an addict who injects drugs into the vein. (Source: Landy, E. E. 1971. The Underground Dictionary. Simon and Schuster, New York.)

Table 2. Causative Organisms of Bacterial Endocarditis
in Two Antibiotic Periods, 1958 and 1964 (3)

Infective agent	1944 to June, 1958	July, 1958 to June, 1964
Alpha-hemolytic streptococci	117	39
Beta-hemolytic streptococci, Group A	3	5
Nonhemolytic streptococci	0	3
Streptococcus, Group G	0	2
Enterococcus, Group D	5	6
Staphylococcus aureus	34	23
Staphylococcus albus	4	2
Pneumococci	9	2
Friedlander-like organisms	0	1
Proteus	1	1
Escherichia coli	4	0
Haemophilus influenzae	2	0
Brucella	1	0
Pseudomonas aeruginosa	1	0
Unknown	47	14
Uncertain cases	0	2
Total Cases	228	100

MORBIDITY AND MORTALITY

Virulent organisms appear to cause more florid clinical symptoms and signs; conversely, the less virulent organisms cause minimal symptoms and signs.

The diagnosis in virulent endocarditis is based upon fever, pathologic murmurs, positive blood cultures, and the embolic manifestations, such as splinters, petechiae, Roth's spots, splenomegaly, and Osler's nodes; it may also be made by surgical confirmation or autopsy.

Table 3. Studies of Causative Organisms of Bacterial Endocarditis, 1961 to 1972, in Two Hospitals

Infective agent	L.A. County-USC Medical Center July 1, 1971–June 30, 1972 (1 year) Total Cases: 63				Hospital of the Good Samaritan Jan. 1, 1961–Dec. 30, 1971 (10 years) Total Cases: 35	
	35 Addicts		28 Nonaddicts		Nonaddicts	
	Cases	Deaths	Cases	Deaths	Cases	Deaths
Group D streptococcus	12	2	6	2	9	2
Candida	8	4	0	0	0	0
Staphylococcus aureus	7	0	0	0	7	3
Pseudomonas	4	1	0	0	0	0
Pneumococcus	2	0	5	4	2	1
Klebsiella	1	0	0	0	0	0
Beta streptococcus	0	0	1	0	2	0
Unspecified	0	0	5	4	0	0
Non Group D streptococcus	0	0	5	2	3	1
Staphylococcus albus	0	0	1	0	7	1
Staphylococcus epidermidis	0	0	0	0	5	2
Serratia	0	0	2	1	0	0
Bacteroides	0	0	1	1	0	0
Aerobacter	0	0	1	0	0	0
Haemophilus	0	0	1	0	0	0
Totals	35	7 (20%)	28	14 (50%)	35	10 (28.6%)[a]

aWhen compared to the lower mortality in addicts (20%), the high mortality in nonaddicts in both hospitals probably reflects overwhelming infection in an older age group, undiagnosed clinical endocarditis (determined only at autopsy), and association with advanced debilitating disease such as neoplasms.

In the indolent type of endocarditis, the diagnosis is made by a high index of suspicion and positive blood culture. Embolic secondary signs are infrequent.

Prior to the antibiotic age, the mortality was 99%. Now the mortality has varied between hospitals: for example, 6 deaths in 35 cases (17.1%) in the private hospital studied; 21 deaths in 63 cases (33.3%) in the general hospital studied. Morbidity and mortality are increased in patients who are debilitated either by age, addiction, malignancy, or leukemia. In the private hospital, 13 patients had rheumatic heart disease, 2 had congenital heart disease, 2 exhibited Marfan's syndrome, and 13 had atherosclerotic heart disease. Of the 13 patients with rheumatic heart disease, 7 had prosthetic valvular implants; 4 of the 7 died when the prosthetic valve was not replaced, and 3 recovered following prosthetic valve replacement. In the general hospital, 35 of the 63 cases were addicts. Group D streptococcus occurred in 12 addicts, 10 of whom recovered with antibiotic therapy. *Candida* infection resulted in the most fatalities, with 4 deaths in 8 patients. All were treated with amphotericin; the 4 survivors were successfully operated on for removal of the nidus. Of the 28 nonaddicts treated with antibiotics, 16 survived.

The source of infection varies with the socio-economic status of the population. In the private and semiprivate hospitals, the most frequent antecedent factors are dental surgery, urinary tract surgery, and cardiac surgery. In the general hospitals, the most frequent antecedent factor is drug addiction.

OBSERVATIONS AND CHANGES

The total yearly incidence of infective endocarditis, as recorded by Weinberg at Massachusetts General Hospital (4), and by us at the Hospital of the Good Samaritan and Los Angeles County-USC Medical Center, has remained relatively constant since 1944.

The infecting organisms have changed, with a shift toward the gram-negative type—especially *Candida.*

The incidence of infection in rheumatic and congenital heart disease is decreasing. The frequency of infection is increasing in the older age group, especially in those older patients subjected to dental, urinary tract, and cardiac surgery. In patients with normal hearts, the incidence of infective endocarditis is greatly increased by drug addiction, malignancy, and the leukemias.

The mortality has decreased since the pre-antibiotic age, when infective endocarditis was 99—100% fatal. In the late 1940's and 1950's there was a very marked decrease in the mortality—to 20%—attributable to the use of potent antibiotics and to a spectrum of bacteria which was nonresistant.

In the last decade the mortality has again increased, caused largely by increased infection with gram-negative resistant organisms as well as by the very

high incidence of infection brought about by drug addiction among the young
people in a low socio-economic group.

REFERENCES CITED

1. Mackenzie, Sir James. 1913. Diseases of the heart, 5th ed., p. 287. Oxford Medical
   Publications, London.
2. White, P. D. 1931. Heart disease, p. 343. Macmillan, New York.
3. Uwaydah, M. M., and Weinberg, A. N. 1965. Bacterial endocarditis: a changing pattern.
   New Engl. J. Med. 273:1231–1235.
4. Symposium on infective carditis. Scientific Session, American Heart Association, Dallas,
   Texas, November 16, 1972. Participants: Humphries, J. O., Weinberg, A. N., and Roberts,
   W. C.

New Paths of Investigation
in Atherosclerosis

A NEW CONCEPT IN ATHEROGENESIS AND THROMBOGENESIS, AND THE TREATMENT OF ATHEROSCLEROSIS WITH AN ENDOTHELIAL CELL RELAXANT

TAKIO SHIMAMOTO

Haust and More (1) have said that "it is still unknown just how a high level of certain plasma lipids initiates the lesions; it has been universally accepted on the other hand that once in the intima, the large molecular complexes of beta- and prebetalipoproteins contribute to a chain of reactions that culminate in lesions."

In this chapter, I will offer my own elucidation of the unknown factors in their theory. The subject of this presentation involves primarily the contracting and swallowing activity of endothelial cells (2–5), specifically induced by atherogenic stress.

ACUTE HYPERLIPIDEMIA AND ITS EFFECT ON THE ARTERY

It is possible to raise temporarily the level of serum cholesterol or saturated fatty acids in animals by simple administration of cholesterol or animal fats in sufficient amounts. For instance, the oral administration of 1 g of cholesterol per kg of body weight may raise the serum cholesterol level in rabbits by at least 2–3 mg/100 ml, and the daily repetition of this procedure for several weeks induces the formation of atheromatous lesions. This is the well-known classical method, first reported by Anitschkow (6) in 1913, for producing atherosclerosis.

I (7–9) discovered that a single administration of cholesterol, or of animal fat such as lanolin or butter, produces a spotty and sometimes diffuse edema in the subendothelial space and inner layer of the media of the artery in animals such as rabbits and rhesus monkeys. The edematous fluid was found to contain acid mucopolysaccharide, as in the case of "das initiale fettfreie Ödem" of the human artery, believed by the German school to be the initial stage of atherosclerosis. With this as a clue, I identified the induced condition as the same "edematous arterial reaction" that has been subjected to such extensive analysis during the past 14 years (Plate 1).

Using an immunofluorescent technique, I (4, 9) found that the edematous fluid also contains plasma proteins such as β-lipoprotein, fibrinogen, and γ-globulin. By sacrificing rabbits or rhesus monkeys serially after a single administration of cholesterol (1 ~ 2 g/kg, P.O.), lanolin (1 ~ 2 g/kg, P.O.), or butter (2 g/kg, P.O.), I found that the plasma proteins first entered the subendothelial space, which was temporarily dammed by the internal elastic lamina. The plasma proteins then penetrated the fenestrations of the lamina into the inner layers of the media, and then escaped from the medial layers, probably through lymphatic ducts, which eliminated them from the arterial wall (Plates 2 and 3).

OTHER RISK FACTORS

Several unsaturated fats or unsaturated fatty acids, as well as glucose, starch, casein, and ethanol, had no such effect. However, epinephrine (0.1 ~ 1 μg/kg, I.V.), norepinephrine (1 ~ 10 μg/kg, I.V.), angiotensin II (1 μg/kg, I.V.), brady-kinin (0.1 μg/kg, drip infusion for 10 min), histamine (10 μg/kg, I.V.), inhalation of cigarette smoke, and traumatization (crushing of thigh muscles) have been shown to produce the same response in the arterial wall as observed following cholesterol feeding. We also noted that a combined challenge with cholesterol and epinephrine, or with cholesterol and angiotensin II, markedly increased the infiltration of plasma proteins into the arterial wall and strengthened the barrier function of the internal elastic lamina, causing plasma proteins such as β-lipo-proteins to stagnate in the subendothelial space (Fig. 1). It is important to note in this regard that hypercholesterolemia or hyperlipidemia, hypertension, and cigarette smoking—the so-called three major risk factors, according to Stamler, Berkson, and Lindberg (10)—are all associated with similar vascular changes. Also, Laragh (11) reported the dangerous outcome in hypertensives with normal or elevated serum renin concentrations. On the other hand, he reported the absence of apoplexy or heart attack among hypertensives with low serum renin concentrations. The same harmlessness of low-renin hypertension and the danger of high- or normal-renin hypertension were independently reported by Kaneko et al. (12) at the annual meeting of the Japan Heart Association in 1971.

TRIGGER MECHANISM IN ATHEROGENESIS AND THROMBOGENESIS

In 1969, I and my collaborators (13) analyzed the transendothelial transport of high-molecular substances in the aorta with a marker, horseradish peroxidase. We found that the transendothelial transport of this large particle (25 ~ 30Å) occurred mainly through the intercellular junctions of the endothelial cells. The enzyme was also transported through the vesicular system, but this was a rather minor part of the process. To investigate the mechanisms of transendothelial infiltration by large particles, I (2–5) studied the behavior of contractile proteins of arterial endothelial cells (14).

For this study, it was necessary to design a suitable method (2) of vital

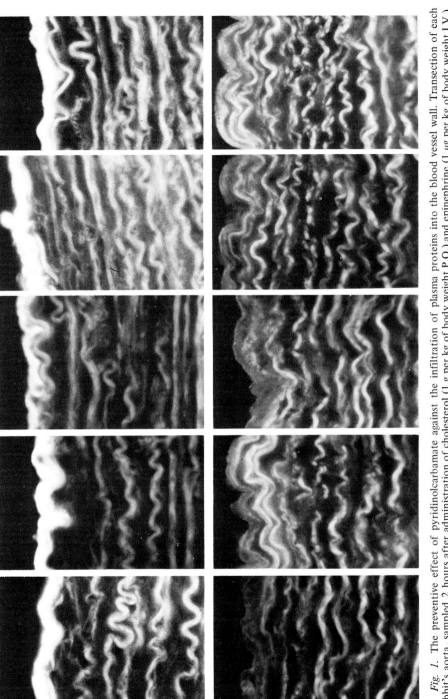

Fig. 1. The preventive effect of pyridinolcarbamate against the infiltration of plasma proteins into the blood vessel wall. Transection of each rabbit's aorta, sampled 2 hours after administration of cholesterol (1 g per kg of body weight P.O.) and epinephrine (1 μg per kg of body weight I.V.). The infiltration of γ-globulin into the subendothelial space is induced in all five animals pretreated with placebo (*top*). It is prevented in all five animals pretreated with pyridinolcarbamate (5 mg per kg of body weight P.O.) given 2 hours before the challenge (*bottom*).

fixation. The fixation of living endothelial cells without changing their shape was successfully performed in the capillary of frog mesentery by Landis (15) and in the capillary of the skin of rat scrotum by Majno et al. (15). My method (2) is a surgical procedure under anesthesia and fixes the living endothelial cells of the artery.

As shown in Table 1, the strong contraction of endothelial cells was induced by single-dose treatment of rabbits with cholesterol (1 g/kg, P.O.), epinephrine (1 μg/kg, I.V.), and angiotensin II (1 μg/kg, I.V.). Under the scanning and transmission electron microscope, endothelial cells of treated animals revealed the typical unevenness seen in Figure 2, and their nuclei exhibited more conspicuous indentations and often pinches, as shown in Figure 3. In the endo-thelium of thoracic aorta, the proportion of cells showing pinches was $6.2\% \pm 1.1$ ($p < 0.001$) in animals sacrificed two hours after challenge with cholesterol, $4.1\% \pm 1.2$ ($p < 0.01$) and $4.3\% \pm 1.2$ ($p < 0.01$), respectively, in those sacrificed 10 min after administration of epinephrine and angiotensin II. Endothelial cells showing pinches were absent in 826 specimens of endothelial cells from the same part of the aorta in all eight rabbits treated with placebo. It is reasonable to assume that such a contraction of endothelial cells widens the intercellular space, permitting the entrance of large particles such as β-lipoprotein, fibrinogen, and γ-globulin from the blood into subendothelial spaces, especially in the vasodila-tive stage of arterial pulsation (Plate 4), because ferritin or carbon particles entered the subendothelial space right through the intercellular space serially widened by cholesterol or epinephrine or angiotensin II challenge.

This phenomenon was relatively long in duration, and the contraction of endothelial cells showing pinch and blebbing by single-dose treatment with cholesterol lasted at least 6 hours. It was also shown to be quite unrelated to

Table 1. Contraction of Endothelial Cells

| Challenge | Pretreatment | SEM | TEM | | Infiltration of β-lipoprotein |
			Indentations/1μ	Pinches	
no	no	1/10	1.73 ± 0.15	0	━ ⌒ ±
	no	9/10	2.43 ± 0.17	6.2 ± 1.1	╫╫╫
Cholesterol 1gm/kg p.o.	Premarin 5mg/kg i.v.	0/10	1.88 ± 0.08	0	━ ⌒ ±
	Pyridinolcarbamate 10mg/kg p.o.	0/10	1.71 ± 0.11	0	━ ⌒ ±
Adrenaline 1μg/kg i.v.	Placebo	8/10	2.04 ± 0.20	4.1 ± 1.2	╫╫╫
	Pyridinolcarbamate 10mg/kg p.o.	2/10	1.60 ± 0.06	0	━ ⌒ ±
Angiotensin 1μg/kg i.v.	Placebo	10/10	2.61 ± 0.21	4.3 ± 1.2	╫╫╫
	Pyridinolcarbamate 10mg/kg p.o.	2/10	1.82 ± 0.08	0	━ ⌒ ±

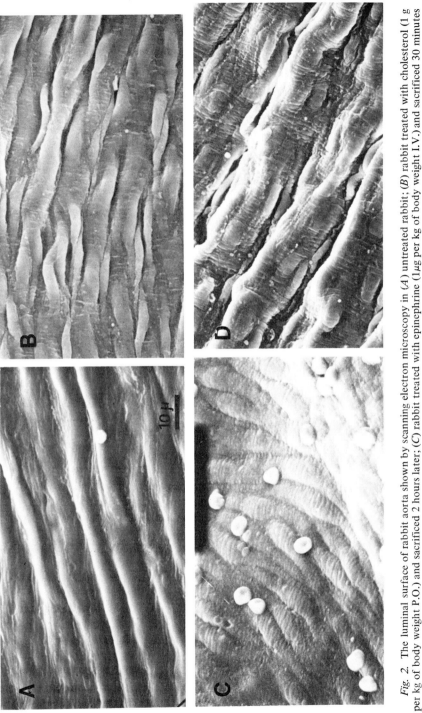

Fig. 2. The luminal surface of rabbit aorta shown by scanning electron microscopy in (*A*) untreated rabbit; (*B*) rabbit treated with cholesterol (1 g per kg of body weight P.O.) and sacrificed 2 hours later; (*C*) rabbit treated with epinephrine (1 μg per kg of body weight I.V.) and sacrificed 30 minutes later; and (*D*) rabbit treated with angiotensin II (1 μg per kg of body weight I.V.) and sacrificed 30 minutes later. The endothelial surface of untreated animal shows the endothelial folds with relatively smooth surface (*A*), while the surface of each endothelial fold shows many fine and horizontal lines at quite regular intervals (*b,c,d*) and is marked in (*d*), showing the contraction of endothelial cells.

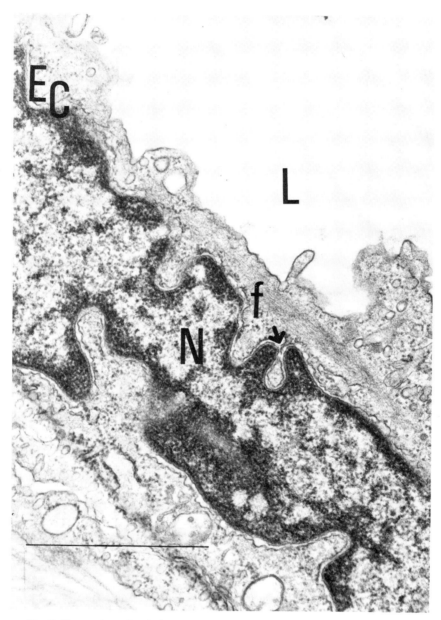

Fig. 3. Transection of endothelial cells (*EC*) contracted by cholesterol challenge. Pinch (*arrow*), deep indentation of the nuclei (*N*), and many filaments (*F*) concentrated in definite tracts in the cytoplasm close to the indentations of nuclei are seen. *LL,* vessel lumen.

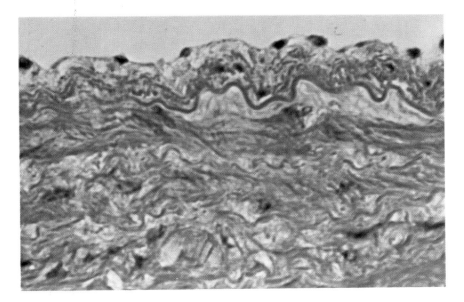

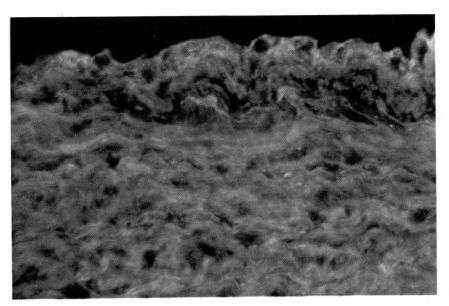

Plate 1. Transection of thoracic aorta of rhesus monkey given cholesterol (1 g per kg of body weight P.O.) and sacrificed 6 hours later. *Top,* hematoxylin-eosin stain shows the edematous arterial reaction in the subendothelial and inner medial layers. *Bottom,* immuno-fluorescent photograph shows the presence of β-lipoprotein in the edematous parts of the subendothelial and inner medial layers.

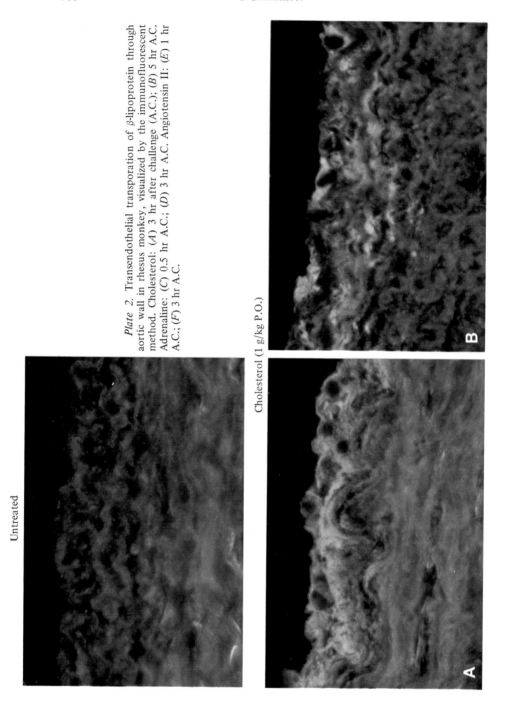

Untreated

Cholesterol (1 g/kg P.O.)

Plate 2. Transendothelial transporation of β-lipoprotein through aortic wall in rhesus monkey, visualized by the immunofluorescent method. Cholesterol: (*A*) 3 hr after challenge (A.C.); (*B*) 5 hr A.C. Adrenaline: (*C*) 0.5 hr A.C.; (*D*) 3 hr A.C. Angiotensin II: (*E*) 1 hr A.C.; (*F*) 3 hr A.C.

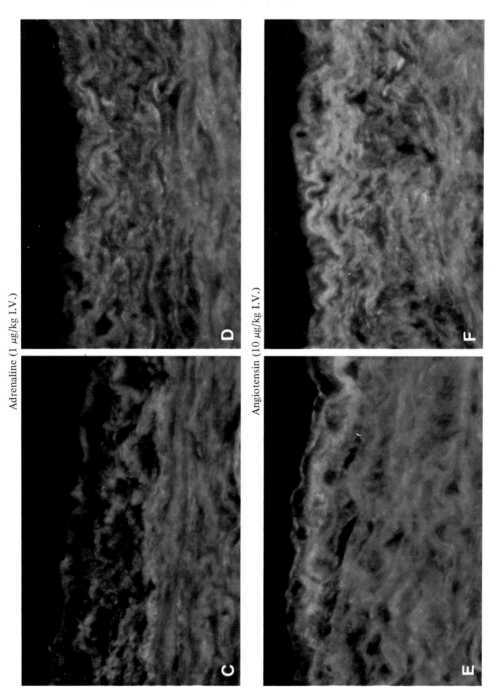

Adrenaline (1 μg/kg I.V.)

Angiotensin (10 μg/kg I.V.)

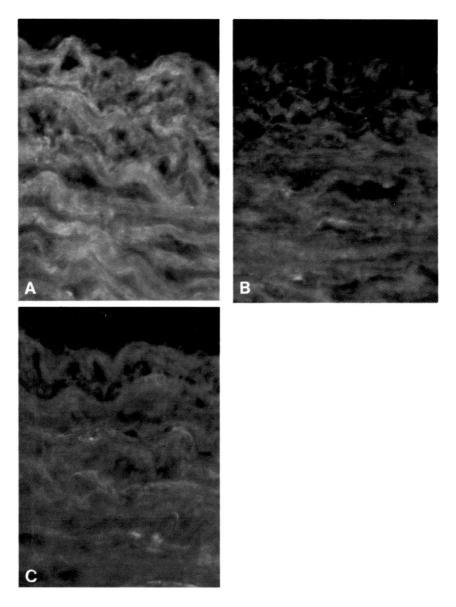

Plate 3. Transection of the aorta of rhesus monkey challenged with (*A*) cholesterol (1 g per kg of body weight P.O.); (*B*) epinephrine (1 μg per kg of body weight I.V.); and (*C*) angiotensin II (1 μg per kg of body weight I.V.) after pyridinolcarbamate-pretreatment (10 mg per kg of body weight P.O.) given 2 hours before the challenge. The animal was sacrificed 3 hours after the challenge with cholesterol. The fact that no fluorescence is found shows the preventive effect of pyridinolcarbamate.

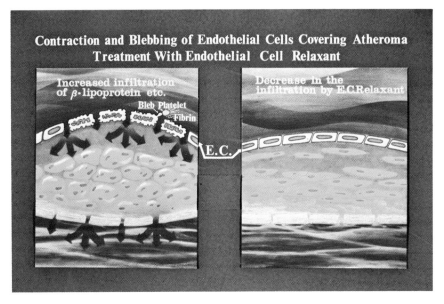

Plate 4. Infiltration of β-lipoprotein, etc., into arterial wall because of contraction of endothelial cells.

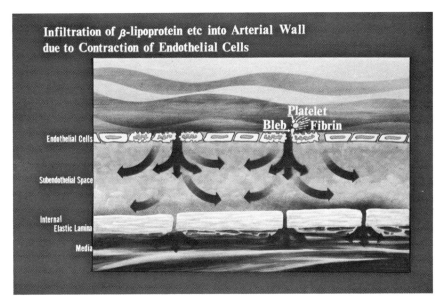

Plate 5. Left, contraction and blebbing of endothelial cell covering atheroma. *Right,* treatment with endothelial cell relaxant.

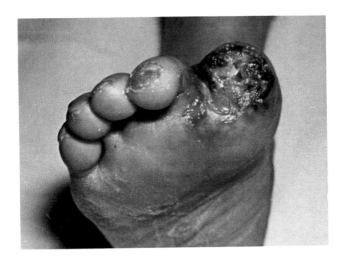

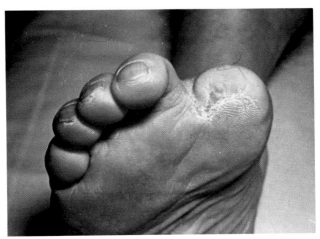

Plate 6. This 43-year-old male complained of paresthesia and intermittent claudication in his right leg for 3 years. He experienced pain in his right calf after walking about 100 meters. In September, 1966, he developed an ulcer on his right first toe which did not heal after lumbar sympathectomy. The toe was amputated, but the wound did not heal, and the patient complained of severe pain which disturbed his sleep. The patient received 1.5 g of pyridinolcarbamate daily after he visited our clinic. After 5 days of treatment with this drug, the severe pain began to decrease, and it completely disappeared after 2 weeks of treatment. After 6 months of treatment, the ulcer had healed completely.

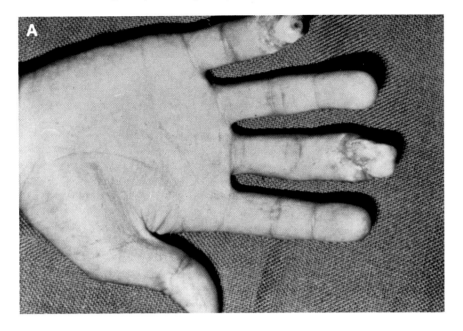

Plate 7. A, ischemic ulcer, which was painful and resistant to 8 months of treatment with vasodilators and antibiotics in a 29-year-old male suffering from atherosclerosis obliterans. Note the pale color with poor granulation. *B,* after 4 weeks of treatment with pyridinolcarbamate (1.5 g per day). Note the definite pink color of the granulation. *C,* after 4 months of treatment with pyridinolcarbamate. Note the healing of the ulcer. All fingers still were not warm enough because of the atherosclerotic change of local arteries.

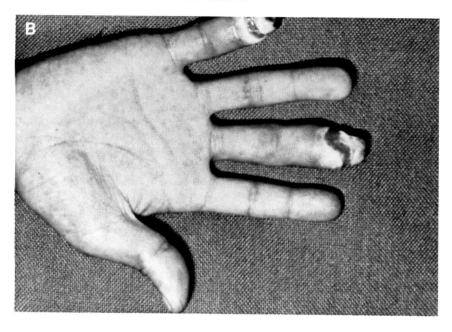

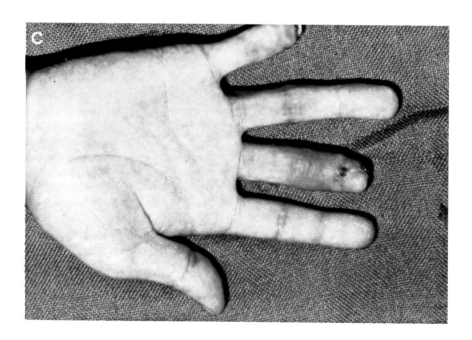

blood pressure. For instance, the cholesterol challenge did not change the blood pressure of animals challenged. Even 30 minutes after the intravenous injection of epinephrine or angiotensin II, the number of highly contracted endothelial cells amounted to 2.4% ± 2.1 and 1.6% ± 0.4, respectively. On the other hand, the hypertensive response was brief and ceased within one minute after the injection, demonstrating that the response of contractile protein of endothelial cells to the injection of epinephrine and angiotensin II is both long-lasting and entirely different from that of contractile protein of the smooth muscle of the arterioles. The distribution of highly contracted endothelial cells with nuclear pinch was neither normal nor of Poisson distribution, and the fact that there were so many nuclei without pinches also suggests the existence of more than one population of endothelial cells. A spotty distribution of endothelial cells with pinches actually would help to explain the focal, rather than diffuse, distribution of the edematous arterial response, as well as atherosclerosis in its initial stage.

Becker and Murphy (14) demonstrated the immunobiological similarity of contractile protein from vascular endothelial cells and smooth muscle of parturient uterus. I first succeeded in visualizing the real contraction of endothelial cells challenged by cholesterol, epinephrine, or angiotensin II. The contraction of arterial endothelial cells induced by angiotensin II and serotonin was also shown recently by Robertson et al. (16).

Pyridinolcarbamate (PDC), EG467, and estrogen have been shown by me (8, 17) to inhibit the edematous arterial reaction and atherosclerosis in cholesterol-fed rabbits. Usually, concomitant conditions, namely, acute infiltration of plasma proteins such as β-lipoprotein into the subendothelial space (9) and a thrombogenic tendency in the edematous arterial reaction (7), were also inhibited by these substances. Other studies (2–5) showed that PDC (10 mg/kg, P.O.), EG467 (1 mg/kg, P.O.), and estrogen (Premarin, 5 mg/kg, I.V.) perfectly prevent the strong contraction and nuclear pinching of arterial endothelial cells induced by the above-mentioned challenge with cholesterol, epinephrine, or angiotensin II. Such evidences show that the prevention of the severe contraction and blebbing of endothelial cells induced by atherogenic stress is the essential procedure in the prevention of atherosclerosis and thrombosis. Actually, PDC has been shown to inhibit significantly atherosclerosis in cholesterol-fed rabbits (18) and in cholesterol-fed cockerels (19), as well as arteriosclerosis induced by calciferol (20) and angiolathyrism (21).

It is important to note, in addition, that administration of these substances in the above-mentioned doses provokes neither vasodilative nor hypotensive responses in animals. Vasodilators, namely, nicotinic acid (1, 10, 20, and 50 mg/kg, P.O.) and papaverin (1 ～ 10 mg/kg, S.C.), were tested but produced no noticeable effect on the edematous arterial reaction. The excessive vasodilation may stretch the endothelial lining, resulting in the widening of intercellular spaces, and may be harmful.

ENDOTHELIAL CELLS COVERING ATHEROMA

In atheromatous lesions, the increased influx of cholesterol has been well known, but the reason for such an enhancement of transendothelial infiltration of cholesterol-bearing plasma proteins remained unknown. However, I found highly contracted endothelial cells with pinches in the arterial wall of hyper-cholesterolemic rabbits (Fig. 4), even in the elevated lesions, which are placed under the stretching force from the growing atheroma. In some specimens from atheroma, the population of endothelial cells with pinches amounted to 21.2% of all endothelial cells counted, but the percentage was more typically around 5.2%±2.6. Even after withdrawal of cholesterol feeding and 48 hours of feeding on normal pellets without cholesterol, highly contracted endothelial cells with pinches could be seen in the endothelial cells covering atheroma of all animals tested.

The endothelial lining covering atheroma certainly is stretched by growing atheroma and, in addition, the contraction of endothelial cells undoubtedly contributes to widening the intercellular junctions, thus permitting the passage of large particles from the plasma, especially in the vasodilative stage of arterial pulsation. Such evidence indicated clearly the need for an endothelial cell relaxant for the prevention and treatment of atherosclerosis.

PDC (10–30 mg/kg, P.O.), EG467 (10 mg/kg, P.O.), and Premarin (5 mg/kg, I.V.) were tested for their inhibitory effect on the contraction of endothelial cells covering atheroma, and their definite relaxing effect has been established. This fact suggests their efficacy in the repair of atheromatous lesions; actually, PDC (7) and Premarin (17) have been shown to enhance the histologic repair process and the withdrawal of cholesterol from the affected arterial wall. The repair of fibrinoid degeneration of arterioles in hypertensive rabbits also has been shown to be significantly enhanced by PDC (22). In addition, Numano et al. (23) have shown that PDC enhances the glycolytic and tricarboxylic acid cycle enzyme activities and the regeneration of smooth muscle. Kritchevsky and Tepper (24) showed that PDC significantly accelerates the oxidation of choles-terol by rat liver mitochondria. Such effects also may be involved in the enhancement of the repair process. As shown in Plate 5 and Figure 5 the relaxation of endothelial cells makes it possible not only to prevent atherosclero-sis, but also to produce a curative effect. This is the principle of the treatment of atherosclerosis with an endothelial cell relaxant.

Blebbing of the endothelial cells of blood vessels has been shown by Willms-Kretschmer and Majno (25) to be induced by ischemia. The author and his collaborators (2, 4, 5) demonstrated further that blebbing can be induced by

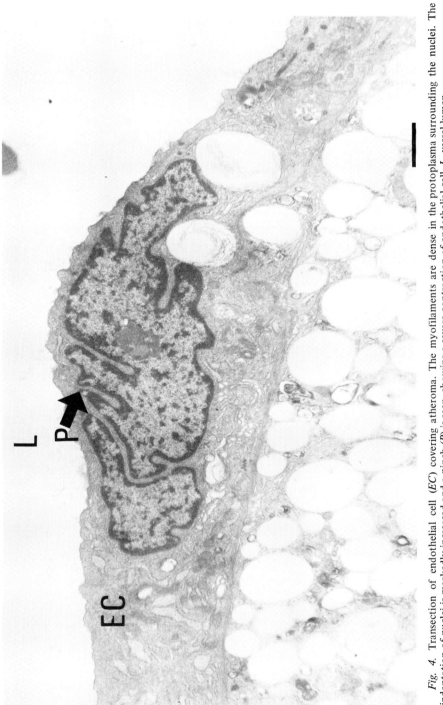

Fig. 4. Transection of endothelial cell (*EC*) covering atheroma. The myofilaments are dense in the protoplasma surrounding the nuclei. The indentation of nuclei is markedly increased and a pinch (*P*) is seen, showing a severe contraction of endothelial cell. *L*, vessel lumen.

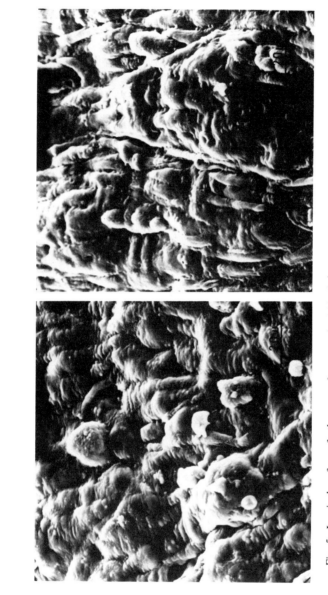

Fig. 5. Luminal surface of atheroma of untreated rabbit (*left*) and rabbit treated with pyridinolcarbamate (10 mg per kg of body weight P.O.) 2 hours before sacrifice (*right*). Untreated animals (*left*): vertical wrinkles are abundant, showing the contraction of endothelial cells. Each elevated and longitudinally long structure roughly represents the nuclear part of each individual cell. Treated animals (*right*): vertical wrinkles are markedly less, showing the relaxing effect of pyridinol-carbamate.

atherogenic stress, such as the administration of cholesterol (1 g/kg, P.O.), epinephrine (1 μg/kg, I.V.), and angiotensin II (1 μg/kg, I.V.). Platelets commonly stick to blebs, and it is not rare to find fibrin forming around such platelets, showing clearly the thrombogenic significance of the blebbing (Fig. 6).

The administration of even the above-mentioned single doses of epinephrine (26, 27), cholesterol (26, 28), or angiotensin II (29) in rabbits has been shown to enhance platelet aggregability significantly, to shorten clotting times, and to reduce temporarily the adhesive platelet count (26). Such hematologic changes have been shown to be significantly inhibited by PDC and EG467.

CLINICAL TRIALS OF ENDOTHELIAL CELL RELAXANTS: PDC AND EG467

The familiar clinical signs and symptoms of atherosclerosis are caused by the narrowing or occlusion of an artery, which causes an inadequacy in the blood supply to the affected organ; this results in aneurysm formation or rupture of the artery with hemorrhage into the surrounding tissues, depending on the organ or tissue affected. Such drugs as PDC and EG467, which are capable of preventing the acute infiltration of plasma into the vessel wall because of their

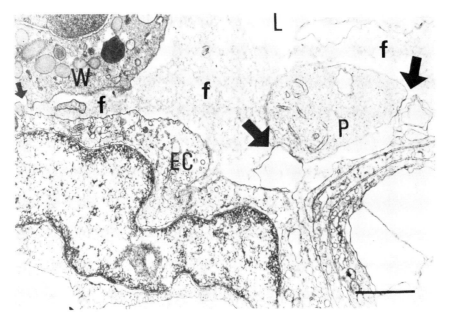

Fig. 6. Blebs (*arrows*) stuck by platelet (*P*) with fibrin (*f*). The severe contraction always accompanies the blebbing of endothelial cells. The bleb is often stuck by platelets with formed fibrin, showing the thrombogenic significance.

relaxing and protective effect directly on the endothelial cells and platelets, seem to inhibit the occlusion, aneurysm formation, and rupture of the artery.

In established atherosclerotic plaques, which are composed mainly of scar tissue, it is impossible to reopen arteries occluded by atherosclerosis with drug therapy, and surgery is indicated. However, PDC makes it possible, at least in experimental animals, to expand the narrowed lumen of arteries partially obstructed by atheromatous lesions with edematous fluid, atheromatous mass, and endothelial cells with thrombotic tendency. This is possible because PDC reduces the infiltration of plasma lipoproteins into the arterial wall by relaxing endothelial cells, and prevents the adhesion of platelets to endothelial surfaces or to each other (2–5, 28, 29), thus maintaining a smooth microcirculatory flow. PDC also makes it possible to prevent or retard the further accumulation of fatty substances in the arterial wall and the formation of thrombosis, as shown (8, 17–23) in experimental atherosclerosis. Such facts have led to the use of PDC in the clinic.

PDC and EG467 were synthesized originally by myself and my collaborators to prevent the acute infiltration of cholesterol-bearing lipoproteins of the plasma into the arterial wall (2–5) and to reduce the thrombotic activities of the vessel wall and platelet (2, 3, 28, 29), as detailed in this article. However, these facts were not widely known in the United States until Professors Henry I. Russek and Walter Redisch of New York Medical College conducted clinical trials of PDC.

PDC has been tested by specialists of many countries, and numerous clinical trials have been conducted by means of modern statistical techniques under double-blind testing (4). Here I summarize the results of the tests and the most recent findings from clinical trials, as well as some data concerning EG467.

Basic Clinical Evidence

Since it is impossible to obtain arterial specimens from living human patients, the immediate effects of PDC and EG467 have been inferred from hematologic changes accompanying responses of patients to atherogenic stress, such as oral administration of large amounts of animal fat (30, 31), injection of epinephrine (30–32), or exercise tests (33, 34) in coronary patients. Years of study have confirmed the fact that hematologic changes accompanying atherogenic stress in man are similar to those observed in animals, so that clinical findings can be supported by experiments in vivo. It was also found by our group (33) that hematologic responses are much more easily induced in patients suffering from atherosclerotic diseases than in healthy subjects. Thus, the effect of PDC in preventing hematologic responses induced by atherogenic substances, shown experimentally in animals, has been confirmed by clinical tests. Such evidence has suggested reasonably that the alteration of the vascular endothelial function in man, provoked by atherogenic stress resulting in the severe contraction and blebbing of endothelial cells, is the same as that observed experimentally in rabbits and monkeys.

Evidence of the antithrombotic effect of PDC is shown easily in patients suffering from atherosclerosis. With Master's two-step test (33, 34), coronary patients with exertion angina exhibited positive ECG changes and anginal pain, accompanied by transient shortening of clotting times, reduction in adhesive platelet count (33), and enhancement of ADP-induced platelet aggregability (34). Such a thrombogenic tendency and clinical and ECG changes have been prevented to a statistically significant degree by pretreatment of patients with PDC (33, 34).

A single injection of epinephrine or oral administration of 50 g of butter in 100 ml of cream in man (30, 31) induced hematologic changes similar to those accompanying the edematous arterial reaction in experimental animals (26). Such changes were prevented significantly by pretreatment of test subjects with PDC (30, 31).

Pyridinolcarbamate and EG467 as a So-Called Platelet Drug (Fig. 7)

As shown by Didisheim et al. (35), Sano and Yokoyama (36), and Yamazaki et al. (37), both substances have a powerful, direct, inhibitory effect against the primary as well as secondary aggregation of human platelets to ADP, epinephrine, and collagen, while aspirin has no inhibitory effect against the primary aggregation of platelets.

SUMMARY OF THE RESULTS OF PDC TREATMENT

In the early period of PDC treatment, adequate dosages and duration of treatment were unknown and the symptoms to be evaluated were not yet understood; thus, many errors were made. For instance, even the angiographic reopening of arteries occluded with atheromatous scar was erroneously reported, despite the fact that such scar tissue calls for surgical treatment rather than drug therapy.

The overall effectiveness rates reported from various institutions were 62.6% in cerebral atherosclerosis, 44.1% in the improvement of the resting ECG, 69.5% in the disappearance or definite improvement in the frequency and severity of anginal attacks in coronary atherosclerosis, and 68.7% in peripheral atherosclerosis. Needless to say, effectiveness varies with conditions; however, PDC has been shown to be significantly effective in comparison to treatment with vasodilators, nicotinic acid, or placebo treatment.

The daily dosage used was 20 mg/kg of the body weight, three times a day. It was often 15 mg/kg and was found to be satisfactory, and sometimes it was 30 mg/kg. Minor side-effects, such as gastrointestinal disturbance, were encountered in less than 5%. In Japanese patients, jaundice was reported on rare occasions.

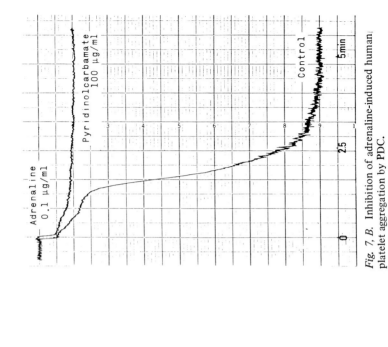

Fig. 7, B. Inhibition of adrenaline-induced human platelet aggregation by PDC.

Fig. 7, A. Inhibition of ADP-induced human platelet aggregation by PDC.

Careful observations recently have been made on hepatotoxicity, including other side-effects in the United States of America and European countries during the past four years, and the results have been collected and published in connection with the international congress held in Tokyo on May 19–21, 1972, but no case of hepatotoxicity was reported, only minor side-effects. More than 30 patients who had received from 1,005–2,483 g of PDC for 5–7 years in my hospital were subjected to various organ function tests, and analysis disclosed no abnormality that could be attributed to the drug.

Cerebral Atherosclerosis

Atherosclerosis of a given cerebral vessel causes no symptoms if the area of the brain supplied by the diseased artery receives adequate compensatory blood supply from other arteries or through collateral circulation. In the treatment of cerebral atherosclerosis, the prevention of acute infiltration of plasma into the cerebral arteries because of the contraction of endothelial cells by stress is also important as a precaution against further narrowing and the progress of athero-sclerosis. At the same time, the microcirculation of the brain, especially its collateral circulation, should be protected from mural thrombosis, i.e. the adhesion of platelets to endothelial cells with blebbing and the aggregation of platelets as a result of stress. For such a purpose, PDC treatment has been applied extensively. There are already many reports on its administration under open or double-blind trials as summarized by myself, and its therapeutic efficacy has been confirmed statistically.

Patients who had survived a first stroke (mainly from cerebral thrombosis) were subjected to controlled clinical trials by Murase et al. (38) for two years. There were 27 patients in the control group and 29 in the PDC group. The age, sex, symptoms, complications, early case history, onset, and duration of observation were well matched in both groups. During 31.6 ± 4.8 months and 31.4 ± 5.9 months of the observation period of the control and PDC treatment groups, respectively, relapse in apoplexy occurred in four of the PDC group and nine of the control group, and the statistically significant effect of PDC in preventing relapse was observed. Fukui (39) reported the statistically significant preventive effect of PDC against relapse in apoplexy and heart attack among his 4,083 postapoplectic patients, and Yoneda et al. (40) reported the same effect of PDC in their 159 postapoplectic patients.

Coronary Atherosclerosis

Angina pectoris is believed to be induced by ischemia of the heart muscle because of narrowing of the coronary arteries. This symptom usually occurs only intermittently from physical exertion or emotional stress, which temporarily increases the need of the heart muscle for blood beyond the available supply delivered by the affected coronary artery. As a rule, such pain subsides promptly with rest or drug therapy. The usual treatment of angina pectoris is designed to relieve chest pain either by avoidance of activities which produce the discomfort or by the use of nitroglycerin.

Using the double-blind cross-over technique with PDC and placebo in one group of 40 patients suffering from angina pectoris (33) and in another such group of 13 patients (34), I found that, besides the well-known clinical responses such as anginal pain and ECG changes, the above-mentioned hematologic changes, such as a transient reduction of adhesive platelet count, a shortening of clotting times, and the enhancement of ADP-induced aggregability of platelets, were induced by Master's two-step exercise test, and that such changes are inhibited to a statistically significant degree after pretreatment of patients with PDC. Russek (41) tested the effect of PDC in patients suffering from coronary atherosclerosis and observed exercise-ECG changes. In the course of treatment, the exercise test improved significantly in a number of his patients with refractory angina pectoris.

Controlled clinical trials in the treatment of coronary atherosclerosis with angina pectoris have been tried under the double-blind technique and have shown the favorable effect of PDC. Figure 8 summarizes results obtained by Shkhvatsabaya (42) at the Central Institute of Cardiology, USSR, showing the representative pattern of PDC treatment of coronary patients. In my experience, PDC treatment of the intermediate form (coronary insufficiency or preinfarction angina) often seemed to prevent infarction. Such clinical evidence (43) suggests the favorable effect of PDC on the affected coronary arteries and on microcirculation, including that of the collaterals in the myocardium.

As shown by Haerem (44), sudden death often is induced by a hampering of

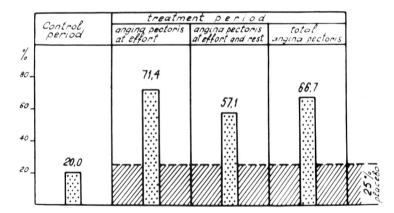

Fig. 8. Effect of the treatment by pyridinolcarbamate (Anginin) of chronic coronary insufficiency (double-blind test). From Ref. 42.

the intramyocardial circulation by platelet aggregation without major acute lesions in the epicardial arteries. Even in thrombosis of epicardial arteries, which is the most common cause of acute myocardial infarction, the above-mentioned hampering of local intramyocardial circulation because of platelet aggregation may contribute to the slowdown and stasis of the local upper stream in the atherosclerotic epicardial artery, thus inducing thrombosis. When such a condition exists, it is feasible to use PDC for the prevention of sudden death or acute myocardial infarction, as suggested by the preventive effect of PDC.

Peripheral Atherosclerotic Disorders

The morbid conditions known as arteriosclerosis obliterans and thromboangitis obliterans have been subjected to PDC treatment since 1963 in Japan and abroad, and many controlled clinical trials (45) have been successfully conducted under the double-blind technique (46). Improvement was noted mainly in the crest time of toe plethysmography, in ischemic signs such as cyanosis and ulcer of the affected fingers and toes (Plate 6), and in intermittent claudication. In the treatment of ischemic ulcer with this compound alone, almost all investigators have experienced a relatively high rate of cure, which averages about 75% in 250 cases. Cyanosis and rest pain of affected feet are also good targets. In aged patients more than 90 years old, these symptoms disappeared with PDC treatment. There was relapse after several weeks without the medication, but recovery from the relapse occurred after the restart of PDC treatment. Such evidence, in addition to statistical evaluation under the double-blind method, has been accepted by examiners.

The slowly appearing effect of PDC in patients suffering from arteriosclerosis obliterans is illustrated in Figure 9. This figure summarized the representative result of long-term PDC treatment of patients suffering from arteriosclerosis obliterans with claudication. As shown in Figure 5, claudication time improved steadily in the course of 20–50 weeks, and statistically significant improvement

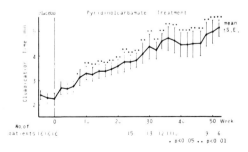

Fig. 9. Improvement in claudication time in patients with atherosclerosis obliterans treated on long-term basis with pyridinolcarbamate.

was shown after 22 weeks of the treatment. After that period, the steady prolongation of claudication time continued to 50 weeks, showing the importance of long-term medication in the treatment of atherosclerotic diseases. In an open study, Cotton (47) treated 13 cases of arteriosclerosis obliterans with PDC (1.5 g daily) for many weeks and observed clinical improvement while measuring the change of platelet aggregability by ADP using his filtration pressure method. He observed that the PDC treatment normalized slowly but steadily the elevated ADP-induced platelet aggregability of patients in the course of 5–6 weeks, and that the improvement of clinical signs followed.

In the PDC treatment of arteriosclerosis obliterans, a favorable response started at the end of the first week in some cases, and the intolerable pain of arteriosclerotic ulcer subsided within 1–3 weeks. Pale ischemic ulcers with poor granulation turned pink after 1 or 2 weeks, and the growth of healthy granulation started relatively soon thereafter (Plate 7). Definite improvement of some other symptoms—notably, a distinct reduction in the crest time of toe plethysmography—started in the course of 4–6 weeks of treatment in quite a number of cases.

PDC treatment seems to increase the blood flow, not only in the skin of the ulcer but in the muscles of the affected extremities as well. Atsumi et al. (48) actually measured the blood flow in anterior tibial muscles of affected legs in patients suffering from arteriosclerosis obliterans by the ^{133}Xe-injection method. Even with such an insensitive method, a definite increase of blood flow at the height of reactive hyperemia was serially demonstrated in the course of PDC treatment in some of the patients, and the increase in blood flow was accompanied by clinical improvement.

Follow-up Study on Patients Suffering from Arteriosclerosis Obliterans under PDC Treatment and under Non-PDC Treatment

One hundred five male patients suffering from arteriosclerosis obliterans were divided into two matched groups of 45 and 60 patients, respectively. The first group of 45 patients received PDC treatment and was observed for 211.5 ± 17.4 weeks, while the second group of 60 patients received various other drugs and was observed for 165.4 ± 13.0 weeks. Among both groups, the age, blood pressure, blood cholesterol level, duration, and severity of arteriosclerosis obliterans as well as complications from diabetes mellitus and myocardial infarction at the start of the treatments were comparable, as shown in Table 2.

It is important to note that deaths attributable to myocardial infarction and apoplexy number six and two, respectively, in patients treated with the other drugs, while among patients receiving PDC treatment, there was only one case of apoplectic attack and no deaths from any cause. The difference is statistically significant ($p < 0.05$).

Table 2. Follow-up Study on Patients Suffering from Arteriosclerosis Obliterans under Pyridinolcarbamate Treatment and Other Treatment*

Category	Pyridinolcarbamate group	Non-Pyridinolcarbamate group
Total number of patients	45	60
Age (years)	50.7 ± 2.4	53.0 ± 1.5
History of disease (months)	50.0 ± 10.9	48.9 ± 6.8
Severity of disease (types)		
II	39	57
IV	6	3
Blood cholesterol level (mg/dl)	198.8 ± 8.7	187.2 ± 5.2
Blood pressure (mmHg)		
Systolic	149.4 ± 5.0	152.9 ± 5.1
Diastolic	83.5 ± 2.7	90.4 ± 2.4
Complications		
Diabetes mellitus	6	4
Myocardial infarction	2	2
Observation period (weeks)	211.5 ± 17.4	165.4 ± 13.0
Number of deaths by apoplectic and heart attacks	0	8 ($p < 0.05$)
Apoplectic attacks	(1) Survived	2
Heart attacks	0	6

* Courtesy of Atsumi, T., Honda, Y., and Matsuda, M.: J. Jap. Coll. Angiol., in press.

DISCUSSION

The experimental evidence shows clearly that the trigger mechanism in athero-genesis by one of the "three major risk factors," hypercholesterolemia, is initiated by the contraction of endothelial cells accompanied by blebbing. The atherogenic property of the remaining two major risk factors, cigarette smoking and hypertension, may be related to epinephrine secreted as a response to smoking, and also to angiotensin II production (11) provoked by certain types of hypertension (except low renin hypertension). These two hormones make arterial endothelial cells contract, as in the case of cholesterol challenge. Stamler, Berkson, and Lindberg (10) showed that the impact on risk of the major risk factors such as hypercholesterolemia, cigarette smoking, and hypertension is additive. Actually, combined challenge with cholesterol, epinephrine, or angiotensin II markedly increased the contraction of endothelial cells, and at the same time the acute infiltration of plasma proteins into the subendothelial space and the barrier function of the internal elastic lamina were enhanced. These facts show clearly that the contraction of arterial endothelial cells is the trigger mechanism in atherogenesis and thrombogenesis.

In this experimental observation, the importance of relaxing the highly contracted endothelial cells accompanied by blebbing was emphasized as a means of inhibiting the infiltration of cholesterol-bearing plasma protein into the arterial lesions, and preventing the progress of atherosclerosis. At the same time, the preventive effect of PDC and EG467 was shown. The direct inhibiting effect of these substances on platelet aggregability also may be beneficial for the prevention of thrombosis and atherosclerosis, but the main effect of these drugs is on the contraction and blebbing of endothelial cells. The presence of highly contracted endothelial cells accompanied by blebbing covering atheroma is clearly the highly important aggravating mechanism of atherosclerosis. It is most urgent that such a condition be relieved by an endothelial cell relaxant such as PDC or EG467 for the prevention of transendothelial infiltration of cholesterol-bearing plasma proteins through widened intercellular spaces, and for inhibiting the progress of atherosclerosis and preventing dangerous consequences such as apoplexy and heart attack. We already know of a similar condition in the treatment of malignant hypertension; needless to say, it is of paramount importance and urgency to relax highly contracted arteriolar smooth muscles to lower the blood pressure and to save the life in such a case. The elimination of risk factors such as hypercholesterolemia, hypertension, and cigarette smoking is, of course, important in the treatment of atherosclerotic diseases, but by the time they are recognized, it is often too late for such conventional measures. I have emphasized the paramount importance of endothelial cell relaxants in the treatment of atherosclerosis and in the prevention of its dangerous outcome. On the basis of solid evidence and experience, it is reasonable to assume that premature death from atherosclerosis can be prevented by controlling the severe contraction of endothelial cells, and that such a procedure will be perfected in the near future.

SUMMARY

Single-dose treatment of rabbits and monkeys was performed with cholesterol, angiotensin II, and epinephrine, which are related to or included as active participants in the so-called three major risk factors: hypercholesterolemia, hypertension, and cigarette smoking (10). The appearance of an edematous arterial reaction was observed, accompanied by a series of characteristic hematologic changes induced by these challenges. In this response, it was found that the arterial endothelial cells show a strong contraction with nuclear pinch in certain groups of cells characteristically appearing spottily. This contraction is accompanied by the infiltration of plasma proteins into subendothelial and inner medial layers dammed temporarily by internal elastic lamina. The severely contracted endothelial cells show bleb formation, and the blebs often are adhered to by platelets with fibrin formation, suggesting a thrombogenic property. Several findings show that the severe contraction is the trigger mechanism in atherogenesis and thrombogenesis, and I proposed it as an explanation of the unknown factor previously mentioned by Haust and More (1).

The severe contraction of endothelial cells was found in large arteries of hypercholesterolemic animals and also in endothelial cells covering atheroma. The need for endothelial cell relaxants in the treatment of atherosclerosis was proposed for the first time in the history of atherosclerosis. In addition, the urgent importance of its application to advanced atherosclerotic patients was emphasized for the prevention of such dangerous outcomes as apoplexy and heart attack.

Accumulated clinical results from the treatment of atherosclerotic diseases with one of the endothelial cell relaxants, pyridinolcarbamate, offer evidence supporting the above-mentioned observations and have been summarized briefly.

Notably, a single-dose treatment of man with epinephrine or animal fat, or Master's exercise test performed by coronary patients, induced characteristic hematologic changes similar to those observed in animals in which atherogenic stress had been induced. Such changes, as in the case of animals, were prevented by pretreatment of test subjects with an endothelial cell relaxant.

The treatment of patients suffering from cerebral, coronary, and peripheral atherosclerosis, performed in many countries, has been summarized. The favorable clinical response of these patients to long-term treatment with an endothelial cell relaxant was reported, and promising results in the prevention of apoplexy and heart attack were also detailed.

Particular emphasis was placed on the importance of further research on the treatment of atherosclerosis with endothelial cell relaxants.

REFERENCES CITED

1. Haust, M. D., and More, R. H. 1972. Development of modern theories on the pathogenesis of atherosclerosis. Pages 1–19 *in* R. W. Wissler and J. C. Geer (eds.), The pathogenesis of atherosclerosis. Williams & Wilkins, Baltimore.
2. Shimamoto, T., and Sunaga, T. 1972. Contraction of endothelial cells as a key mechanism in atherogenesis. Proc. Jap. Acad. 48:633.
3. Shimamoto, T., and Numano, F. 1972. Preventive effect of estrogen against cholesterol-induced contraction of arterial endothelial cells. An electron microscopic observation. Proc. Jap. Acad. 48:742.

4. Shimamoto, T. 1972. New concept on atherogenesis and treatment of atherosclerotic diseases. Jap. Heart J. 13:537.
5. Shimamoto, T., and Numano, F. 1973. Endothelial-cell contraction covering atheroma and its relaxation. Proc. Jap. Acad. 49:77.
6. Anitschkow, N. 1913. Uber die Veränderungen der Kaninchenaorta bei experimenteller Cholesterinsteatose. Beitr. Pathol. Anat. 56:379.
7. Shimamoto, T. 1963. The relationship of edematous reaction in arteries to atherosclerosis and thrombosis. J. Atheroscler. Res. 3:87.
8. Shimamoto, T. 1969. Experimental study on atherosclerosis—An attempt at its prevention and treatment. Acta Pathol. Jap. 19:15.
9. Shimamoto, T., Kobayashi, M., and Numano, F. 1972. Infiltration of γ-globulin, fibrinogen and β-lipoprotein into blood vessel wall by atherogenic stress visualized by immunofluorescence. Proc. Jap. Acad. 48:336.
10. Stamler, J., Berkson, D. M., and Lindberg, H. A. 1972. Risk factors: Their role in the etiology and pathogenesis of the atherosclerotic diseases. Pages 41–119 in R. W. Wissler and J. C. Geer (eds.), The pathogenesis of atherosclerosis. Williams & Wilkins, Baltimore.
11. Laragh, J. H. 1971. Biochemical profiling and the natural history of hypertensive diseases: Low-renin essential hypertension, a benign condition. Circulation 44:971.
12. Kaneko, Y., Takeda, T., Ikeda, T., Yagi, S., Ishii, M., Ebihara, A., Tagawa, H., Nishiyama, K., and Ohno, K. 1972. Plasma renin activity and prognosis of essential hypertension. Jap. Circ. J. 36:995.
13. Yamashita, Y. 1969. Electron microscopic analysis of aortic wall permeability—Visualization of the transendothelial passage through intercellular junctions in endothelial cells of aortic wall and vasa vasorum using peroxydase as a tracer. Jap. Circ. J. 33:1395.
14. Becker, C. G., and Murphy, G. E. 1968. Demonstration of actomyosin in cells of heart valve, endothelium, intima, the arteriosclerotic plaque, and endocardial and myocardial aschoff bodies. Amer. J. Pathol. 52:220.
15. Majno, G., Shea, S. M., and Leventhal, M. 1969. Endothelial contraction induced by histamine-type mediators. An electron microscopic study. J. Cell Biol. 42:647.
16. Robertson, A. L., Khaivallah, P. A., and Kyncl, J. 1972. Role of endothelial contraction and platelets in atherogenesis [abstr.]. Circulation 46(Suppl. II):252.
17. Pick, R. 1952. Estrogen-induced regression of coronary atherosclerosis in cholesterol-fed chicks. Fed. Proc. 11:122.
18. Perrin, A., and Loire, R. 1969. Bilan d'une première experience clinique et expérimentale avec le pyridinolcarbamate. Pages 71–74 in T. Shimamoto and F. Numano (eds.), Atherogenesis. Excerpta Medica, Amsterdam.
19. Wu, C. C., Huang, T. S., and Hsu, C. J. 1969. Prevention of experimental atherosclerosis with pyridinolcarbamate. Amer. Heart J. 77:657.
20. Grafnetter, D., Shimamoto, T., and Numano, F. 1973. Blood and tissue lipids during the treatment of rats with high fat diet, calciferol and pyridinolcarbamate. Tokyo Conference on Atherogenesis, Thrombogenesis and Pyridinolcarbamate Treatment. May 18-20, 1972. Pages 122–128 in T. Shimamoto, F. Numano, and C. M. Addison (eds.), Atherogenesis II. Excerpta Medica, Amsterdam.
21. Yamamura, T. 1969. Inhibitory effects of pyridinolcarbamate in angiolathyrism and osteolathyrism. Pages 29–36 in T. Shimamoto and F. Numano (eds.), Atherogenesis. Excerpta Medica, Amsterdam.
22. Ooneda, G., Yoshida, Y., Kojimahara, M., and Fukushima, T. 1969. Effect of pyridinolcarbamate on arterial lesions in hypertensive rats. Pages 47–52 in T. Shimamoto and F. Numano (eds.), Atherogenesis. Excerpta Medica, Amsterdam.
23. Numano, F., Katsu, K., Takenobu, M., Sagara, A., and Shimamoto, T. 1971. Comparative studies on the preventive effect of pyridinolcarbamate and estrogen against aortic and coronary atherosclerosis of cholesterol-fed rabbits. Part II. Histoenzymatic studies. Acta Pathol. Jap. 21:193.
24. Kritchevsky, D., and Tepper, A. 1971. Influence of pyridinolcarbamate on oxidation of cholesterol by rat liver mitochondria. Arzneim.-Forsch. 21:146.

25. Willms-Kretschmer, K., and Majno, G. 1969. Ischemia of the skin. Electron microscopic study of vascular injury. Amer. J. Pathol. 54:327.
26. Yamazaki, H., Sano, T., Kobayashi, I., Takahashi, T., and Shimamoto, T. 1973. Enhancement of ADP-induced platelet aggregation by adrenaline and cholesterol in vivo and its prevention. Pages 177–194 in Atherogenesis II. Excerpta Medica, Amsterdam.
27. Sano, T. 1964. An immediate and transient thrombocytopenic reaction by adrenaline. Jap. J. Med. 3:357.
28. Sano, T., Yamazaki, H., and Shimamoto, T. 1973. Enhancement of ADP-induced platelet aggregation by cholesterol and its prevention by pyridinolcarbamate. Thrombos. Diathes. Haemorrh. (In press).
29. Sano, T., Shimamoto, T., Yamazaki, H., and Shimamoto, T. 1973. Enhancement of ADP-induced platelet aggregation by angiotensin in vivo. Thrombos. Diathes. Haemorrh. (In preparation).
30. Odakura, T. 1965. Preventive effect of pyridinolcarbamate against decrease of adhesive platelet count by adrenaline and animal fat in man. Ochanomizu Med. J. 13:309.
31. Takeuchi, K. 1965. Antithrombotic property of pyridinolcarbamate in man. Increase of blood coagulation by adrenaline or high fatty meal in man and prevention by pyridinolcarbamate. Ochanomizu Med. J. 13:310.
32. Yamazaki, H., Sano, T., Odakura, T., Takeuchi, K., Matsumura, T., Hosaki, S., and Shimamoto, T. 1971. Appearance of thrombogenic tendency induced by adrenaline and its prevention by β-adrenergic blocking agent, nialamide and pyridinolcarbamate. Thrombos. Diathes. Haemorrh. 26:251.
33. Yamazaki, H., Sano, T., Odakura, T., Takeuchi, K., and Shimamoto, T. 1970. Electrocardiographic and hematological changes by exercise test in coronary patients and pyridinolcarbamate pretreatment—A double blind crossover trial. Amer. Heart J. 79:640.
34. Yamazaki, H., Kobayashi, I., and Shimamoto, T. 1970. Enhancement of ADP-induced platelet aggregation by exercise test in coronary patients and its prevention by pyridinolcarbamate. Thrombos. Diathes. Haemorrh. 24:438.
35. Didisheim, P., Sturm, R. E., and Owen, C. A., Jr. 1971. Experiments on thrombosis and its prevention, current concepts of coagulation and haemostasis. Pages 177–184 in R. Losito and B. F. K. Longpré (eds.), Schattauer Verlag, Stuttgart-New York.
36. Sano, T., and Yokoyama, M. 1971. Effect of pyridinolcarbamate on platelet aggregation. Amer. J. Med. Sci. 262:205.
37. Yamazaki, H., Sano, T., and Shimamoto, T. 1972. Enhancement of ADP-induced platelet aggregability by adrenaline and cholesterol and its prevention. Third Congress, International Society on Thrombosis and Haemostasis, August, 1972, Washington, D. C.
38. Murase, H., Odakura, T., Takeuchi, K., Yamazaki, H., Shimamoto, T., and Shimamoto, T. 1969. The effect of pyridinolcarbamate on cerebral vascular disease. Pages 245–248 in T. Shimamoto and F. Numano (eds.), Atherogenesis. Excerpta Medica, Amsterdam.
39. Fukui, K. 1969. Clinical results of pyridinolcarbamate treatments of hemiplegics in Kakeyu Hospital. Pages 239–244 in T. Shimamoto, and F. Numano (eds.), Atherogenesis. Excerpta Medica, Amsterdam.
40. Yoneda, T., Date, T., Sasaki, S., and Suzuki, S. 1967. Anginin in the treatment of postapoplectic patients. Diagnosis Treatment 55:1228.
41. Russek, H. I. 1973. Evaluation of anginin in the treatment of patients with angina pectoris. Tokyo Conference on Atherogenesis, Thrombogenesis and Pyridinolcarbamate Treatment, May 18–20, 1972. Pages 354–362 in T. Shimamoto, F. Numano, and C. M. Addison (eds.), Atherogenesis II. Excerpta Medica, Amsterdam.
42. Shkhvatsabaya, I. K. 1973. Anginin in treatment of chronic coronary insufficiency. Tokyo Conference on Atherogenesis, Thrombogenesis and Pyridinolcarbamate Treatment, May 18–20, 1972. Pages 347–350 in T. Shimamoto, F. Numano and C. M. Addison (eds.), Atherogenesis II. Excerpta Medica, Amsterdam.
43. Yamazaki, H., Murase, H., and Shimamoto, T. 1965. Effect of pyridinolcarbamate on angina pectoris. Ochanomizu Med. J. 13:283.
44. Haerem, J. W. 1972. Platelet aggregates in intramyocardial vessels of patients dying suddenly and unexpectedly of coronary artery disease. Atherosclerosis 15:199.

45. Shimamoto, T., Atsumi, T., Yamashita, S., Motomiya, T., Isokane, N., Ishioka, T., and Sakuma, A. 1970. Clinical pharmacologic evaluation of the antiatherosclerotic agent, pyridinolcarbamate. A double-blind crossover trial in the treatment of atherosclerosis obliterans. Amer. Heart J. 79:5.
46. Atsumi, T., Motomiya, T., Isokane, N., and Shimamoto, T. 1971. Treatment of atherosclerosis obliterans with pyridinolcarbamate. Jap. Heart J. 12:335.
47. Cotton, R. C., Bloor, K., and Archibald, G. 1972. The effect of pyridinol carbamate treatment on the platelet response to ADP in patients with peripheral atherosclerosis. Brit. J. Surg. 59:313.
48. Atsumi, T., Isokane, N., Honda, Y., Matsuda, M., and Shimamoto, T. 1971. Studies on atherosclerosis obliterans, tibialis anterior blood flow measured by Xe-133 clearance method and its clinical evaluation. Jap. Circ. J. 35:1220.

IS THERE A PREVENTIVE THERAPY FOR PROGRESSION OF ATHEROSCLEROSIS?

HENRY I. RUSSEK, WALTER REDISCH, ERWIN N. TERRY,
and ROY H. CLAUSS

Physicians have long dreamed of the day when a "magic" drug might reverse the atherosclerotic process or at least arrest its progression. Although drugs of this type already exist for the experimental lesion in some species, to date none has proved beneficial in retarding atheromatosis in the human subject. Indeed, in a recent study by one of us (H. I. R.) employing W-1372, a promising new agent which has proved remarkably effective in animal trials, progression of coronary lesions was observed in all patients evaluated by repeat cineangiography after a period of six months to one year of continuous therapy. Despite such failure, effective prophylaxis in clinical coronary disease remains a realistic objective in current scientific research.

It hardly seems necessary to point out that a rational approach to preventive action against any disease requires, first of all, some rudimentary insight at least into those basic pathogenetic factors at which such measures are specifically to be aimed. Myocardial infarction once was considered to be synonymous with acute coronary thrombosis. The traditional concept held that atheromatosis was caused by elevated levels of cholesterol which infiltrated the vessel wall to cause partial obstruction to blood flow, but ultimate cessation of perfusion was dependent on the development of a thrombus at the site of the obstructing lesion. Contrary to expectation, however, neither the reduction of cholesterol by diet and drugs nor the use of anticoagulant agents has thus far appeared to exert any significant impact in secondary prevention or in the reduction of mortality risk from ischemic heart disease. Moreover, despite the continuing crusade for decades against the evils of obesity, lipid abnormalities, hypertension, physical inactivity, and the cigaret habit, heart attack fatalities have risen by 14% since 1950 in the United States among men between the ages of 25 and 44 (1). It therefore appears logical to question whether we really have been addressing ourselves to basic pathogenetic mechanisms in our efforts to prevent, reverse, or contain this devastating disease (2).

CONTRADICTIONS TO CLASSIC
CONCEPTS OF BASIC MECHANISMS

It is now widely recognized that a large segment of patients with unequivocal coronary atherosclerosis and myocardial infarction have *normal lipid values* by

American standards. This has been "explained" by emphasis on the multifac-
torial nature of the pathogenesis of atherosclerosis. Nonetheless, the gross
discrepancies frequently observed between the incidence, degree, and location of
coronary vascular lesions and those of myocardial structural lesions have challenged the crucial significance of atherosclerosis per se in the genesis of ischemic
heart disease. Certainly, the occurrence of angina pectoris in the absence of
demonstrable angiographic evidence of atherosclerotic lesions is no longer an
uncommon observation, and cases of myocardial infarction in this setting currently are being reported with increasing frequency. Such observations are in
accord with the pioneer research of the late Wilhelm Raab (3). His historic
investigations clearly have demonstrated that catecholamines and adrenal corticoids, by affecting the oxygen economy and electrolyte balance of the myocardium, may produce actual necrosis either through this mechanism alone or by
increasing the vulnerability of the heart muscle to an already diminished coronary blood flow. Traditional concepts have been further challenged by the
frequency with which thrombosis is found to be absent in cases of acute
myocardial infarction examined at necropsy. Thus, various reports indicate that
more than 50% of recent infarctions observed postmortem are unassociated with
fresh thrombosis. Furthermore, it also has appeared likely that even when
thrombosis is present, it may well be a consequence rather than a cause of
myocardial infarction (4). The conclusion therefore seems evident that the
etiology of atherosclerosis still remains obscure and that we do not as yet possess
either a rational concept of basic pathogenetic factors or a promising approach
to their control.

More recently, hope for the resolution of this impasse has arisen from the
studies of Shimamoto and associates (5). These investigators have conceptualized
a specific mechanism of pathogenesis involving both the vessel wall and cellular
elements of the circulating blood. Their intriguing observations appear to have
established an important link between cholesterol, catecholamines, and other
stressors and the metabolism of vascular endothelial cells and blood platelets.
That an acute rise of catecholamines is the characteristic response of man and
animal to physical and mental stress has long been recognized. While such
response obviously was intended by nature to protect the organism, hyper-
response or undue prolongation of physiologic stress mechanisms has been
suspected in the pathogenesis of a variety of disorders. Selye (6) has asserted
repeatedly that the time has come to lay aside the idea that stress does not cause
myocardial infarction.

While emphasis has been placed on the adverse direct effects of catecholamines and other stressors upon the heart muscle (3), their harmful influence on
blood platelets and vessel wall is gaining increasing attention. Indeed, recent
studies have shown that infusion of epinephrine in dogs for several hours

regularly precipitates myocardial necrosis caused by the aggregation of platelets undergoing viscous metamorphosis in the capillaries of the heart (7). These changes, however, are prevented readily when the animals are pretreated with aspirin or dipyridamole. Shimamoto and collaborators (5) have demonstrated similar effects in animals, including the rhesus monkey, and have shown that in addition to such changes, "stressors" increase the intercellular spaces of vascular endothelium and permit a greater influx of lipoprotein material for entrapment in the intima. They also have shown that changes in the cellular elements of the blood and in the vessel wall itself that are evoked by an epinephrine challenge can be blocked completely in the experimental animal by the prior administration of pyridinolcarbamate (PDC) (Anginin). Favorable reports also have appeared in the world literature attesting to the benefit obtained from treatment with PDC in patients with coronary disease, cerebrovascular disorders, and occlusive atherosclerosis involving vessels of the lower extremities. The value of such therapy as a preventive in atherogenesis and thrombogenesis is currently under clinical investigation in this country. The purpose of this presentation, therefore, is to record some preliminary observations by our group in the use of pyridinolcarbamate for the therapy of occlusive atherosclerosis involving the bifurcation branches of the abdominal aorta and for the treatment of angina pectoris, respectively.

PERIPHERAL OCCLUSIVE ATHEROSCLEROSIS

In a two-year double-blind study now in progress, patients who have had reconstructive vascular surgery for occlusive atherosclerosis involving the bifurcation branches of the abdominal aorta currently are receiving either pyridinolcarbamate or an identical placebo. (This investigation is being conducted by Drs. Redisch, Terry, and Clauss at the New York Medical College.) Since vein grafts placed on the arterial side of the circulation are particularly prone to the development of atherosclerotic lesions and since restenosis or reocclusion may be anticipated in 40%–50% of all reconstructed vessels within a two-year period from the time of surgery, careful follow-up of these cases may be expected to shed light on the efficacy of PDC in retarding the development and progression of atherosclerosis.

At the present time, it is possible to record the results in only 19 patients of the series who have undergone repeat angiography, plethysmographic blood flow studies, and measurements of controlled claudication distance after one year of therapy. Since the results of the objective measurements to be presented were compiled by an observer not involved with the care of patients in the study, the introduction of bias has been avoided and the double-blind nature of the continuing study has been preserved.

Methods

Each patient was seen at four-week intervals in the research clinic, where, after clinical examination, pulses were recorded and claudication determined. For those receiving PDC, the daily dosage was 2 g divided into four equal doses. All subjective responses and experiences throughout the treatment period were recorded. Plethysmography was performed at six-month intervals. Angiography was performed one year after surgery unless indicated earlier on clinical grounds.

Angiography

Standard procedures were carried out by the Department of Radiology. The films were reviewed independently by the radiologist and the investigators.

Blood flow determinations

Venous occlusion was chosen as the most accurate and convenient method in spite of the various difficulties involved. Studies were carried out in the constant temperature-humidity laboratory. Patients always were brought into the laboratory at the same time of the day and then rested in supine position to adjust to the ambient temperature of $23°C$. Pulses were recorded with a mercury-in-silastic (Whitney) strain gauge applied around the maximum circumference of the calf, while venous occlusion was accomplished with a pneumatic cuff of appropriate size applied just above the knee. Upon inflation of the cuff to a pressure 10 mm. Hg. below diastolic blood pressure, the recorded plethysmogram deviates from the baseline and initially rises in proportion to perfusion. A slope is constructed along the peaks of the first pulsations recorded after occlusion which may be joined by a straight line, and a segment of the baseline representing 10 seconds is measured from the point at which it is intersected by the slope. The altitude between the baseline and the slope at the point on the graph 10 seconds after occlusion together with the initial circumference of the calf and the strain gauge calibration factor constitute the variables used to calculate perfusion.

Exercise blood flow

The patients exercised by performing dorsal-plantar flexions at a rate of one flex per second against a hinged spring "pedal board." The resistance offered by the spring was 4 lbs. After 2 minutes, exercise was stopped and perfusion was measured at 5–10 seconds, 30 seconds, and at 1 minute. Subsequently, measurements were made at 1-minute intervals until the flow had returned to the previously established resting levels for a period of 10 minutes.

Walking test

An electrically driven treadmill with adjustable elevation was used. Speed and angle of inclination of the treadmill were adjusted to individual patients and maintained until absence of a reaction to walking indicated the need to increase workload.

Results

Evidence of visualized vascularization in the one-year postoperative angiogram compared to the immediate postoperative pretreatment angiogram was judged as "increased," "unchanged," or "decreased" (Table 1). Although it is seen that the results obtained with PDC do not differ significantly from those observed with placebo, it is of interest that deterioration was noted in proportionately fewer patients on the active drug. Obviously, the series is at present too small to state whether the slight differences noted represent a trend or are purely accidental. Because vein grafts tend to develop atherosclerotic plaques, the finding of "unchanged" vascularization after one year of follow-up must be considered to represent a highly desirable and beneficial result of treatment in the patient with reconstructive vascular surgery. Comparable findings were observed when comparisons were made between the results of blood flow and treadmill studies, respectively, in the placebo and treated groups (Tables 2 and 3). Obviously, only the passage of an adequate length of time and inclusion of other patients in the series currently under investigation will assist in the interpretation of the final results.

Table 1. Visualized Vascularization (Angiography)

	Pyridinolcarbamate	Placebo
Increased	3	1
Unchanged	2	4
Decreased	3	6
Total	8	11

Table 2. Blood Flow (Venous Occlusion Plethysmography)

	Pyridinolcarbamate	Placebo
Increased	3	
Unchanged	7	8
Decreased		3
Total	10	11

Table 3. Claudication Distance (Treadmill)

	Pyridinolcarbamate	Placebo
Increased	4	
Unchanged	5	4
Decreased	1[a]	5
Total	10	9

[a]Caused by angina.

ANGINA PECTORIS

PDC or a placebo has been administered by a single-blind technique in six patients with severe angina pectoris and advanced triple coronary artery disease proved angiographically. All patients had been rejected for surgical revascularization because of the diffuse nature of their coronary vascular involvement and poor peripheral runoff.

Case 1

In the case of a 56-year-old male patient whose exercise-electrocardiographic tests are shown in Figure 1, propranolol and isosorbide dinitrate (ISD) administered sublingually had been associated with significant symptomatic improvement, yet the patient remained markedly disabled and dependent on the repeated use of nitroglycerin. The patient had not slept in his bed for more than one year because the supine position produced repetitive attacks of angina pectoris. Administration of propranolol and Isordil could not be terminated during the therapeutic trial of PDC because of the severity of symptoms. In all of the tests shown, therefore, ISD was administered sublingually 10 minutes before exercise and propranolol 1 hour before testing. In addition, the patient was given either Anginin placebo or Anginin itself. After recording the response to Anginin placebo, Anginin was administered in a 2-g daily dose for four days when the tests were again repeated. Little or no change was observed when comparison was made with the placebo control. The patient continued on Anginin for two weeks in the dosage of 2 g per day. At the end of that time, an improved response was noted compared with the control (Fig. 1). Improvement was demonstrable in all tests performed to the tenth week of observation. While on therapy, this patient volunteered the information that for the first time in a year he had been able to sleep in his bed without the need to sit up in a chair. When placebo was substituted for the active drug, aggravation of symptoms occurred within one week and the patient was again unable to assume the supine position in bed.

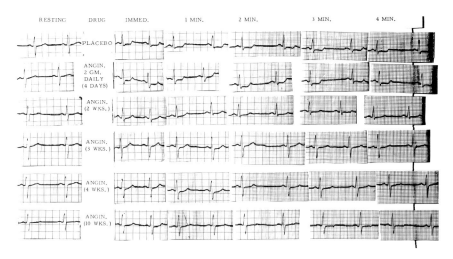

Fig. 1. Exercise-electrocardiographic tests (30 trips) showing lead V_4 in 56-year-old male patient (R. M.) with angina pectoris receiving placebo or Anginin (*Angin.*).

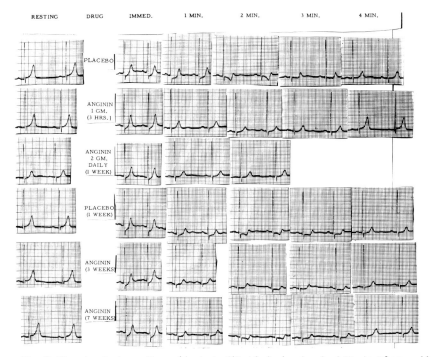

Fig. 2. Exercise-electrocardiographic tests (40 trips) showing lead V_4 in 53-year-old male patient (A. K.) with angina pectoris receiving placebo or Anginin.

Case 2

The second patient in the series was a 53-year-old male with severe angina pectoris and triple coronary artery disease of a diffuse nature reported in angiography. Exercise to the point of pain after administration of placebo characteristically produced ischemic S-T segment depression and T-wave inversion in the postexercise electrocardiogram (Fig. 2). After a one-shot dose of 1 g of Anginin given orally, a repeat test 3 hours thereafter showed an almost normal response. When Anginin was administered to this patient in a 2-g daily dose for one week, the response continued to be favorably maintained. With the institution of placebo, deterioration in the electrocardiographic response was recorded. After restarting Anginin therapy, after one week on placebo, the tests were repeated after three weeks and seven weeks, respectively, but the exercise-electrocardiographic responses did not appear as favorable as when the drug was administered during the initial period of one week.

Case 3

Figure 3 shows the responses in the case of a 61-year-old male who manifested marked ischemic changes after placebo. Anginin was given in a 1-g dose, and

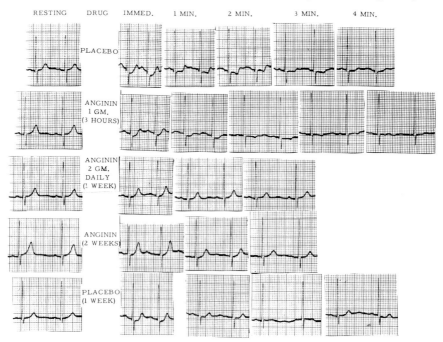

Fig. 3. Exercise-electrocardiographic tests (26 trips) showing lead V_4 in 61-year-old male patient (R. S.) with angina pectoris receiving placebo or Anginin.

when the patient was tested 3 hours later, some improvement occurred but a normal pattern was not recorded. Anginin then was given in a dose of 2 g daily for one week, and upon retesting the patient a completely normal response was obtained. The same finding was observed after two weeks of Anginin therapy. When the tests were repeated after the substitution of placebo for one week, deterioration was noted in the electrocardiographic pattern.

In the remaining three patients who have been studied thus far in a similar manner, minimal alterations have been observed without significant change in clinical manifestations.

DISCUSSION

Inasmuch as pyridinolcarbamate has no known hemodynamic influence on the systemic or coronary circulation and is not a beta-blocking agent, the findings suggest that favorable therapeutic response may arise from effects on vascular endothelium and cellular elements in the blood, as postulated by Shimamoto (5). Although adverse effects were uncommonly observed in these studies, gastrointestinal symptoms do occur from pyridinolcarbamate and may require discontinuation of therapy.

Atherosclerosis is a systemic condition progressing relentlessly and presenting with varied symptoms. Although atherosclerotic plaques are found very rarely in the venous portion of the vascular bed, when vein grafts are put into the arterial side of the circulation they become prone to the development of atherosclerosis even more than does the vessel into which they have been grafted. If it is ultimately shown that vein grafts in the peripheral circulation are protected by pyridinolcarbamate, the same might be expected in saphenous vein bypass grafts for coronary artery disease. Confirmation of favorable effects in angina pectoris would suggest comparable benefits in the arterial circulation. Continued studies with large groups of patients over an adequate period of time will be necessary to provide answers to these questions.

REFERENCES CITED

1. Moses, C. 1972. Heart attacks. *The New York Times,* April 4.
2. Russek, H. I. 1971. "Progress" in the treatment and prevention of coronary heart disease. Amer. Fam. Physician, p. 68.
3. Raab, W. 1972. Cardiotoxic effects of emotional, socioeconomic and environmental stresses. Page 707 *in* E. Bajusz and G. Rona, eds. Myocardiology. University Park Press, Baltimore.
4. Roberts, W. C. 1972. Coronary arteries in fatal acute myocardial infarction. Circulation 45:p215.
5. Shimamoto, T., and Sunaga, T. 1973. The contraction and blebbing of endothelial cells accompanied by acute infiltration of plasma substances into the vessel wall and their

prevention. Page 3 *in* T. Shimamoto, F. Numano, and G. M. Addison, eds. Atherogenesis. Excerpta Medica, Amsterdam.

6. Selye, H. 1972. Stress, hormones and cardiovascular disease. Page 701 *in* E. Bajusz and G. Rona, eds. Myocardiology. University Park Press, Baltimore.

7. Haft, J. I. 1972. Platelet aggregation and myocardial infarction. Med. World News, March 10.

Advancing Frontiers
in Surgical Treatment
for Cardiovascular Disease

Valve Replacement or Repair?

HEART VALVES: PROSTHESES AND PROSPECTS

DWIGHT EMARY HARKEN

> The great ceremonial occasions of life are so endlessly repeated that the more important the comment they evoke—the more hackneyed they seem.
>
> *Adapted from* VERMONT ROYSTER

So have we argued the virtue of biologic versus mechanical valves versus repair. So did we beat that poor horse, closed versus open correction of mitral stenosis, only to discover that with proper case selection and surgical experience there was a valuable and proper place for both.*

It turns out that biologic or mechanical valves, or occasionally a perfect repair of the patient's own valve, can be the proper choice (1,3,12,30,34,44). Therefore in this article I will try to define the place for each and attempt to point up potential shortcomings of my own as well as other persuasions. By expressing a strong personal preference for mechanical valves when the patient's tissue is destroyed beyond reconstruction, I am obligated to set up standards by which the awesome variety of mechanical valves can be measured in the aortic and atrioventricular positions. The two anatomic areas currently involve quite different standards.

AORTIC VALVES

The options with aortic valves are biologic or mechanical valves, versus reconstruction. The problems and selection factors are quite distinct from the atrioventricular positions, as discussed below.

Biologic Valves

In the child with relatively small aortic base and valve but pure noncalcific aortic stenosis there remains a place for valvuloplasty. This accepts the probability of another operation subsequently. If the base is too small to accept one of the

---

*Laurence B. Ellis' report of the 15–20 year followup on D. E. Harken's first 1,000 closed operations for mitral stenosis shows that more than 30% of patients with pure tight noncalcific mitral continued to flourish at the end of the followup.

nonthrombogenic, covered, nonvariant, caged ball valves (i.e., Starr covered stainless steel chassis and hollow ball or Harken Dacron-covered titanium chassis and hollow titanium ball), there is justification for the biologic valve replacement. These biologic valves, like the modern covered caged ball valves, do not require anticoagulation procedures. They avoid the all but prohibitive physical and emotional dangers of anticoagulating a child. It is much better to accept the real hazards of another operation than those of constant medications and restriction of activities.

There possibly is an area of controversy with biologic valves. Tilting disc (10) valves can be placed in smaller people with smaller aortic bases and therefore are more likely to continue to serve as the patient grows. However, none has yet proved to be nonthrombogenic, and all require anticoagulants. There is a message here for surgeons operating on adults with congenitally small aortic bases or constricting aortic waists immediately above the valve area. In the adult with such a configuration, the larger orifice-to-outside-base diameter coupled with a low profile justifies the use of the Björk-Shiley or Lillehei-Kaster valves (10,11). Indeed, time and/or further modifications of these valves may establish designs with good flow properties that do not require anticoagulation.

The problem of a narrow or constricting supravalvular aortic waist should be clarified. If there is narrowing of the aorta at the level of the top of the cage of a ball valve, supravalvular obstruction can result when the ball rises in systole, occluding the raceway, and the narrow aortic waist tightly encircles the cage. In such situations the aorta must be enlarged by a plastic procedure or by the insertion of a gusset. Such procedures are time consuming and leave suture lines, so a low profile, central flow, tilting disc valve may be preferable (10).

Mechanical Valves

In the aortic portion, except for the situations enumerated above, the choice comes down to biologic versus ball valves. A number of excellent surgeons have espoused biologic valves. The latter embrace homografts (55,68), xenografts (57), and utilization of the patient's own tissue (18,59). Homografts have been extended by Zerbini (70) to include biologic valves fashioned on struts from dura mater. Autografts include Ross' transplantation of the patient's own pulmonary valve for the aortic replacement followed by substitution of a homograft for the lost pulmonary valve. This constitutes a technical tour de force which few surgeons have the appetite or skill to execute. At the other end of the spectrum is the autograft fascia lata particularly identified with Senning (57). Somewhere within the spectrum is the growth of the patient's own tissue on implanted fabric skeletons. To oversimplify criticism of biologic valves (with partial to complete validity in each type, however), problems in harvesting, preserving, sterilization, insertion, and uncertainty of long term results have tempered wide usage. Even so, we must salute Ross (55), Barratt-Boyes (4,5),

Merendino (50), Kirklin (51), Ionescu (40), Yacoub (55,67,68), Wooler (18), and indeed a host of others (9,18,23) whose care I would accept should the need arise. However, my preference in that unlikely situation would be for my own Dacron-covered titanium cage and base with a hollow titanium ball (Fig. 1). The reasons are straightforward:

1) Ball variance is almost impossible.
2) Fabric wear has been demonstrated only twice, and only on early models.
3) Base variance (irregular proliferation of tissue on the ball seat producing hemodynamic effects similar to those caused by ball variance) is prevented by a narrow outflow orifice seating rim of ultra high molecular weight polyethylene.
4) The ratio of orifice to outside diameter of the base allows a larger orifice than some of the other popular ball valves. Minor to minimal

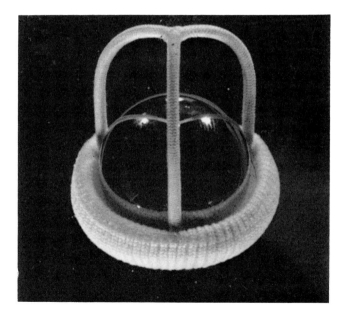

Fig. 1. The Harken Dacron-covered aortic caged ball valve has the largest orifice-to-base dimension. Ball and chassis are made of titanium. The seating rim is formed of ultra high molecular weight polyethylene. Anticoagulation is not necessary with this valve. (Made by Surgitool, Pittsburgh, Pa.)

gradients, even with high cardiac output and systolic rates ranging to 180/min, have been established.

5) Low thrombogenicity when patients were carried for six months on anticoagulants was experienced. Paradoxically it must be emphasized that we and also Dr. Starr have had no known thromboembolic complications when *no* anticoagulants have been used.

The current Starr valve would appear to share most of these advantages except:

1) The larger struts and fabric outflow tract might be expected to produce more hemolysis.
2) The cloth outflow tract might propagate irregular neointimal tissue growth with hemodynamic results somewhat like ball variance.
3) The metal studs on the base to prevent fabric shift also produce metal ball contact in diastole with consequent wear potential (metal to metal) and increased sound level.

The above points merely represent questions raised. The Starr-Edwards quality control, design genius, and reporting accuracy are all exemplary.

In short, there are available fabric-covered light weight chasses with nonvarying metal balls that offer signal advantages in most adult situations. These advantages include low thrombogenicity without anticoagulation, low late hemolysis, good hemodynamic qualities, and lack of ball variance.

In the near future we will probably see improved low profile, covered, tilting disc valves that will be only slightly hemolytic or nonhemolytic, nonthrombogenic without anticoagulation, and with nonvariant hinges that can neither wear, stick, nor propagate pannus. Such valves of the tilting disc variety are not known to exist presently. However, use of the excellent ball valves for the aortic area is currently greatly preferable to the risks of delay in patients with symptomatic aortic valve disease. The surgical risk is low; the risk of delay is great.

MITRAL VALVES

Options with mitral valves are similar to those with aortic valves, but the advantages and disadvantages are quite dissimilar. Once again we can choose between biologic versus mechanical valves (ball or low profile) and reconstruction. Reconstruction is clearly more widely applicable in the mitral than in the aortic areas. Good competent valves may often be created. The seduction is to overuse reconstruction. Bailey, Kay, Rumel, Gerbode, Kerth, and others have found a wide application for reconstruction. Bailey (2) has treated valve tissue with the versatility of the dressmaker but has failed to accept the fact that his materials (tissues) change character (stiffen and contract) in a way quite as fickle as the dressmaker's product!

We still use closed mitral valvuloplasty in noncalcific pure stenosis. This is always used with pump standby; and if any compromise with quality is encountered, open operation is immediate. Then, if open reconstruction of insufficiency and stenosis is at all incomplete, the option of *low* profile mechanical prosthesis is exercised.

Biologic mitral valves are even more speculative than aortic. The outstanding men cited as espousing biologic aortic valves would agree that their biologic aortic replacements have been more successful. However, the lesson from open reconstruction is that, no matter how well the normal appearing tissue is reefed and approximated to resemble and function like normal valves *initially*, the tissue has with disappointing consistency failed during the long term followup. Even though the reefing sutures hold perfectly, even when the inserted elongation tissue or fabric functions as intended, the leaflets tend to contract and stiffen (2,43). The implication is that the coaptation was unlike the natural contact surfaces. If the patient's own tissue changes after the surgeon's best efforts at reconstruction, why should we expect a more favorable fate from homografts, inverted aortic human grafts, porcine or dura mater grafts, or autografts of fascia lata? The patient's reconstructed valve should represent the ideal autograft. Why then should we expect more of the psychedelic changes in the spectrum of biologic valves paraded before us?

However, mechanical valves in the mitral and tricuspid areas present quite different problems than they do in the aortic position:

1) The sheer volume of a caged ball valve in the atrioventricular position can reduce stroke volume.
2) The cage can irritate the septum.
3) The ball, though isobaric, can obstruct by opening inertia.
4) The caged ball may obstruct the left ventricular outflow tract.
5) In our experience with caged *ball* mitral valves, the cardiac output has in most instances remained low, the gradient over the valve has been considerable, and the pulmonary vascular resistance has remained elevated. This experience has been shared by surgeons and confirmed by hemodynamic studies at the Massachusetts General Hospital and the Mayo Clinic (31,36,37). More favorable results have been enjoyed by Starr (61), Tubbs (28), and others. Presumably the different results reflect heart chamber size and the relevant size selected for the ball prosthesis.

Many surgeons have become disenchanted with ball valves and biologic valves in the mitral position. Many large series of low profile valves of varying quality have resulted. Prominent among these have been the valves from Hufnagel (39), Gott (27), Kay-Shiley, Beall (6), and our own valves (36). The Kay-Suzuki valve was the first that we found to have essentially physiologic function. Those valves with wide exposed areas of nonwettable parts seem more embolus-prone, particularly some of the tilting disc hingeless hinged valves; e.g., Wada, Björk-Shiley, and Lillehei-Kaster (10,11). Furthermore, when one considers the near physiologic function of a valve used in these cases there seems to be a loss of rationale to the "central flow" concept in the mitral position (10,11).

Our own valve (Fig. 2) does require anticoagulation. Whether platelet antiadhesive agents, salicylates, and dipyridamole alone will prove as effective as combinations with warfarin has not yet been established (49,63,64). The thromboembolic potential does remain, even though the excellent valve demonstrated has shown:

1) No gradient even at high cardiac output and pulse rates.
2) Prompt increase in cardiac output after surgery.
3) Prompt and dramatic fall in pulmonary vascular resistance (20,36). The extra sewing skirt affords simplified insertion and protection against paravalvular leak (the bete noire of any valve replacement).

Prospects

I hope the excellent hemodynamic qualities of the low profile valves such as the one illustrated, or the improved Beall valve (6) and possibly the Lillehei-Kaster valve, can be modified to embrace the nonthrombogenic qualities of the aortic ball valve now available.

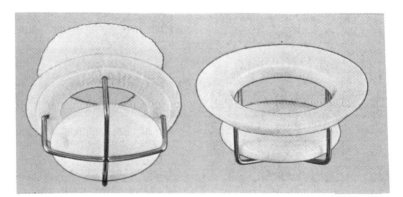

Fig. 2. (Right) The Harken low profile mitral valve. Dacron covered offset seat prevents "cocking." Titanium struts form a frustrum area that provides physiologic function. *(Left)* Alternative extra sewing skirt to protect against paravalvular leak. (Made by Surgitool, Pittsburgh, Pa.)

CONCLUSIONS

The *aortic valve* replacement of choice for most adults is the covered hollow metal ball valve. Its limitations remain as follows: 1) possibility of fabric cover wear; 2) hemolysis (severe degree generally transient); 3) technical problems when the aortic base or neck is small in which case the low profile valves can then be used to advantage.

The *mitral valve* replacement of choice is a low profile valve embracing the principles incorporated in the valve illustrated in Figure 2. This valve has excellent physiologic properties. Its residual disadvantage is that it requires anticoagulation. What form of pharmacologic protection against thromboemboli is best has yet to be determined. I hope a nonthrombogenic, nonvarying lens (fused carbon) can be developed in a covered chassis and offset base configuration similar to the preferred valve.

REFERENCES CITED

1. Bailey, C. P. 1949. The surgical treatment of mitral stenosis (mitral commissurotomy). Dis. Chest 15:377.
2. Bailey, C. P. 1972. Reconstruction of the mitral valve. Presented at the meeting of the American College of Chest Physicians, Denver, Colorado, December 1972.
3. Baker, C., Brock, R. C., and Campbell, M. 1950. Valvulotomy for mitral stenosis. Report of six successful cases. Brit. Med. J. 1:1283.
4. Barratt-Boyes, B. G., Rocke, A. H. G., Brandt, P. W. T., Smither, J. C., and Lowe, J. B. 1969. Aortic homograft valve replacement: A long term follow-up of an initial series of 101 patients. Circulation 40:763.
5. Barratt-Boyes, B. G. 1971. Long-term follow-up of aortic valvar grafts. Brit. Heart J. 33 (Suppl.):60.
6. Beall, A. C., Jr., Bloodwell, R. D., Bricker, D. W., et al. 1969. Prosthetic replacement of cardiac valves. Five and one-half years' experience. Amer. J. Cardiol. 23:250.
7. Beach, P. M., Jr., and Malm, J. R. 1971. Homologous aortic valve replacement. *In* M. I. Ionescu, D. N. Ross, and G. H. Wooler, eds: Biological tissue in heart valve replacement. Butterworths, London.
8. Bernheim, B. M. 1909. Experimental surgery of the mitral valve. Bull. Johns Hopkins Hosp. 20:107.
9. Bigelow, W. A., Yao, J. K., Aldridge, H. E., Heimbecker, R. O., and Murray, A. D. W. 1964. Clinical homograft valve transplantation. J. Thorac. Cardiov. Surg. 48:333.
10. Björk, V. O. 1970. A new central-flow tilting disc valve prosthesis. One year's clinical experience with 103 patients. J. Thorac. Cardiov. Surg. 60:355.
11. Björk, V. O., Olin, C., and Astrom, H. 1970. Haemodynamic results of aortic valve replacement with the Kay-Shiley disc valve. Scand. J. Thorac. Cardiov. Surg. 4:195.
12. Black, H., and Harken, D. E. 1958. Mitral valvuloplasty in patients past fifty. New Engl. J. Med. 259:361.
13. Bozer, A. Y., and Karamehmetoglu, A. 1972. Thrombosis encountered with Björk-Shiley prosthesis. J. Cardiov. Surg. 13:141.
14. Braunwald, N. S., and Bronchik, L. I. 1967. Prevention of thrombus formation on rigid cloth covered Starr-Edwards prosthesis. J. Thorac. Cardiov. Surg. 54:630.
15. Braunwald, N. S., Tatooles, C., Turina, M., and Detmer, D. 1971. New developments in the design of fabric-covered prosthetic heart valves. J. Thorac. Cardiov. Surg. 62:673.

16. Brunton, T. L. 1902. Preliminary note on the possibility of treating mitral stenosis by surgical methods. Lancet 1:352.
17. Bush, V. Personal communication.
18. Carpentier, A., and Dubost, C. 1971. From xenograft to bioprosthesis: Evolution of concepts and techniques of valvular xenografts. *In* M. I. Ionescu, D. N. Ross, and G. H. Wooler, eds: Biological tissue in heart valve replacement. Butterworths, London.
19. Collins, J. J., Jr., and Cohn, L. H. 1973. Reconstruction of the aortic valve; correcting valve incompetence due to acute dissecting aneurysm. Arch. Surg. 106:35.
20. Dalen, J. E., Matloff, J. M., Hoppin, F. G., Jr., Evans, G. L., Bhardwaj, P., Harken, D. E., and Dexter, L. 1967. Early reversibility of pulmonary vascular disease after mitral valve replacement. Clin. Res. 25:344.
21. Edwards, J. E. 1961. Calcific aortic stenosis; pathologic features. Proc. Mayo Clin. 36:444.
22. Ellis, L. B., and Harken, D. E. 1964. Closed valvulopasty for mitral stenosis; a 12-year follow-up study of 1571 patients. New Engl. J. Med. 270:643.
23. Gerbode, F. L. A. 1971. Discussion of Shumacker, H. D., Jr.: Autogenous tissue cardiac valves. Surgery 70:848.
24. Gonzalez-Lavin, L., and Ross, D. N. 1971. Biologic aortic valve repair or replacement. *In* D. E. Harken, ed. Cardiac Surgery I. Davis, Philadelphia.
25. Gorlin, R., and Goodale, W. T. 1956. Changing blood pressure in aortic insufficiency—its clinical significance. New Engl. J. Med. 255:77.
26. Gorlin, R., McMillan, I. K. R., Medd, W. E., Matthews, M. B., and Daley, R. 1955. Dynamics of circulation in aortic valvular disease. Amer. J. Med. 18:855.
27. Gott, V. L., Rowe, G. G., Daggett, R. L., Whiffen, J. D., Koepke, D. E., and Young, W. P. 1965. Preoperative and postoperative hemodynamic data in patients with a prosthetic hinged-leaflet aortic valve. Circulation 31:1.
28. Hamer, J., Boulton, T., Fleming, J., Hayward, G. W., Hill, I. M., Monro, I., Simon, G., and Tubbs, O. S. 1968. Mitral valve replacement. Thorax 23:1.
29. Harken, D. E., Black, H., Taylor, W. J., Thrower, W. B., and Ellis, L. B. 1961. Reoperation for mitral stenosis. A discussion of postoperative deterioration and methods of improving initial and secondary operation. Circulation 23:7.
30. Harken, D. E., Ellis, L. B., Dexter, L., Farrand, R. E., and Dickson, J. F. 1952. The responsibility of the physician in the selection of patients with mitral stenosis for surgical treatment. Circulation 5:349.
31. Harken, D. E. 1971. Mitral and aortic valve surgery. *In* P. Cooper, ed. The craft of surgery, 2nd ed. Little, Brown, Boston.
32. Harken, D. E. 1965. A new caged-ball aortic and mitral valve. J. Mount Sinai Hosp., N.Y. 32:95.
33. Harken, D. E., Soroff, H. S., Taylor, W. J., Lefemine, A. A., Gupta, S. K., and Lunzer, S. 1960. Partial and complete prostheses in aortic insufficiency. J. Thorac. Cardiov. Surg. 40:744.
34. Harken, D. E., and Curtis, L. E. 1967. The Lawrence Brewster Ellis lecture—Heart surgery, legend and a long look. Amer. J. Cardiol. 19:393.
35. Harken, D. E. 1971. Surgery of the mitral valve. *In* D. E. Harken, ed. Cardiac Surgery I. Davis, Philadelphia.
36. Harken, D. E., Matloff, J. M., Zuckerman, W., and Chaux, A. 1968. A new mitral valve. J. Thorac. Cardiov. Surg. 55:369.
37. Harken, D. E. Valvular heart disease. *In* B. Blades, ed. Surgical diseases of the chest, 3rd ed. Mosby, St. Louis.
38. Hodam, R., Anerson, R., Starr, A., Wood, J., and Dobbs, J. 1971. Further evaluation of the composite-seat, cloth-covered aortic prosthesis. Presented at Seventh Annual Meeting, The Society of Thoracic Surgeons, Dallas, Texas, January 18, 1971.
39. Hufnagel, C. A., and Conrad, P. W. 1962. Calcific aortic stenosis. New Engl. J. Med. 266:72.
40. Ionescu, M. I., Pakrashi, B. C., Holden, M. P., Mary, D. A., and Wooler, G. H. 1972.

Results of aortic valve replacement with frame-supported fascia lata and pericardial grafts. J. Thorac. Cardiov. Surg. 64:341.

41. Kay, E. B., Mendelsohn, D., Jr., and Zimmerman, H. S. 1962. Surgical treatment of aortic valvular disease by prosthetic replacement. Amer. J. Cardiol. 9:284.

42. Kloster, F. E., Farrehi, C., Mourjinis, A., Hodam, R. P., Starr, A., and Griswold, H. E. 1970. Hemodynamic studies in patients with cloth-covered composite-seat Starr-Edwards valve prostheses. J. Thorac. Cardiov. Surg. 60:879.

43. Lillehei, C. W., Gott, V. L., DeWall, R. A., and Varco, R. L. 1957. Surgical correction of pure mitral insufficiency by annuloplasty under direct vision. Lancet 77:446.

44. Logan, A., and Turner, R. 1959. Surgical treatment of mitral stenosis with particular reference to the transventricular approach with a mechanical dilator. Lancet 2:874.

45. Lown, B. D., Perlroth, M. G., Kaidbey, S., Tadaaki, A., and Harken, D. E. 1963. "Cardioversion" of atrial fibrillation. A report on the treatment of 65 episodes in 50 patients. New Engl. J. Med. 269:325.

46. Lown, B., Amarasingham, R., and Neuman, J. 1962. New method for terminating cardiac arrhythmias; use of synchronized capacitor discharge. J.A.M.A. 182:548.

47. McEnany, M. T., Ross, D. N., and Yates, A. K. 1972. Cusp degeneration in frame-supported autologous fascia lata mitral valves. Thorax 27:23.

48. Magovern, G. J., Kent, E. M., Cromie, H. W., Cushing, W. B., and Scott, S. 1964. Sutureless aortic and mitral prosthetic valves; clinical results and operative technique on sixty patients. J. Thorac. Cardiov. Surg. 48:346.

49. Matloff, J. M., Collins, J. J., Jr., Sullivan, J. M., Gorlin, R., and Harken, D. E. 1969. Control of thromboembolism from prosthetic heart valves. Ann. Thorac. Surg. 8:133.

50. Merendino, K. A., and Bruce, R. A. 1957. One hundred seventeen surgically treated cases of valvular rheumatic heart disease with preliminary report of two cases of mitral regurgitation treated under direct vision with aid of a pump-oxygenator. J.A.M.A. 164:749.

51. Pacifico, A. D., Karp, R. B., and Kirklin, J. W. 1972. Homografts for replacement of the aortic valve. Circulation 46 (Suppl. 1):36.

52. Parker, R., Jr., and Weiss, S. 1936. The nature and significance of the structural changes in the lungs in mitral stenosis. Amer. J. Path. 12:573.

53. Reis, R. L., Glancz, D. L., O'Brien, K., Epstein, F. E., and Morrow, A. G. 1970. Clinical and hemodynamic assessment of fabric covered Starr-Edwards prosthetic valves. J. Thorac. Cardiov. Surg. 59:84.

54. Roberts, W. C., Lambird, P. A., Gott, V. L., and Morrow, A. G. 1966. Fatal aortic regurgitation following replacement of the mitral and aortic valves. A mechanical complication of double valve replacement. J. Thorac. Cardiov. Surg. 52:189.

55. Ross, D., and Yacoub, M. H. 1969. Homograft replacement of the aortic valve. A critical review. Prog. Cardiov. Dis. 11:275.

56. Sakakibara, S. 1955. A surgical approach to the correction of mitral insufficiency. Ann. Surg. 142:196.

57. Senning, A., and Turina, M. 1971. Aortic valve replacement with free fascia lata grafts: Clinical experience and after evaluation of 141 consecutive cases. In M. I. Ionescu, D. N. Ross, and G. H. Wooler, eds. Biological tissue in heart valve replacement. Butterworths, London.

58. Shean, F. C., Austen, W. G., Buckley, M. J., et al. 1971. Survival after Starr-Edwards aortic valve replacement. Circulation 44:1.

59. Shumacker, H. B., Jr. 1971. Autogenous tissue cardiac valves. Surgery 70:848.

60. Smithy, H. G., and Parker, E. F. 1947. Experimental aortic valvulotomy—a preliminary report. Surg. Gynec. Obstet. 84:625.

61. Starr, A., and Edwards, M. L. 1961. Mitral replacement: Clinical experience with a ball-valve prosthesis. Ann. Surg. 154:726.

62. Stein, P. D., Harken, D. E., and Dexter, L. 1966. The nature and prevention of prosthetic valve endocarditis. Amer. Heart J. 71:393.

63. Sullivan, J. M., Harken, D. E., and Gorlin, R. 1969. Effect of dipyridamole on the

incidence of arterial emboli after cardiac valve replacement. Circulation 39 (Suppl. 1):149.

64. Sullivan, J. M., Harken, D. E., and Gorlin, R. 1973. Pharmacologic control of thromboembolic complications of cardiac valve replacement—Prevention of arterial emboli. New Engl. J. Med. In press.

65. Taylor, W. J., Black, H., Thrower, W. B., and Harken, D. E. 1958. Valvuloplasty for mitral stenosis during pregnancy. J.A.M.A. 166:1013.

66. Tubbs, O. S. 1962. Transventricular mitral valvotomy. Nederl. T. Geneesk. 106:355.

67. Yacoub, M. H., and Kittle, C. F. 1969. A new technique for replacement of the mitral valve by a semilunar valve homograft. J. Thorac. Cardiov. Surg. 58:859.

68. Yacoub, M. H., and Kittle, C. F. 1970. Sterilization of valve homografts using antibiotic solutions. Circulation 41 (Suppl. 2):29.

69. Young, W. P., Gott, V. L., and Rowe, G. G. 1965. Open heart surgery for mitral valve disease with special reference to a new prosthetic valve. J. Thorac. Cardiov. Surg. 50:827.

70. Zerbini, E. J. 1972. Discussion of Ionescu, M. I., Pakrashi, B. C., Holden, M. P., et al. Results of aortic valve replacement with frame-supported fascia lata and pericardial grafts. J. Thorac. Cardiov. Surg. 64:353.

RECONSTRUCTION OF THE MITRAL VALVE BY CREATION OF A "COMMISSURAL CUSP"

CHARLES P. BAILEY, TERUO T. HIROSE,
FRANK S. FOLK, and SANSERN HASTANAN

During the past 12 years, certain of us have been concerned with reconstruction of the cardiac valves with grafts of autologous tissue. Pericardium, aortic wall, vein wall, full-thickness left atrial wall, and central tendon of the diaphragm have been tried successively, both in animals (mongrel dogs) and in man. However, pursuant to the suggestion of Senning (1, 2) that fascia lata be used for this purpose, we have come to recognize the superiority of that tissue for this purpose over all of those mentioned.

During the past eight years, we have reported a number of advances in the correction of mitral insufficiency by using the successively innovated techniques of "patching" (Fig. 1), "cusp lengthening" (Fig. 2), "skirt lengthening" (Fig. 3), and resuspending (Fig. 4) of the "flail" portion of the valve margin in cases of rupture of the chordae tendineae (3–10). In the same articles, we have described comparable advances in the treatment of mitral stenosis (Figs. 5–7).

All of these developments were aggregated in the form of a scientific exhibit called "Reconstruction of the Cardiac Valves with Autologous Fascia Lata," which was awarded the Hektoen Gold Medal for original investigation at the 120th Convention of the American Medical Association at Atlantic City, New Jersey, on June 23, 1971.

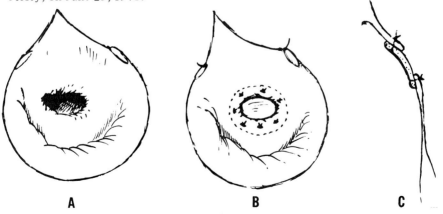

A   **B**   **C**

Fig. 1a–c. Patching a perforation of the mitral valve with a graft of autologous tissue.

417

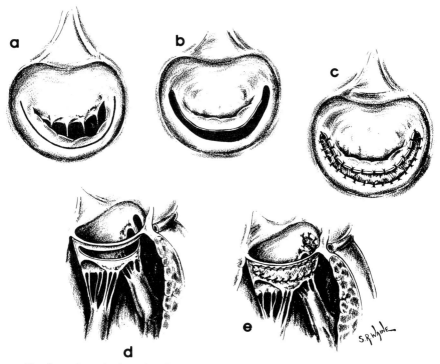

Fig. 2a–e. Lengthening of a shrunken and retracted mitral cusp by interposition of a crescentic graft of autologous tissue.

However, our own demonstration of the early hemodynamic benefits obtained in a consecutive series of 41 patients operated on for predominant mitral stenosis by the latest of these techniques clearly indicated that the described procedures, while undeniably beneficial (Fig. 8), had not been successful in abolishing the diastolic transmitral pressure gradient completely in even a *single* instance.

Of all the commonly studied physiologic parameters, the recorded transmitral diastolic gradient most directly reflects the existence of an impedance to left ventricular filling. This gradient, therefore, was a clear-cut measure of the degree to which we had benefited the patient, or conversely, the degree to which we had failed completely to correct the abnormal pathophysiology in each one of these patients.

Reflection upon the possible cause or causes for this failure led inexorably to the conclusion that the effective "caliber" of the mitral valve "skirt" had become significantly reduced because of the disease and that our corrective techniques had not sufficiently enlarged it. Had our grandmothers encountered such a difficulty with a too-small skirt, they surely would have enlarged its

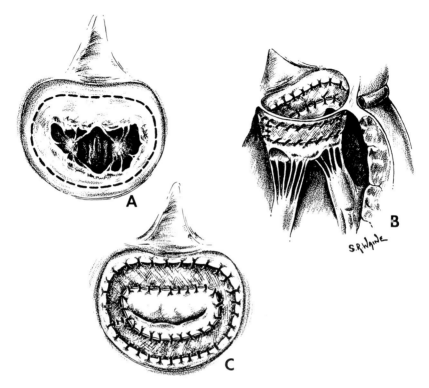

Fig. 3a–c. Lengthening of the mitral skirt with a circumferential strip of fascia lata.

caliber by inserting a widening "piece" (or gusset). The thought occurred that this same principle might be applicable to the shrunken mitral valve. Perhaps a gusset of flexible membranous tissue might be interposed into the circumference of the diseased mitral valve, with or without prior excision of a portion of that circumference. The next question to arise was: where in the valve circumference should such a widening gusset be introduced?

In May, 1954, at the meeting of the American Association for Thoracic Surgery in Montreal, one of the present authors (CPB) had become engaged in a controversy with Dr. Dwight Harken of Boston (11) about the number of "leaflets" existing in the normal mitral valve. While Dr. Harken argued that the number was four, and the present author contended that there were only two (the conventional view, then and now), more recent anatomical investigations by Zimmerman (12, 13) have clearly established that the mitral valve is composed of a continuous "sleeve" of membranous tissue. Its structure is similar to that of a feminine girdle, with numerous garter-like chordae tendineae attaching its "hemline" to the two leg-like papillary muscles (Fig. 9a).

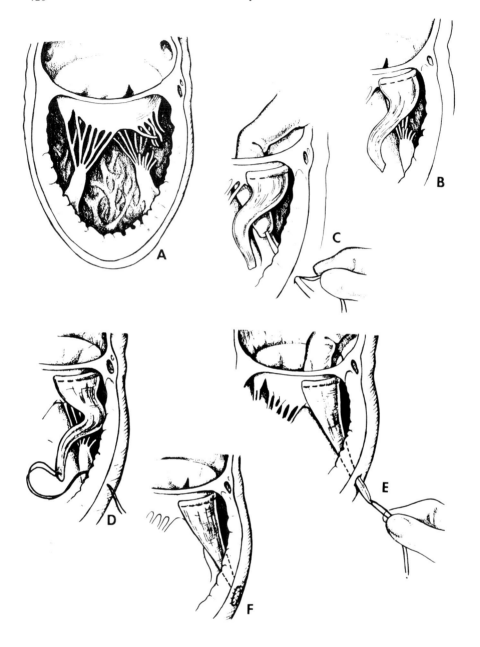

Fig. 4a–f. Resuspension of the flail margin of the mitral valve caused by chordal rupture. Note that the amount of tension to be applied to the extracardiac portion of the wedge-shaped fascial graft is determined by the intra-atrial (digital) examination of the functioning valve.

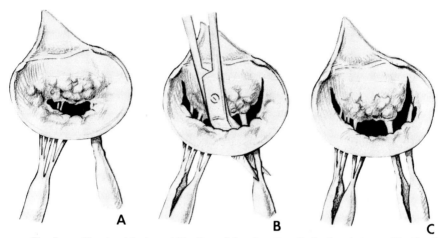

Fig. 5a–c. Neostrophingic mobilization of the stenotic mitral valve. A tongue-like flap is created by mobilizing the septal component of the valve up to the flexible subaortic curtain. While initially an effective procedure, restenosis must be expected eventually.

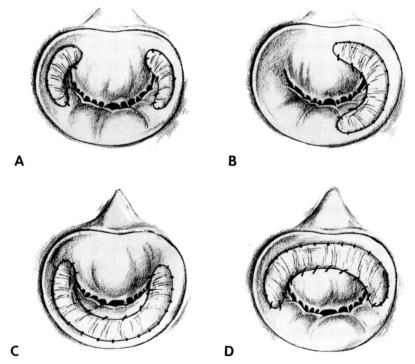

Fig. 6a–d. Permanent resuspension of the completely separated mural and septal valve components by separate reattachment to a span of normal fascia lata. This may be in the form of polar fascial inserts (*a,b*) or by reattachment to a custp-lengthening crescent of this material which has been caused to extend beyond the lines of the surgical valve cleavage (*c,d*).

C. P. Bailey *et al.*

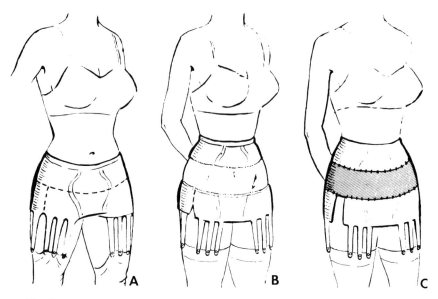

Fig. 7a–c. Prototype procedure for shrinkage of the valve girdle combined with harden-ing of the tissues at the hemline (mitral stenosis and insufficiency). *b.* Circumferential interposition of a lengthening fascial graft. *c.* Separate resuspension of the surgically separated valve "lips" from the lower margin of the lengthening graft.

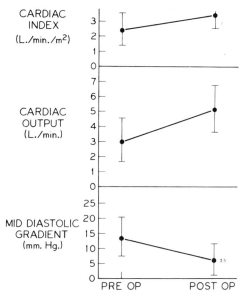

Fig. 8. Graphic depiction of the hemodynamic benefit achieved in 41 consecutive patients treated for mitral stenosis by the previously described techniques. Note that the transmitral gradient is consistently improved, but never completely abolished.

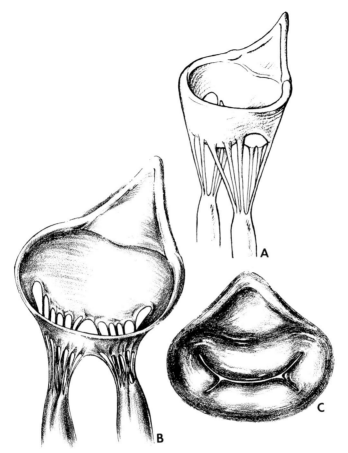

Fig. 9a. Diagrammatic representation of the entire mitral valve structure (after Zimmerman 12, 13). *a.* Note similarity to a girdle (see Fig. 7). *b.* Actual representation of the mitral valve in the fully opened position. Note distribution of chordae of the first order about the margin of the valve orifice. *c.* Representation of the mitral valve in the closed position. Note that the valve does not close simply by the linear approximation of the edges of the septal and mural components. The "junctional" tissues, which sometimes are seen to be widened into intermediate or accessory cusps (constantly in bovine species), also become bulged-in during systole, contributing to formation of a line of closure which is H-shaped. Harken has called these junctional areas the "commissural cusps."

While both of these adversaries were completely incorrect in their views of the anatomy of the normal mitral valve, there can be no doubt Dr. Harken was essentially right in his concept of valve physiology. During systole, the margin of the normal mitral valve becomes infolded (or bulged-in) from both "extremities" as well as from "top-to-bottom" (Fig. 9*b,c*). This produces the "quadricuspid" appearance Dr. Harken was trying to describe. He designated these infoldings of the valve "poles" (extremities) as the "intermediate" or "commissural" cusps.

It would seem that great advantages could accrue from interposing the gusset of new valve material in the position of one (or both) of the commissural cusps. Brock (14) had previously (1952) demonstrated that the presence of the under-lying papillary muscles, with their radiating "crowns" of chordae tendineae beneath the two valve poles, interposed significant impedance to the free flow of blood through these portions of the open valve area (Fig. 10). Hence, placement of one (or two) commissural cusps in these regions would introduce very little interference to the natural pattern of transvalvular blood flow. On the other hand, interposition in the region of the "septal" or "aortic" leaflet would cause maximum interference.

These commissural cusps, unlike simple widening gussets which might be interposed into the circumference of a woman's skirt, would require a "chordo-papillary" type of suspension of the "hemline" if the valve were to remain competent. It was reasoned that a mechanism similar to that employed in resuspending the flail margin of the valve, incompetent because of chordal rupture (see Fig. 4), might be suitable. Thinking that such a tapering "tail" of margin-supporting fascia lata should be made to traverse the ventricular wall in close proximity to the ventricular origin of the appropriate papillary muscle led us to feel that the similar supporting tail of the commissural cusp also should be located at such a site. Today, however, we believe that simple passage of the tail through the apical portion of the ventricular wall will suffice.

It should be recognized that the development of rheumatic mitral stenosis is almost always associated with a "purse-stringing" of the valve orifice, with the

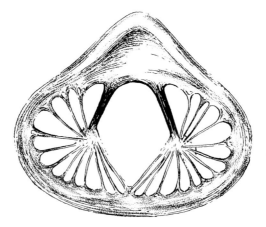

Fig. 10. Note that the mitral subvalvular area is significantly encumbered at both poles by the presence of the two papillary muscles with their radiating chordae tendineae. Free flow of blood cannot take place through the mesh of the chordae tendineae. Note the two unusually heavy chordal supports *arcuately* suspending the septal margin. These consisute Brock's direct line of tendinous support.

marginal chordae then becoming aggregated about the now-diminutive opening (Fig. 11). This is the explanation for the frequently observed lack of peripheral chordal support of the extremities of the "anatomically" mobilized stenotic mitral valve (neostrophingic mobilization).

OPERATIVE TECHNIQUE

In January of 1972, while reoperating on a 44-year-old female patient (L.M.) who had developed mitral restenosis five years following an open-heart type of valve mobilization (for pure stenosis), the orifice was found to be eccentrically located—displaced toward the left fibrous trigone. This portion of the valve was "leathery." The right pole, however, had become infiltrated (actually partially replaced) with readily fragmentable, calcific material. Incisional cleavage of this portion of the valve resulted in fragmentation of the valve substance and in the creation of two long, irregular valve "lips" without significant underlying chordal support (Fig. 12).

It was obvious that a major degree of valvular incompetence thereby had been produced. It appeared that nothing less than replacement with a prosthetic

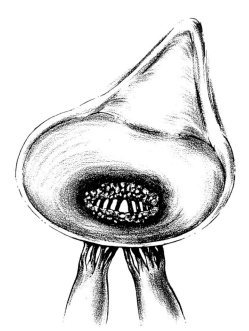

Fig. 11. With the development of severe mitral stenosis, the orifice becomes purse-stringed and the chordal supports become aggregated about the diminutive orifice. The remainder of the valve expanse then is essentially unsupported.

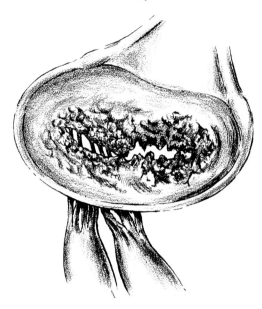

Fig. 12. Anatomically accurate surgical cleavage of the eccentrically located, calcified, and restenosed valve orifice in L. M. led to fragmentation and detachment of friable, calcific material located about the retion of the right, inadequately supported commissure. This created valve "deficit" would have caused severe valvular imcompetence.

device would ensure the patient's operative survival. Reluctant as we always are to introduce such a foreign body into the valvular area of a young person (for the approximately five years of life which it may offer), it was thought that this might be a suitable case to try the introduction of a commissural cusp of fascia lata. After all, the valve function could be evaluated digitally (immediately after closing the left atriotomy and defibrillating the ventricles). If it were not satisfactory, a prosthetic device still could be introduced, thus ensuring immediate survival.

Accordingly, that portion of the septal leaflet which lies to the right of the heavy pair of chordae tendineae which constitute Brock's "direct lines of tendinous support" (14) was excised back to the subaortic curtain [spacium intervalvulare of Henle (15)]. The line of valve incision then was directed to the right, passing in close proximity to the right fibrous trigone, running along the origin of the "mural" leaflet from the atrioventricular junction, to a site along the mural continuity exactly opposite the original line of section of the septal leaflet (there are no especially heavy chordae tendineae similar to the direct line of tendinous support arising from the margin of the mural leaflet). The mural leaflet was transected at this point. All chordae tendineae arising from the detached portion of the valve then were cut away, permitting removal of the specimen (Fig. 13*a,b*).

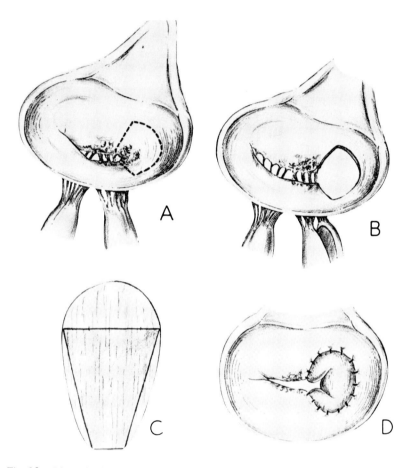

Fig. 13a. Line of valve excision in patient. *b.* Deficit created in the valve. *c.* Creation of a large isosceles fascial triangle (with a truncated tail) by trimming the entire excised fascia lata. Note that the entire width of the fascia is used for the base of the graft. The stronger longitudinal fibers run down to the very tip of the fascial tail. *d.* Note the characteristically convoluted atrial appearance of the finally inserted commissural cusp. The technique of ventricular attachment is the same as that depicted in Fig. 4d,e,f.

The sheath-like tendon of the entire left tensor fascia lata muscle had been removed earlier during the course of the operation, anticipating the possibility of the need for a significant but surely less extensive reconstruction of the valve. The elliptical fascial segment now was trimmed to produce a long, tapering isosceles triangle of tissue, the base of which consisted of the maximum cross-section of the fascia lata (Fig. 13c).

The graft was so oriented that its smoother aspect presented toward the atrium. Beginning at the cut edge of the margin of the septal leaflet, the base of the graft was joined successively (by a continuous displacement mattress-suture technique) to the ventricular aspect of the line of valve excision. To our amazement, the 3-1/3-inch-wide base of the graft proved to be exactly the length needed for the cut edge of the valve remnant, so that no excess fascial tissue had to be cut away.

Now the operator's right index finger was introduced through the valve orifice to identify the site of origin of the appropriate papillary muscle. The tip of the pointed probe, bearing a heavy silk suture in its terminal eye, then was made to pierce the ventricular epicardium exactly over the fingertip and was caused to follow the fingertip as it retreated from the ventricular chamber, emerging within the atrium. The suture was grasped and the probe was withdrawn.

The suture was threaded upon a curved cutting-edge needle, and the latter was passed through the tapering extremity (tail) of the fascial triangle. After the suture was tied securely, the suture end that emerged from the ventricular epicardium was drawn upon, thus causing the tip of the fascial tail to traverse the transventricular probe track and finally to emerge upon the epicardial surface of the heart (see Fig. 4).

The atriotomy was closed in three layers, up to the base of the stump of the appendage. The latter was controlled by an encircling purse-string suture. After defibrillating the ventricles, the operator introduced his index finger into the atrium, and the function of the reconstructed mitral valve was evaluated with the heart beating. Release of traction applied to the extracardiac portion of the

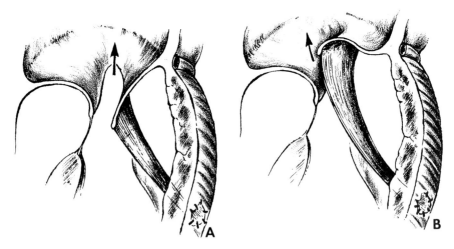

Fig. 14a,b. Demonstration of the effects of greater or lesser tension being applied to the extracardiac end of the commissural cusp. While the functioning valve becomes demonstrably incompetent when the fascial tail is drawn upon either too tightly or too loosely, it is completely competent at any intermediate range of tension.

graft permitted the tail to be drawn into the ventricle and the base to bulge excessively into the atrial chamber. An increase in the traction upon the suture in the tail caused the intra-atrial bulge to become less prominent (Fig. 14a,b). At either extreme of tension, the valve became noticeably incompetent, but over an intermediate range of more than 4 cm of variation in the legnth of the portion of the graft drawn out of the ventricle, the valve remained fully competent.

Finally, the extraventricular portion of the graft was affixed at near maximum effective tension to the ventricular epicardium with one traversing mattress suture and several interrupted ones. The finger was removed from the stump of the appendage, and the latter was tied off and oversewn.

Pressures within the left atrium and ventricle were obtained by simultaneous needle punctures. No transmitral gradient could be detected! One month later, at conventional cardiac catheterization, we were able to confirm the abolition of the transmitral gradient (Table 1).

Rather remarkably, the state of chronic atrial fibrillation which had been present for more than six years spontaneously became converted to a sinus type of rhythm nine days after the operation. We have ascribed this happy occurrence to the unusually great restoration of a "normal" physiological state.

Since that time, 21 additional patients have been submitted to this procedure or a close modification thereof. There have been 16 survivors. One obvious modification was the insertion of a commissural cusp with extensions at its base (created by appropriate tailoring of the original full-sized fascial triangle), so that the shrunken remaining portions of the valve leaflets could be lengthened effectively to overcome a significant element of coexisting mitral insufficiency (Fig. 15a,b,c). However, the effective size of the widening gusset is significantly reduced by this tailoring, and the reduction of the transmitral gradient may not reach the normal level (Table 2). It was suggested that the simultaneous insertion of two such gussets (at both valve poles) might eliminate this residual gradient, and this modification has been used (Fig. 16a–d). In theory, one might well argue that two commissural cusps should always be preferable to one. However, this would imply a double technical procedure which necessarily would prolong the operation and might be unduly taxing in many patients. Moreover, our early experience suggests that it may not prove necessary in every case.

Table I. Abolition of transmitral gradient (patient L.M.)

Date	PAP mm/Hg	PVR dynes/sec/cm^{-5}	CO l/min	CI 1/min/m^2	MDG mm/Hg
4/12/67	40/25 m32	729	3.48	2.07	18 mm
10/29/71	40/25 m32	384	3.70	2.15	10 mm
2/7/72	38/15 m24	341	5.60	3.55	0 mm

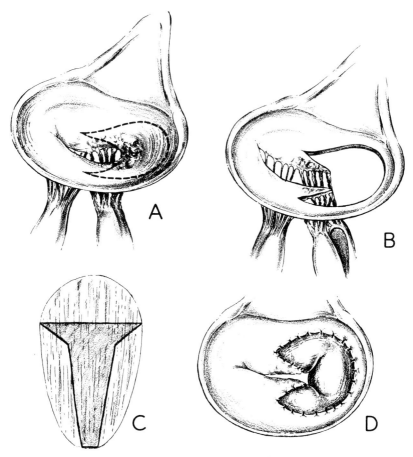

Fig. 15a–d. Modification of the commissural cusp by basal trimming to provide two lengthening fascial extensions. These basal extensions are then interposed into the continuity of the apico-basally "shrunken" remaining valve to overcome an element of coexisting insufficiency.

Table 2. Reduction of Transmitral Gradient (Patient E.S., 38-Year-Old Female; Mitral Insufficiency, 2½ +)

Date	PAP mm/Hg	LVP mm/Hg	CO l/min	CI l/min/m²	MDG mm/Hg
3/16/72	35/14	80/8	3.33	1.96	9
7/14/72	23/12	100/7	3.92	2.28	5
			ex 4.67	(No M. I.)*	

* M. I., mitral insufficiency.

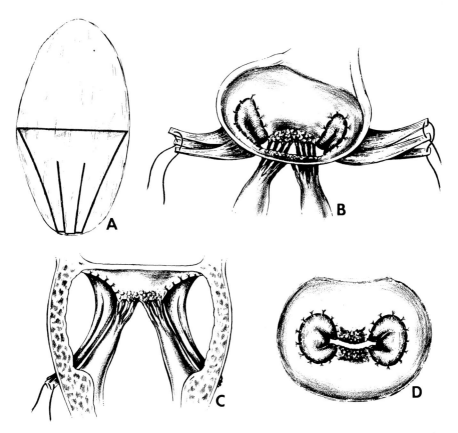

Fig. 16a–d. Steps in creation and interposition of two commissural cusps (at the respective valve poles) by appropriate tailoring of the single entire removed fascia lata.

DISCUSSION

Although our experience with this procedure is short and the number of cases in the series is relatively few, the consistent and rather remarkable improvement which it provides in basic cardiac physiology is a new phenomenon in mitral valvular surgery. Certainly, neither the mobilization procedures (commissurotomy, valvotomy, valvuloplasty, or neostrophingic mobilization) nor the various types of prosthetic replacement are capable of abolishing completely the transvalvular gradient. Neither type of procedure is associated with a high incidence of reversal of chronic atrial fibrillation, whereas 6 of 16 patients surviving the introduction of a commissural cusp have undergone spontaneous conversion. We attribute this to the unusually high grade of restoration of cardiac physiology which is achieved. The actual operative steps are no more taxing to the technical skill of the surgeon than is ordinary prosthetic replacement. Our surgical residents have proved adept in mastering it. While initially it was thought that this type of procedure might be unusually time-consuming (and at first it was), we are now able to carry out the definitive portion of this procedure (when uncomplicated and when limited to insertion of a single commissural cusp) in less than one hour. Obviously, the necessary operative time would be extended if two such cusps were to be inserted.

As in other reconstructions of the cardiac valves with fascia lata, there has proved to be no need for anticoagulant therapy either postoperatively or on a long-term basis.

Gross and histological examination of fascial grafts introduced into the continuity of the mitral valve as long as five years previously indicates good preservation of tissue integrity and no evidence of shrinkage and fibrosis. Senning (1) has had considerably greater experience and reports similar findings.

While the long-term results with particular procedures are not yet ascertainable, our six-year-long experience with that very method of resuspension of the flail margin of the valve for cases of rupture of the chordae tendineae which led us to try the presently employed technique for suspension of the commissural cusp suggests that here there is nothing to be unduly concerned about. A recent six-year follow-up on the second of these particular patients reveals a fully competent and fully functional valve in a vigorous man engaged in heavy outdoor work (professional gardening). Obviously, there has been neither significant shortening nor significant elongation, nor shrinkage in width, of the suspending fascial graft. And initially, the suspending fascial triangle was made essentially the same length as the present-day commissural cusp, subtracting, of course, the perhaps 1.5 cm of apico-basal length which the residual natural valve membrane itself may measure.

SUMMARY

A new type of mitral reconstruction has been designed by which the effective caliber of the shrunken valve skirt is increased by the introduction of a "papillary-supported" gusset of fascia lata at one or both valve poles, after excision of a sizeable amount of pathological valve substance. These operations have proved to be capable of providing an unusually high grade of restoration of those physiological parameters which indicate normal valve function. The clinical response has been correspondingly gratifying.

A number of individuals with unusual pathological findings at operation have been submitted to this type of procedure when no other seemed ideally indicated.

Because the tissue employed is autologous, no problems of immunological incompatibility are involved. Long-term experience (more than six years) with this same tissue used for a very similar purpose in valvular reconstruction (resuspension of the flail valve margin in cases of chordal rupture) has revealed no unexpected or disturbing late development.

The operative procedures proposed have not proved unduly time-consuming or otherwise excessively taxing to the patient. No early or late anticoagulant therapy has been needed.

All of the mobilization types of procedures, many of the other reconstructive operations, and the various types of prosthetic replacement having been shown to be essentially of partial or even of frankly palliative effect, we propose the surgical introduction of commissural cusps of fascia lata for the treatment of stenotic lesions of the mitral valve in younger patients as basically and permanently "curative" operations.

REFERENCES CITED

1. Senning, A. 1967. Fascia lata replacement of aortic valves. J. Thorac. Cardiov. Surg. 54:65.
2. Senning, A. 1970. Reconstruction of the aortic valve with patient's own tissue. Pages 186–194 *in* C. P. Bailey, S. Gollub, and A. G. Shapiro, eds. Therapeutic advances in the practice of cardiology. Grune & Stratton, New York.
3. Bailey, C. P., Zimmerman, J., Hirose, T., and DeVera, E. 1967. Mitral valvular reconstruction with human tissues. Pages 105–126 *in* C. P. Bailey, ed. Rheumatic and coronary heart disease. Lippincott, Philadelphia.
4. Bailey, C. P., Zimmerman, J., and Hirose, T. 1968. Reconstructing cardiac valves with patient's own tissues. N.Y. State J. Med. 1835.
5. Bailey, C. P., Vera, C. A., and Hirose, T. 1969. Mitral regurgitation from rupture of chordae tendineae due to "steering wheel" compression. Geriatrics 24:90.
6. Bailey, C. P., Zimmerman, J., Hirose, T., and Folk, F. S. 1970. Reconstruction of the mitral valve with autologous tissue. Ann. Thoracic Surg. 9:103.
7. Bailey, C. P., Zimmerman, J., and Hirose, T. 1970. Graft reconstruction of the mitral valve. Pages 141–162 *in* C. P. Bailey, ed. Therapeutic advances in the practice of cardiology. Grune & Stratton, New York.
8. Bailey, C. P., Zimmerman, J., Hirose, T., and Folk, F. S. 1970. Use of autologous tissue in mitral valve reconstruction. Geriatrics 25:119.
9. Bailey, C. P., Hirose, T., and Folk, F. S. 1972. Autologous tissue repair in mitral and aortic valvular disease. Pages 406–443 *in* H. I. Russek, ed. Changing concepts in cardiovascular disease. Williams & Wilkins, Baltimore.
10. Bailey, C. P., Hirose, T., and Folk, F. S. 1973. Autologous tissue repair in valvular surgery. Proceedings of the American College of Cardiology and St. Barnabas Hospital Symposium, December, 1971. Williams & Wilkins, Baltimore. (In press.)
11. Harken, D. E., Black, H., Ellis, L. B., and Dexter, L. 1954. Surgical correction of mitral insufficiency. J. Thorac. Surg. 28:604.
12. Zimmerman, J., and Bailey, C. P. 1962. The surgical significance of the fibrous skeleton of the heart. J. Thorac. Cardiov. Surg. 44:701.
13. Zimmerman, J. 1967. New concepts of the anatomy of the mitral and aortic valves. Pages 63–72 *in* C. P. Bailey, S. Gollub, and A. G. Shapiro, eds. Rheumatic and coronary heart disease. Lippincott, Philadelphia.
14. Brock, R. C. 1952. Surgical and pathological anatomy of the mitral valve. Brit. Heart J. 14:489.
15. Henle, J. 1867. Handbuch der Gefasslehre des Menschen. Braunschweig.

Coronary Bypass Grafts–
Artery or Vein?

LONG-TERM RESULTS OF INTERNAL MAMMARY-CORONARY ARTERY ANASTOMOSIS FOR ANGINA PECTORIS

GEORGE E. GREEN

Microsuture anastomosis of the internal mammary artery to coronary arteries was introduced in 1968 (1). From February of 1968 through September of 1972, I performed internal mammary anastomosis in 326 patients. In order to estimate long-term clinical results, this total group of patients was subdivided so that the group operated upon prior to July of 1971 was subjected to special scrutiny. This group afforded a minimum follow-up period of 12 months per patient and a cumulative follow-up period of approximately 5,000 patient months.

MATERIALS AND METHODS

Internal mammary anastomosis was one of the first methods of direct coronary arterial surgery to be applied to large numbers of patients. Although the surgical technique of microsuture of the internal mammary artery to coronary arteries did not vary during the period, patient selection did vary. During the earliest period no patient was rejected because of extent of vascular disease or compromise of ventricular function. This was conspicuously modified later. Also, when the operation was first introduced only single vessel anastomosis was performed. As time went on and experience accumulated, the need for multiple grafts in the majority of patients was increasingly appreciated. Therefore, in the most recent groups of patients to be operated, it has been the exception rather than the rule to perform single vessel anastomosis.

Technique of anastomosis did not vary and has been previously described (2). I consider the high magnification available only with an operating microscope to be an important aspect of this surgery (Fig. 1). Other than the increasing use of multiple grafts and the tendency to eliminate patients with more serious impairment of ventricular function, technical changes that took place were the following: beginning in 1969 the operating microscope was used for all anastomoses, venous as well as arterial; beginning in 1970 all venous grafts were taken from the lower limb rather than from the thigh (3).

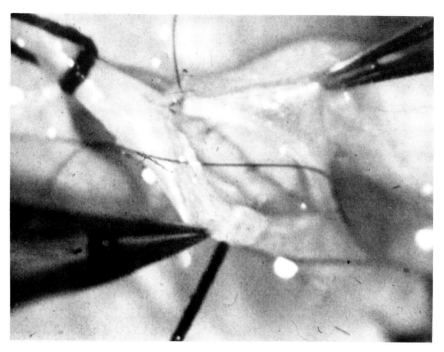

Fig. 1. View of anastomosis through the operating microscope.

RESULTS

Clinical results are presented in detail only for the first group of patients operated upon. It should, however, be noted that of 161 patients operated upon from July of 1971 through September of 1972, there were no hospital deaths. In other respects, the clinical course of the second group of patients was very similar to the subgroup operated upon through June of 1971 and this course is presented in detail. Figure 2 summarizes the clinical course of 156 patients (follow-up data were unavailable for 9 patients) operated upon between 1968 and June of 1971. An important factor accounting for the absence of operative mortality in the group operated upon after 1971 was that patients with far advanced impairment of ventricular function were not considered surgical candidates. An important factor in avoiding sepsis was the giving of more careful attention to the possibility of late cardiac tamponade. The patient who died of sepsis in 1971 did so because late cardiac tamponade, occurring on the tenth day following operation, was unrecognized until the patient was in shock. Sepsis developed after unsterile sternotomy was performed as an emergency. Reference to Table 1 further shows that propranolol cardiac arrest, which accounted for 2

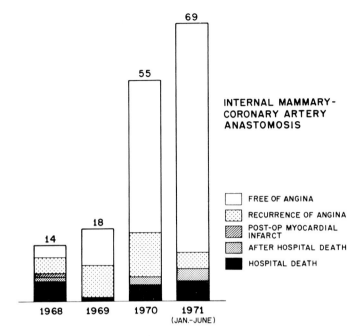

Fig. 2. Long-term results of internal mammary artery-coronary artery anastomosis.

Table 1. Hospital Deaths After Internal Mammary
Artery-to-Coronary Artery Anastomosis

Cause of death	1968 (5/14)[a]	1969 (1/18)	1970 (4/61)	Jan–June, 1971 (3/70)
Unexplained cardiac arrest 6–10 days postoperation	2	–	1	–
Sepsis	2	–	–	1
Irremediable ventricular impairment	–	–	–	2
Faulty anastomosis	1	–	1	–
Propranolol arrest during operation	–	–	2	–
Mesenteric artery thrombosis	–	1	–	–

[a]Total annual hospital deaths/total annual number of patients operated upon.

deaths in 1970, did not occur thereafter. This is because patients who have taken propranolol within 7 days of the time of the projected operation are no longer operated upon.

Unexplained cardiac arrest occurring 6–10 days following operation accounted for 3 of 13 deaths in the early group of patients. This has not occured since 1971. It is believed that wider use of multiple grafts has afforded greater safety. Reference to Figure 2 shows there were 7 deaths in patients after leaving the hospital. Two of these were caused by hepatic failure following viral hepatitis. One death occurred in 1968 and one in 1970. The reduced utilization of blood in recent years (averaging 5.5 units per patient) and the wider availability of volunteer blood accounts for the lack of deaths from hepatitis, and within the past 12 months for the absence of any clinically recognized transfusion hepatitis. One late death in a patient operated upon in 1970 was attributable to gradual closure of a vein graft (the patient had aortic valve replacement, internal mammary anastomosis to the anterior descending artery, and saphenous vein graft to the right coronary artery) resulting in fibrous replacement of the posterior papillary muscle and massive mitral valve insufficiency. The patient died before mitral valve replacement could be performed.

Four late deaths occurred in patients who were operated upon during the first half of 1971. One of these was caused by cancer of the lung. Another was caused by pulmonary embolism in a patient with previous history of thrombophlebitis. Because of previous obliteration of his lower leg veins, it was necessary to use a segment of saphenous vein from the thigh. It has been my consistent experience that phlebothrombosis and pulmonary embolus had been much more frequent when veins were removed from the thigh. One death occurred approximately 18 months after operation, from massive gastrointestinal hemorrhage. Finally, one sudden death occurred 14 months after operation. This probably represents the only late cardiac death in the entire series. The patient, at the time of operation, had far advanced diffuse triple vessel disease. Two grafts were performed: an internal mammary anastomosis to the left anterior descending artery and a saphenous vein graft to a lateral branch of the circumflex coronary artery. The totally occluded and diffusely diseased right coronary artery was not protected by a graft.

RECURRENCE OF ANGINA

Reference to Figure 2 shows that the incidence of recurrent angina progressively diminished to 5% as experience accumulated. The predominant reason for this is that multiple vein grafts were used with increasing frequency. Table 2 shows that the most common cause of recurrent angina is progression of disease in unoperated vessels. In 1971, as a general rule all lesions that appeared to compromise

Table 2. Recurrence of Angina After Internal
Mammary-to-Coronary Artery Anastomosis

Description	1968	1969	1970	1971
Number of patients with angina	4	7	11	3
Number of surviving patients	8	18	55	69
Time of recurrence (months postoperation)	3–12	1–30	1–6	0.5–2
Average	7.8	8.5	3.4	1
IMA[a] angiogram	4	5	6	2
Good IMA anastomosis	4	5	3	1
Thrombosed IMA	0	0	1	1
Stenosed IMA	0	0	2	0
Progression of disease in operated vessels[b]	0	3	0	2
Progression of disease in unoperated vessels	4	0	4	2

[a]IMA = internal mammary artery.

[b]Documented progression of disease in operated vessels was always proximal to site of anastomosis.

the vessel by 50% or more were bypassed. In this series of patients, late angiograms have not suggested that such prophylactic bypasses contribute to closure of partial occlusions. Progression of disease proximal to the site of anastomosis in operated vessels can cause diminished perfusion of myocardium and has accounted for a substantial proportion of recurrences of angina. The angina has not usually, in this setting, been a clinical problem. The smallest proportion of cases of recurrent angina were caused by closure of internal mammary artery anastomoses, this having occurred in 2 patients, representing an incidence of 3% in a group of 70 patients examined by angiography following operation. In contrast, closures of vein grafts accounted for a total of 30% of the patients having vein grafts who were examined by postoperative angiography. This 30% is a higher figure than would be obtained in patients who had been studied at routine intervals by angiography. It represents closures discovered in predominantly symptomatic patients.

EARLY MYOCARDIAL INFARCTIONS

Seven of the 326 patients operated upon developed new Q waves after operation and while in the hospital—an incidence of 2%; however, 3 of these patients underwent early postoperative cardiac catheterization which demonstrated patent grafts and no change in the preexisting coronary circulation or ventricular function.

LATE MYOCARDIAL INFARCTIONS

No patient in the entire series has been observed to have developed transmural myocardial infarction after leaving the hospital. One patient developed subendocardial infarction 18 months following a single graft. One patient sustained a sudden death that was probably caused by a myocardial infarction. This would make for a total of 2 myocardial infarctions in a cumulative follow-up period of approximately 5,000 patient months.

TOTAL OPERATIVE AND POSTOPERATIVE MORTALITY

Table 3 shows that over the 4-year period, a total hospital and late cardiac mortality of 4.2% was observed. This makes for an annual mortality of approximately 1%. When compared with the expected annual mortality (8–12%) from coronary artery disease in patients with either angiographically documented triple vessel disease or in patients with angina and abnormal cardiogram, one sees that an annual reduction of cardiac mortality in the range of 8-fold to 10-fold is achieved by bypass grafting. This, combined with the current elimination of angina pectoris in more than 90% of patients being operated upon, puts the operative procedure on a very sound footing.

Table 3. Hospital Mortality 1968–1972 (September)

1968–1971	(July)	13/165	
1971–1972	(September)	0/161	
		13/326	3.9%
Plus late cardiac deaths (1/326)			0.3%
Cumulative hospital and late cardiac mortality			4.2%

PROSPECTS

Because of the excellent experience with internal mammary artery anastomosis, within recent months both internal mammary arteries have been used in an increasing proportion of patients. Usually the right internal mammary artery is suitable for anastomosis to the anterior descending artery and the left internal mammary artery can be anastomosed to the circumflex vessel. The right internal mammary artery usually is not sufficiently long to reach the distal segment of the right coronary artery but Edward's procedure (4) of splenic anastomosis to the distal right coronary artery shows great promise.

REFERENCES CITED

1. Green, G. E., Stertzer, S. H., and Reppert, E. H. 1968. Coronary arterial bypass grafts. Ann. Thoracic Surg. 5:443.
2. Green, G. E. 1972. Internal mammary artery-to-coronary artery anastomosis. Three-year experience with 165 patients. Ann. Thoracic Surg. 15:260.
3. Green, G. E., Hutchinson, J. E., and McCord, C. W. 1971. Choice of saphenous vein segments for aorto-coronary grafts. Surgery 69:924.
4. Edwards, W. S., Blakeley, W. R., Lewis, C. E., and Abrams, J. 1973. Coronary bypass entirely with arteries. Circulation (in press).

LATE RESULTS IN CORONARY VEIN GRAFTS

W. DUDLEY JOHNSON

Surgical efforts at treating coronary disease during the past many years have been designed primarily for treating the patient with active symptoms. This usually means patients with moderate to severe angina.

Since angina continues to be the major factor leading patients to surgery, it seems reasonable that its relief after surgery should be one of the first factors of importance in evaluating surgical results. To a surgeon, it seems inconsistent for cardiologists to refer patients only for angina and then postoperatively to claim that the loss of angina is no index of surgical success. Catheterization studies have shown a remarkably close correlation between recurrent symptoms and graft failure and/or progression of disease. As a generalization, patients who have lost all of their symptoms nearly always have patent grafts.

Quality of Life

While the quality of life is a subjective matter, 66% of patients questioned in January, 1972, stated they had had no angina since surgery. The questionnaire was returned by 886 patients (91% of the total); all patients were at least six months postoperative, and some were as much as 40 months postoperative. An additional 25% stated they were much better. In 91% of patients, the quality of life was, therefore, significantly improved, even though no basic cure of the underlying atherosclerosis was achieved. Results of surgery during the past two years seem to show an even better clinical response, corresponding to the development of better and more complete surgical revascularization. No methods of medical therapy have achieved this degree and duration of palliation, and this factor is undoubtedly the reason that this surgery has expanded so rapidly.

Exercise Studies

While angina is the first and foremost factor which continues to cause patients to be referred for surgery, many other methods of evaluation, both early and late, have demonstrated significant results following bypass grafts. In our own Center, bicycle ergometry testing has been performed on large numbers of patients during their catheterization procedures. These studies demonstrate marked deterioration of left ventricular function under stress in most patients studied preoperatively. End-diastolic pressure commonly elevates markedly during quantitated amounts of work. The same ergometry studies have been performed on

445

patients early and late following surgery. In patients who have relatively good ventricles, there is a statistically significant improvement in the ability of these hearts to respond to stress following bypass grafting. While deterioration of the end-diastolic pressure under stress to 30 or 40 mm Hg is common preoperatively, after successful grafting the end-diastolic pressure usually remains at normal or nearly normal levels, even though the amount of exercise performed has been increased greatly. The hearts have not shown a tendency to improve further during the year following surgery. Bicycle ergometry studies performed a few weeks following surgery and again one year later rarely show any significant difference.

In patients who previously suffered one or more major infarcts and who have distinctly abnormal ventricular function, the results of surgery as measured by stress testing have been somewhat discouraging. The majority of patients with grossly abnormal ventricular contractility show relatively little change following surgery. The angina is generally relieved, but the heart does not contract normally and the abnormal stress response frequently persists. The occasional dramatic improvement is noted, but as a group there is no statistically significant improvement in the stress response postoperatively. The measurement of end-diastolic pressure by itself is of relatively little help in evaluating the patients for surgery. A moderate to marked drop in the end-diastolic pressure following surgery commonly is observed. The maximum drop noted in the end-diastolic pressure postoperatively has been 40 mm Hg. This degree of improvement is rare, but improvement by a factor of 5–10 mm Hg is seen relatively commonly. While the end-diastolic pressure often is improved, gross improvement in the ventriculogram following surgery is again relatively rarely observed. Minor improvement is often present, but gross improvement usually is confined to the patient who has severely incapacitating angina in addition to a poorly functioning, dilated ventricle.

All of the exercise studies performed on these patients have made one point rather apparent. Coronary bypass surgery is primarily prophylactic in nature. If improvement in ventricular performance is desired, it must be achieved while the myocardium is still viable and functioning. No amount of revascularization can alter the function of fibrotic and scarred myocardium. The best results, both early and late, following this surgery occur in patients who still have relatively well-functioning myocardial tissue.

Rhythm Disturbances

In coronary disease, the development of rhythm disturbances is a relatively common occurrence. Patients often are seen who have chronic premature ventricular beats. Over the years, no patient yet has been observed in whom these chronic premature ventricular beats disappeared following successful revascularization surgery. A number of late deaths have occurred in these patients, and it is strongly recommended that, following surgery, these patients be treated vigorously for their ventricular rhythm problem. Because the chronic premature ventricular beats do not disappear after successful revascularization, it is now felt quite strongly that the mere presence of premature ventricular contractions (PVC's) is not an indication for surgery. If the patients have major obstructing coronary lesions and/or are incapacitated in their ability to perform, they still should undergo surgery. The angina will be relieved and the ventricular performance often improved, as in other patients, but the chronic PVC's have always continued.

While the chronic PVC patient is not a candidate for surgery, another type of ventricular rhythm disturbance is a clear and almost absolute indication for revascularization. This disturbance is in the patient who has runs of several ventricular beats in a row, particularly when this episode of ventricular tachycardia occurs in response to stress. In our experience, these patients are very prone to fibrillation and death. When revascularization is achieved, this type of episodic ventricular tachycardia usually disappears. We now consider the patient who has runs of tachycardia to be a strong preinfarction or pre-sudden death candidate, and surgery in these patients is performed on a relatively urgent basis.

Patency Rates

Of particular concern to surgeons and cardiologists has been the patency rate of the grafts which are inserted at surgery. My own experience from 1968 through 1971 is summarized in Table 1, correlating graft patency with intraoperative flow measurements. This information was compiled from a computer in which surgical and postoperative catheterization studies are tabulated. As can be seen from the data, the early patency rate following surgery consistently has been at the 90–95% level. The patency was tabulated also by the site of the recipient artery, and there appears to be no difference in the patency no matter where the veins from the aorta are attached except for the posterior descending artery. In this locale, the patency has been consistently 10–15% less than in veins placed into the other more proximal and usually larger arteries. Patients are not ordinarily studied in the 3–12 month interval. The patients catheterized at this stage have by and large had some type of recurrent symptoms. This correlates with the relatively high failure rate of patients studied during this interval. When patients are studied after one year, the patency rate is consistently less than the early rate. We estimate that 8–10% of the vein grafts will occlude during the first 12–18 months. Graft failure after 18 months has been remarkably rare, and the early failure of 10–15% is not a continuing yearly problem. Occlusion of one graft in a patient with several grafts does not mean that the other grafts will also close. Closure of all grafts in a given patient has been extremely rare. Furthermore, closure of a graft because of subintimal fibrous hyperplasia does not predispose the patient to the same process in a new vein inserted at a later

Table 1. Patency Related to Flow*

Flow (ml/min)	Total no. of veins	Total no. closed	Total no. patent	% Patent
0–3 months				
20	20	8	12	60.0
21–40	60	2	58	96.7
41–100	106	9	97	91.5
101	17	1	16	94.1
4–12 months				
20	3	1	2	66.7
21–40	19	4	15	78.9
41–100	48	11	37	77.1
101	13	2	11	84.6
13 or more months				
20	6	4	2	33.3
21–40	18	2	16	88.9
41–100	44	7	37	84.1
101	13	1	12	92.3

* Vein graft patency early and late as correlated with intraoperative flow measurements. The critical flow appears to be about 20 cc/min. Above that level, the patency rate is relatively constant, both early and late. Patients are not routinely studied in the 4- to 12-month period. Most of these patients have had recurrent symptoms, hence the higher graft failure rate. The failure rate between the early studies and those after one year is not a continuing yearly process, as failure after one year has been quite rare.

procedure. The subintimal fibrous process usually obliterates the vein within a few months of the initial operation. A number of patients now have had secondary operative procedures for replacement of the first graft, and the new second graft has continued to function satisfactorily for a long period. It is apparent, therefore, that failure of one graft does not necessarily foretell the fate of further grafts inserted at secondary operative procedures.

While the patency rate with the coronary vein graft technique has been encouraging, and the graft failure rate after 18 months has been remarkably rare, a significant percentage of grafts do close during the first one to two postoperative years. Because of this fact, the left mammary artery has been used with increasing frequency during the past two and one-half years. The mammary-coronary bypass procedure is technically more difficult than inserting vein grafts, and the technique is not as versatile as the use of a free vein graft. Nevertheless, the patency rate with the mammary-coronary technique has been extremely high. In our experience, as well as that of several other centers, the patency rate consistently has exceeded that of vein grafts. In my experience, more than 90% of patients now have at least one mammary-coronary bypass procedure, and the majority of patients are receiving two mammary bypass grafts. Additional grafts are constructed with veins and occasionally with the use of radial artery grafts. With more than 350 mammary bypasses performed, late recurrent symptoms or late infarction caused by late failure of a mammary bypass graft have been rare. In my series of patients in whom bypass grafts have been constructed with both mammary arteries and vein grafts, the percentage of veins closed has been twice the percentage of mammary closures. These patients have served as their own controls to compare the success of a vein graft with that of a mammary-coronary bypass. The mammary-coronary bypass technique clearly has been the preferable procedure. It is for this reason that both mammary arteries currently are used for bypasses in the majority of patients.

Mortality

One of the unknown factors related to this surgery is the effect it has on mortality. No comparable surgically and medically treated groups have been described. The surgeon tends to see advanced patients. Most patients have a long history of disease, and the factors finally influencing the practicing physician to refer the patient for surgery are difficult to define. The surgical population has been filtered off by many physicians and further screened by cardiologists. A comparable group of nonoperated patients has not been followed, and comparisons therefore are difficult. From 1969 through 1971, 112 patients were identified in whom surgery was recommended by the cardiologists, yet none of these patients were operated upon (1). Many died waiting for surgery, and many others either declined surgery or were advised to do so by their physician. Sixty-one of the 112 were dead within two years. While heavily biased by those dying on the surgical waiting list, this fact suggests at least that surgical patients are probably a different group from those included in a general medical group. Evaluation of these patients from the time of their catheterization indicated that symptomatology was of minimum help in predicting who would subsequently live or die. The coronary anatomy was of far greater predictive quality. Patients with disease of one artery did well, with only two deaths occurring in this group. With disease of two or three arteries, the mortality rate rapidly increased. As based on the coronary anatomy defined by cine studies, there was a statistically significant difference in one-, two-, and three-artery disease in terms of the patients subsequently living or dead. Good or poor ventricular function was less significant in predicting subsequent death than was the coronary anatomy. It has long been our opinion that the coronary anatomy should be at least as important as the symptoms in selecting patients for surgery.

Of even greater significance in predicting death was the presence of a major obstruction in the proximal left coronary system (greater than 70% obstruction proximal to the first septal and diagonal arteries). Whether there was one-, two-, or three-artery disease, in each category the presence of a high left lesion carried an even further increased risk of death.

While the overall effects of surgery on longevity cannot yet be defined, the above-mentioned patients with a high left lesion fared much worse than those surgical patients who had even worse disease, namely, left main stenosis (2). This series of 56 patients, operated upon in 1970 and 1971, had a 10% operative mortality and a 4% late mortality. With a major proximal left obstruction, especially a left main lesion, surgery does appear to alter mortality favorably. As the disease becomes more diffuse and more peripheral, the effects of surgery are more difficult to evaluate.

In contrast to nonoperated patients, surgical and late postoperative mortality has related more closely to the degree of ventricular function and much less to the extent of coronary disease. Mortality data, early and late, have been tabulated by McRaven (Table 2). These data relate to the first few years of the surgical experience in Milwaukee. Surgical and late mortality steadily increased as the degree of ventricular malfunction increased. In each category of function, the surgical mortality rate has steadily decreased year by year, and the data presented represent the results of the first few years of this surgery. During 1972, the surgical mortality with good ventricular function was less than 2%, regardless of the diffuseness of the disease. Most late deaths have been in patients with damaged hearts to begin with. There appears to be a relatively large increase in mortality in the third year after surgery. Such an increase at this level is difficult to explain. The numbers are small, and thus a very few deaths could cause this apparent result. Further time will be needed to substantiate the

Table 2. Coronary Vein Graft Surgery Mortality by Ventricular Function (March, 1968–June, 1972

Left ventricular angiogram	No. of patients	% Survival			
		1 month	1 year	2 years	3 years
Normal–mild general hypokinesis	433	95	94	91	86
Local hypokinesis, single wall	279	94	87	85	82
Hypokinesis in two walls	121	89	79	79	69
Severe general hypokinesis	91	78	73	64	59

* A composite summary of the early (surgical) and late mortality of the first patients undergoing bypass surgery as correlated by ventricular function. Note that the best early and late results occur in patients with relatively good ventricles. While many with poor function have been greatly improved, it would be preferable to have surgery prior to destructive infarcts. Surgical mortality in each category has been sharply reduced each year, but these data include the first few years of experience.

long-term mortality rate. As more thorough and better revascularization procedures have been developed, current symptoms, late complications, and late deaths appear to be steadily decreasing.

SUMMARY

Coronary bypass surgery has demonstrated the ability to markedly relieve or eliminate anginal symptoms in more than 90% of patients for up to three years after surgery. Ventricular function is usually improved as measured by ventriculography, end-diastolic pressure, or stress testing. The best response to stress testing occurs when surgery is performed prior to extensive myocardial damage. Surgical mortality has steadily decreased, and currently is in the 1% range if resting ventricular function is still relatively normal. Most late deaths have occurred in patients with damaged ventricles preoperatively. Surgical and late mortality correlates better with ventricular function than with the extent of coronary disease. In patients with high anterior descending or left main disease, surgery clearly appears to decrease mortality rates. As the disease becomes more peripheral, the effect on mortality is less clear.

Vein grafts should have an early patency near the 95% level, and an additional 8 or 10% failure occurs the first year. Failure after one year is rare. Mammary-coronary bypass carries a higher patency rate, and where it can be used is the procedure of choice. Surgery should be considered basically prophylactic. It must be performed while the myocardium is still viable. Surgery does nothing for scarred and fibrotic tissue resulting from a series of infarcts.

REFERENCES CITED

1. Johnson, W. D., and Kayser, K. L., 1973. An expanded indication for coronary surgery. Ann. Thorac. Surg. 16:1.
2. Zeft, H. J., Manley, J. C., Huston, J. H., Tector, A. C., and Johnson, W. D. 1972. Direct coronary surgery in patients with left main coronary artery stenosis. Circulation 45, 46 (Suppl. 2).

THE NATURAL HISTORY OF SEVERE ANGINA
PECTORIS WITH MEDICAL THERAPY ALONE

HENRY I. RUSSEK

In the present era of revascularization surgery, the physician is hampered by a lack of knowledge concerning the natural history of angina pectoris. Currently, two divergent views are readily found in the literature: 1) that angina pectoris is a highly lethal disease and 2) that it is a benign disorder compatible with long survival in the majority of cases. Although a number of authors (1-6) have reported on mortality rates in large groups of patients followed for one, two, or more decades (Table 1), the relevance of their data to patient populations under treatment today with modern drugs and new perspectives in management may be readily challenged.

With no specific regimen of therapy, Zukel and co-workers (1), for example, reported the annual mortality rate in a large series of patients with angina pectoris to be only about 3%, while Kannel and associates (2) found the yearly attrition rate in their patients in the Framingham study to approximate 4%. Today, with modern therapeutic approaches consisting of dietary management, weight reduction, hypocholesterolemic drugs, control of hypertension and diabetes, curtailment of stress and tobacco, exercise training, and the use of such agents as propranolol and isosorbide dinitrate, it does not seem unreasonable to

Table 1. Mortality in Angina Pectoris

Authors	Annual mortality (%)	
Zukel and co-workers (1)	3	
Kannel and associates (2)	4	
Parker et al. (3)	6	
Block and co-workers (4)	6	
Moberg et al. (5)	6.4	
	3.3	(1 vessel)
	6.7	(2 vessels)
	10.5	(3 vessels)
Sheldon and associates (6)	8.8	

expect that the outlook has become more favorable. At the present time, however, it cannot be stated unequivocally that the prognosis in 1973 is appreciably better for the anginal patient than it was in former years. This is because the availability of comprehensive measures, even of established value, can afford no assurance that they will be applied on a wide scale and in an effectual manner. The status of treatment for arterial hypertension in this country, for example, provides adequate insight into the wide gulf that may exist between actual results of *casual* management and those potentially attainable under *optimal* therapy. A similar disparity may exist with respect to angina pectoris, since many physicians appear to rely on nitroglycerin alone, despite dramatic advances in treatment. This narrow approach not only has contributed appreciably to the incidence of "refractory" patients but also has led to premature or needless referral for surgical revascularization.

It should be evident that even if accurate statistics were now available to indicate the average annual mortality rate in anginal patients receiving optimal medical care, the physician would gain little help in assessing prognosis for the individual case and in rendering a decision with regard to surgery. Just as average mortality rates for acute myocardial infarction tell little about the actual risk with a mild first attack or with a massive recurrent episode associated with cardiogenic shock, average annual attrition rates for patients with angina pectoris as a group similarly must mask the mortality risk prevalent in various clinical subsets of this syndrome. At the present time, therefore, there is urgent need not only to seek out clinical profiles that may identify anginal patients at varied risk but also to record the natural hazards in these categories under the best available medical care.

Since there is a variety of factors which are known to influence the prognosis in angina pectoris, the classification, intensive treatment, and follow-up of patients in relatively high- and low-risk categories could provide useful data for weighing the hazards of surgery against the natural consequences of the disease. Insight gained from long clinical experience has shown that among the major factors contributing to risk in this disorder are cardiac enlargement, congestive heart failure, multiple myocardial infarctions, hypertension, atrial fibrillation, valvular heart disease, and diabetes mellitus. Since patients suffering from severe angina pectoris frequently possess none of these poor prognostic signs, it seemed that it might be possible to identify "good risk" subjects who, despite severe initial symptoms, could have excellent prospects under appropriate medical therapy for both dramatic clinical improvement and relatively long survival. It is of interest that similar classification has proved useful in selecting patients for anticoagulant therapy in acute myocardial infarction (7). Thus, we have reported that the low morbidity and mortality in patients initially classified as "good risk" on the basis of clinical prognostic signs did not justify even the small hazard attending the use of anticoagulant drugs during the acute phase of myocardial infarction. In contrast, the reverse was found to be true for "poor risk" patients. The question which we sought to answer with respect to severe angina pectoris, therefore, was whether or not similar classification and follow-up could prove helpful in establishing criteria for or against surgical intervention. From the prospective study, which was begun in November of 1966, and which has continued to the present time, useful data appear to be emerging (8−12).

MATERIAL

In all, a total of 133 patients presenting with severe forms of angina pectoris, unresponsive to conventional treatment, have been followed under a well-defined and intensive therapeutic program. Their ages ranged from 29 to 80 years. Of the total, 102 patients were men and 31 were women. In each instance, slight to moderate physical or emotional stress regularly evoked classical episodes of angina pectoris which, until the time of study, could not be adequately controlled or prevented, despite alterations in life style and the customary use of nitroglycerin, long-acting nitrates, sedatives, and other measures. None of the patients had been treated with beta-blocking agents. As a consequence, in many the activities of daily living, occupational performance, and even sleep, frequently were disturbed. The diagnosis was confirmed in each patient by an unequivocal history of the classic symptoms, present for one year or more, and typical ischemic electrocardiographic (ECG) patterns after exercise, previous episodes of myocardial infarction, or cinecoronary angiographic evidence of advanced disease. Thirty-two patients in the series had been studied by angiography, and 26 of this number were found to have severe triple coronary artery disease. A history of one or more myocardial infarctions requiring hospitalization was elicited in 55 of the 133 patients and confirmed by electrocardiography. Seventeen in the series were on digitalis therapy prescribed for previous congestive heart failure. Eight suffered from other complications, such as cerebrovascular insufficiency, previous stroke, or severe and uncontrolled diabetes. Twelve patients were more than 70 years old.

CLASSIFICATION OF PATIENTS

Although all patients suffered from severe and refractory forms of angina pectoris, they were classified as "good risk" or "poor risk" at the time of their initial examinations on the basis of certain clinically recognized poor prognostic signs. Thus a patient was considered to be a poor risk for relatively long survival if he presented any one of the following unfavorable criteria:

1. Congestive heart failure, past or present
2. Significant enlargement of the heart

Table 2. Classification and Characteristics of 133 Patients with Severe Angina Pectoris

Type	No.	Average age	Over 70 yr.	C.H.F.[a]	Previous M.I.[b]	Other complications
Good risk	102	58.8	0	0	28	0
Poor risk	31	65.2	12	17	27	8

[a]C.H.F., congestive heart failure.
[b]M.I., myocardial infarction.

3. Multiple myocardial infarctions
4. Gallop rhythm
5. Severe hypertension
6. Atrial fibrillation
7. Severe and uncontrolled diabetes
8. Previous "stroke" or cerebrovascular insufficiency
9. Advanced age

Of the 133 patients in the series, 102 qualified as "good risk" by manifesting none of the predesignated unfavorable indices, while 31 were identified as "poor risk" on the basis of these criteria (Table 2). Fifteen of 26 patients with severe triple coronary artery disease on angiography were classified in the good risk group because of the presence of good left ventricular function and no adverse clinical signs.

When judged by functional status (New York Heart Association Classification), 87 of the patients were found to be in Class III and 46 were in Class IV.

THERAPEUTIC MANAGEMENT

All patients were placed on a regimen designed to achieve or maintain optimal weight. Serum lipid abnormalities were treated by means of diet and often by hypocholesterolemic agents. Hypertension and diabetes were managed with appropriate drugs with the aim of careful control. Tobacco and stimulants were proscribed. Alterations in life style to minimize stress were adopted where feasible. When left ventricular function was not impaired, graduated exercise on a daily basis, always preceded by prophylactic medication, was encouraged.

Medicinal treatment in all cases consisted of the combined administration of propranolol and isosorbide dinitrate. The dosage of propranolol was determined in each patient by careful titration to discover the amount needed to reduce resting heart rate to a frequency of 55–60 beats/min. The daily dosage of propranolol varied from as little as 10 mg twice daily to 160 mg four times daily.

Isosorbide dinitrate was administered *sublingually* in a dosage varying between 2.5 and 10 mg, according to individual tolerance and response. The dose of propranolol was taken orally *before* each meal and that of isosorbide dinitrate sublingually *after* each meal in order to obtain the longest possible period of synergistic activity during expected times of physical stress (8–11). When congestive heart failure was detected or even suspected, digitalis and an oral diuretic were prescribed prior to the use (or continuation) of propranolol.

RESULTS

Clinical Manifestations

The striking clinical response to propranolol and isosorbide dinitrate observed among subjects in this series has been reported previously (8–11). In 90.2% of the 133 patients, marked amelioration of angina pectoris associated with significant increments in exercise tolerance has been documented by controlled observations. These favorable responses correlate closely with improvement in ischemic ECG patterns evoked by standard exercise. In 50% of 62 patients so tested, there has been complete reversal of exercise ECG abnormalities when evaluations were performed during periods of combined pharmacologic activity of these agents (Fig. 1). It is of interest that no tendency has been observed toward an attenuation of effect with the passage of time.

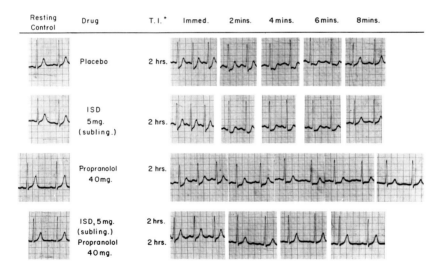

Fig. 1. Comparative ECG responses (lead V_5) to standard exercise (30 trips) following treatment with propranolol and/or isosorbide dinitrate (*ISD*) (A. S., 60-year-old male). *T.I.*, time interval between administration of drug and beginning of test; *subling.*, sublingually.

Table 3. Comparison of New York Heart Association Functional Class Before and After Propranolol-Isosorbide Dinitrate Therapy

Functional class	No. of patients	
	Pretreatment	Posttreatment
I		20
II		81
III	87	23
IV	46	9

Improvement in functional class following the administration of propranolol-isosorbide dinitrate therapy has been most significant (Table 3). Twenty of the 87 patients originally in Class III showed sufficient improvement to be grouped in Class I, while 63 shifted to Class II. Of the 46 patients in class IV at commencement of this study, 18 were judged to be in Class II and 19 were in Class III after the institution of therapy.

Myocardial Infarction

Over the six-year period, 24 of the 102 good risk patients suffered attacks of acute myocardial infarction, and of these 19 recovered and six died. In the poor risk group, myocardial infarction occurred in 24 patients and accounted for death in 17 of the 31 patients during the same period.

Mortality Rate

Only six of the 102 good risk patients followed from three to six years have died. None of the 102 died during the first year, two of the 102 patients died during the second year, one of the 100 surviving patients died during the third year, two of 94 patients died during the fourth year, and one of 85 patients died during the fifth year. A small number have been followed through the sixth year, during which there were no deaths. From the mortality rate experience in this study, the probability of death in good risk and poor risk patients has been plotted in Figure 2. It can be seen that 6% of good risk patients may be expected to die by the end of fifth year of follow-up, indicating an average annual mortality rate of 1.2% for this group. This is in sharp contrast to the rate in poor risk patients, for whom it may be anticipated to exceed 16%, with only about one-third of the patients surviving to the end of the fourth year. It is of interest that no patients in the poor risk group died during the fifth year of observation. Since all of the survivors in the poor risk group were patients over the age of 70

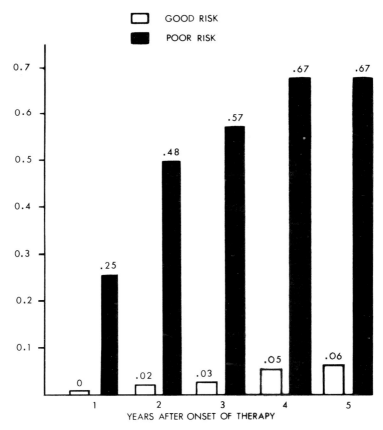

Fig. 2. Probability of death according to clinical status. Propranolol-isosorbide dinitrate therapy of severe angina pectoris.

with good left ventricular function and no adverse clinical signs, it seems apparent that old age per se should not have been used as one of the indices for an unfavorable five-year prognosis. These data make it clear that overall mortality rates in any reported series will depend on the composition of the sample with respect to the numbers of good risk and poor risk patients.

DISCUSSION

In the present era of coronary bypass surgery for angina pectoris, justification for operative intervention often is based on little more than the contention that there is an appalling mortality rate with any form of medical management. Thus, it has been claimed that 50% of patients on conservative therapy die within five years, a decimation rate averaging 10%/year (13). In sharp contradiction to this alleged threat to life even under "optimal" medical care are the more favorable results reported by other investigators. Thus, Zukel and co-workers (1), in a 15-year follow-up study, have shown that about 3% of patients with angina pectoris die each year, while Kannel and associates (2), in the Framingham study, have indicated an annual mortality rate of approximately 4% in this disease. Moreover, since these more favorable results have been reported in large series of patients at varied risk and under no specific program of therapy, an even better prognosis seemed likely for carefully selected good risk patients participating in a modern, comprehensive medical regimen. This was actually the finding in the present study, which has shown that in such patients, the probability of death over a period of five years is only 6%, or approximately 1.2%/year. This rate of mortality is not unlike that found in the general population in the same age groups. The significance of this observation is perhaps more meaningful when it is realized that it has been made in patients who, at the time of entry into this study, were suffering from severe and refractory forms of angina pectoris often associated with severe two- or three-vessel disease but with relatively *normal* left ventricular function. Inasmuch as coronary bypass surgery in similar patients is associated with an immediate operative mortality rate ranging from 2.5 to 10%, as well as with a formidable incidence of nonfatal complications and graft failure, early and late, these data make it difficult to justify surgical intervention unless disabling symptoms persist despite optimal medical care.

The relatively favorable outlook for good risk patients in this study, despite presenting symptoms of severe angina pectoris, undoubtedly is related to comparatively normal left ventricular function in all cases. In this regard, the use of noninvasive measures may prove valuable to identify or confirm those believed to be at minimal risk. Nevertheless, the total medical regimen directed at the removal of coronary risk factors and the utilization of propranolol in combination with isosorbide dinitrate to prevent recurrent bouts of coronary insufficiency may have played an important, although presently undefined, role in determining prognosis in these patients.

When refractory angina pectoris is associated with impairment of left ventricular performance, as observed in poor risk patients of this series, the prognosis appears grave whether medical or surgical therapy is adopted. In spite of excellent symptomatic response to medical treatment in most cases, 25% of these poor risk subjects died within the first year and 67% failed to survive to the end of the fourth year. Equally dismal, however, are the results of surgical therapy in which the immediate mortality rate has been reported to be as high as 40% or more, with the chances of salvage relatively poor. Thus in this category also, operative intervention should be considered only after the most careful clinical assessment.

The overall mortality rate for the 133 patients in this series was approximately 4%/year, which is strikingly similar to that reported by Kannel and associates (2) in the Framingham study. When it is realized, however, that all of the patients in the present investigation suffered from severe symptoms often associated with one or more previous myocardial infarctions, whereas those in the Framingham study were selected anginal subjects without prior infarction, significant benefit from intensive medical therapy is suggested. In this regard, careful attention to risk factors and the administration of propranolol and sublingual isosorbide dinitrate to prevent pain and ischemic changes would appear to be of paramount importance.

Although saphenous vein bypass surgery is a potentially useful procedure in some cases of angina pectoris, it should be recognized that coronary disease is not necessarily ominous without heroic interventions. Indeed, it is possible to identify the large segment of patients who are not only responsive to antianginal therapy but in whom the prognosis for life and prolonged survival is often reasonably good. Certainly, more harm than benefit is likely to ensue when surgery is undertaken without prior consideration of the natural history of the disease and without meticulous selection of patients in whom the risks appear warranted and with whom technical success seems reasonably assured. More frequent and better utilization of available drugs and medical procedures would undoubtedly reduce the incidence of refractoriness and disability and thereby diminish the haste to seek often unattainable surgical solutions.

SUMMARY AND CONCLUSIONS

A prospective study in 133 patients with severe angina pectoris has shown that the prospects for five-year survival are excellent in patients with good left ventricular function and no adverse clinical signs. The annual mortality rate in a group of 102 good risk patients selected in this manner was actually only 1.2%. In sharp contrast, the yearly attrition rate in subjects with poor left ventricular function and/or other adverse signs (poor risk patients) exceeded 16%. Marked amelioration of pain, increase in exercise tolerance, and improvement of ischemic exercise-electrocardiographic patterns were observed in 90.2% of the 133 patients in response to dosages of propranolol and sublingual isosorbide dinitrate, respectively, titrated for the individual patient.

It is concluded that:

1. Severe angina pectoris which is refractory to *casual* methods of management frequently responds to an intensive program of *optimal* medical care.

2. The favorable outlook in good risk patients responding to modern medical therapy does not appear to indicate the need or justify the risk of surgical revascularization. Consideration for surgery seems warranted in this group pri-

marily to improve the quality of life in the relatively small number of patients whose symptoms cannot be controlled by a comprehensive medical regimen.

3. The high mortality rate in poor risk patients, whether they are treated medically or surgically, requires careful clinical assessment and meticulous selection of patients if lives are to be salvaged by surgical intervention.

4. The synergistic action of propranolol and sublingual isosorbide dinitrate, when these agents are employed properly in the treatment of severe angina pectoris, generally affords excellent control in cases previously refractory to traditional management.

5. It is only when medical therapy is pursued with a high degree of enthusiasm and intensity of purpose that the attending physician will be able to gain insight into the true indications for surgical intervention.

REFERENCES CITED

1. Zukel, W. J., Cohen, B. M., Mattingly, T. W., et al. 1969. Survival following first diagnosis of coronary heart disease. Amer. Heart J. 78:159.
2. Kannel, W. B., and Feinleib, M. 1972. Natural history of angina pectoris in the Framingham study. Amer. J. Cardiol. 29:154.
3. Parker, R. L., Dry, T. J., Willius, F. A., and Gage, R. P. 1946. Life expectancy in angina pectoris. J.A.M.A. 131:95.
4. Block, W. J., Crumpacker, E. L., Dry, T. J., and Gage, R. P. 1952. Prognosis in angina pectoris. Observations in 6,682 cases. J.A.M.A. 150:259.
5. Moberg, C. H., Webster, J. S., and Sones, F. M. 1972. Natural history of severe proximal coronary disease as defined by cineangiography (200 patients, seven year follow-up). Amer. J. Cardiol. 29:282.
6. Sheldon, W. C., et al. 1973. Circulation. (In press.)
7. Russek, H. I., and Zohman, B. L. 1957. Limited use of anticoagulants in acute myocardial infarction. J.A.M.A. 162:922.
8. Russek, H. I. 1967. Propranolol and isosorbide dinitrate synergism in angina pectoris. Amer. J. Med. Sci. 254:406.
9. Russek, H. I. 1968. Propranolol and isosorbide dinitrate synergism in angina pectoris. Amer. J. Cardiol. 21:44.
10. Russek, H. I. 1969. New dimension in angina pectoris therapy. Geriatrics 24:81.
11. Russek, H. I. 1970. Intractable angina pectoris. Med. Clin. N. Amer. 54:333.
12. Russek, H. I. 1972. Prognosis in severe angina pectoris: Medical versus surgical therapy. Amer. Heart J. 83:762.
13. Favaloro, R. G. 1971. Surgical treatment of coronary arteriosclerosis by the saphenous vein graft technique: Critical analysis. Amer. J. Cardiol. 28:493.

Cardiac Transplantation
or the Mechanical Heart?

CURRENT STATUS OF HEART TRANSPLANTATION AT STANFORD UNIVERSITY

EUGENE DONG, JR.

The first human heart transplant at Stanford University was done in January of 1968. Since that time 54 transplants have been carried out in 52 patients. We described specific aspects of this experience in a series of prior publications (1–6).

The basic conclusions are that transplantation of the heart in appropriately selected patients with advanced myocardial disease will result in improved quality of life and prolonged survival. This is particularly true in those patients in whom the myocardial disease had advanced to the point where other surgical procedures appeared to be warranted and were carried out, either with temporary or no success in relieving symptoms or cardiomegaly.

The statistics of mortality and morbidity reveal a plateau in our experience and suggest directions of continued effort in both applied and basic research. Nevertheless, the uncertainties do not detract from the therapeutic nature of cardiac transplantation today.

SURGICAL TECHNIQUE

The basic concept for the cardiac transplantation technique has not varied since its first description in the dog in 1960 (7). This concept is the elegantly simple method of decreasing the surgical time for anastomosis and avoiding postoperative thromboses on major venous-cardiac inflow channels by atria-to-atria anastomosis. The decrease in time required for the anastomosis reduces the cardiac ischemic time. Thus, preservation of the heart can safely be achieved by cooling, avoiding the encumbrances of coronary artery perfusion apparatus. The detailed and important steps in cannulation, cardiac excision, and the sequence of atrial repair are given in other publications (8).

OPERATIVE MORTALITY

The immediate circulatory response of the transplanted denervated heart using these surgical techniques varied from good to excellent in all but four cases. One heart was obtained from a patient whose heart was resuscitated using intracardiac epinephrine. Uncontrollable arrhythmias necessitated a second transplant. Examination revealed septal hemorrhage possible caused by the resuscitation effort. In the other three cases extensive pulmonary arteriosclerosis led to severe right ventricular failure and death. An extreme level of increased pulmonary vascular resistance, therefore, is a contraindication to heart transplantation at this time. One patient succumbed to multiple complications 15 days following a bleeding disorder which remotely may be considered operative death. No other patients have died within 24 hours of operation. Thus, the analysis suggests that the degree of heart disease is not related to operative mortality. Indeed, deselection of patients with extreme pulmonary hypertension would probably result in an operative mortality rate close to zero, using the aforementioned techniques.

CARDIAC DONOR

The transplanted heart has in all cases been obtained from patients who have suffered brain death from a variety of causes including vehicular trauma, gunshot wounds, spontaneous hemorrhage, anoxia following respiratory arrests from drug overdosage, and a primary intracranial tumor. The absence of cerebral function is diagnosed by three attending neurosurgeons and neurologists. It is based upon the history of a catastrophic intracranial event known to cause death, apnea at demonstrably normal blood gases, absence of cranial reflexes, a flat EEG, and nondetectable blood levels of drugs which depress the central nervous system.

Obviously, a thorough examination of the donor is required which may include coronary arteriography and cardiac ventriculography. Arteriosclerotic lesions have been noted in relatively young males. Traumatic mitral insufficiency has also developed in potential cardiac donors.

The management of these patients consists of maintenance of artificial respiration and blood pressure during the 8 to 24 hours usually required to mobilize the facilities to carry out the transplant.

Neural regulation of the circulation in the cerebrally dead patient has not been thoroughly investigated. Diabetes insipidus responds to pitressin every four hours, reducing vasopressor and fluid replacement requirements.

TISSUE TYPING

In all cases, organ transplantation followed the rules of red cell transfusions. Lymphocyte typing for the HLA series and direct white cell crossmatch for the detection of preformed antibodies have always been performed (9). Preformed cytotoxic antibodies have not been found, although many patients have been exposed to blood transfusions. We have not had identical donor-recipient HLA pairing in our experience. Further, there does not appear to be a correlation between histocompatibility grade (i.e., 1–4 mismatches) and survival in cardiac transplantation. The degree of recipient illness is the more important determinant in selection for transplant.

PATIENT SELECTION

Sex and Age

Of the 52 patients, 4 were female. The youngest patient was 17 years of age and the oldest 61. Two patients were in the 21–30 year old group, 8 in the 31–40 group, 24 in the 41–50 group, 15 in the 51–60 group, and 2 in the 61–70 group.

Disease

The majority of the patients (36 of 52, 69%) suffered from advanced congestive failure secondary to coronary arteriosclerosis; 28% of the patients suffered from cardiomyopathies; and one patient suffered a coronary embolus two years after successful aortic valve replacement. Fifty patients complained of or presented with severe congestive heart failure, and 2 presented with disabling angina, myocardial infarction, and failure of revascularization. In the first 24 patients none had previous surgical attempts to correct or ameliorate their heart disease. However, 10 patients in the last 28 underwent one or more cardiac procedures.

Additional patients, 29 in all, were accepted for transplantation but died before a donor was obtained. Of these, 55% suffered from coronary arteriosclerosis, 35% from cardiomyopathy, and the remainder from miscellaneous causes.

IMMUNOSUPPRESSION

There has been a progression in the immunosuppressives used. The current protocol begins with a loading dose of azathioprine, 3–4 mg/kg, just preoperatively, to the recipient. This drug is maintained at a level of 2 to 3 mg/kg/day and is adjusted upon the appearance of bone marrow or hepatic toxicity. Cyclophosphamide in doses ranging from 50 to 175 mg/day has recently been substituted for azathioprine in selected patients. Oral prednisone is begun at 1.5 mg/kg/day and is gradually tapered during the first two months to 1 mg/kg/day. Antilymphocyte globulin (ALG) or antithymocyte globulin (ATG) has been used in all but the first two patients.

Treatment for diagnosed cardiac rejection consists of methylprednisolone 1,000–2,000 mg intravenously on a daily basis and three days of actinomycin D until initial reversal of the signs of rejection. Azathioprine has generally been held constant at maintenance dosages. If ATG has been discontinued, it is reinstituted.

REJECTION SURVEILLANCE

Patients are examined frequently for cardiac rejection crises. This involves electrophysiologic, mechanical, and clinical observation. The ECG reveals decreased voltage, right shift in axis, right bundle branch block, and atrial arrhythmias. Mechanical signs include the appearance of 3rd and 4th heart sounds, decreased precordial impulse, and decreased fullness of the pulse. Clinical symptoms and signs may include relative hypotension, hepatomegaly, fatigue, anorexia, and a gain in weight. Chest x-ray may demonstrate increased heart size. Signs of left heart failure such as orthopnea or pulmonary edema appear very late. As a practical matter, the decreased voltage tends to be the major parameter for suspicion of cardiac rejection crisis.

Transvenous endomyocardial biopsy has recently contributed in a large way to diagnostic accuracy (10). A percutaneous sheath technique is used to introduce a locally modified Konno-Sakkabara bioptome through the internal jugular vein. Under fluoroscopic observation, the catheter is manipulated into the apex of the right ventricle. A 1–3 mm biopsy section is retrieved by closing the jaws and withdrawing the catheter. To date, all evidence points to the conclusion that the endomyocardium of the right ventricle reflects accurately the immunological state of the heart.

RESULTS

Fifty-four transplants on 52 patients have been carried out, 9 in 1968, 9 in 1969, 8 in 1970, 12 in 1971, 13 in 1972, and 1 so far in 1973. Eighteen patients were alive on February 1, 1973. Thus, 34 patients have died. Twenty-five have succumbed within the first three months after transplantation: 5 from rejection, 13 from infection, 3 from pulmonary hypertension, 3 from cerebral vascular disease, and 1 from intravascular coagulation (1). Nine patients succumbed after good physiological recovery and discharge from the hospital: 5 from chronic rejection and 4 from late infection.

Using the Cutler life table method, the estimated risks of survival for the entire patient group are 50% at 6 months, 40% at 1 year, 37% at 2 years, and 23% at 3 years. Two patients in the transplant group from more than 4 years ago have survived to 44 months and one patient is still doing well working full time nightly as a professional organist.

Of the 29 patients selected but not transplanted, all but 3 are dead. One was deselected upon recovery from an acute cardiomyopathy and 2 are awaiting their operation. In comparison to the survival figures following transplant, the figures for this nonoperated group are 18% at 3 months, 9% at 6 months, and 4% at 9 months and beyond.

The influence of age on survival is given in Table 1. The general trend is for improved postoperative survival with younger age. There is at present a relatively arbitrary limit of 55 years of age precluding consideration for transplant.

The influence of disease on survival is as follows: with coronary artery disease the survival is 50%, 47%, and 43% at 6, 12, and 24 months respectively; with cardiomyopathies the survival is 50%, 14%, and 14% again at 6, 12, and 24 months.

The one year survival rate has improved. Of the 18 patients transplanted in the first two program years the survival rate was 39%, 33%, and 28% at 6, 12, and 24 months. Of the 34 patients transplanted in the last 3 years, the survival rate was 56%, 44%, and 44% at 6, 12, and 24 months.

Long Term Survival

The period of highest risk has been the first 3 months. If the patient survives this period (and 27 have), he has a 72% chance of surviving to 1 year; a 66% chance of surviving to 2 years; and a 41% chance of surviving to 3 years.

Effect of Previous Surgery

Thirteen procedures have been carried out in 10 patients prior to transplant. They include 4 valve replacements (2 for mitral insufficiency in cardiomyo-

Table 1. Influence of Age on Survival after Heart Transplant

Age (years)	No.	Living 02-03-73	One year survival	Two year survival	Three year survival
11–20	1	0	0% (0)	0% (0)	0% (0)
21–30	2	1	0% (0)	0% (0)	0% (0)
31–40	8	6	75% (8)	50% (4)	66% (3)
41–50	24	9	36% (19)	46% (13)	14% (7)
51–60	15	2	30% (10)	22% (9)	11% (9)
61–70	2	0	0% (2)	0% (2)	0% (1)
	52	18	41% (39)	35% (28)	20% (20)

a ( ) = Number at risk

E. Dong, Jr.

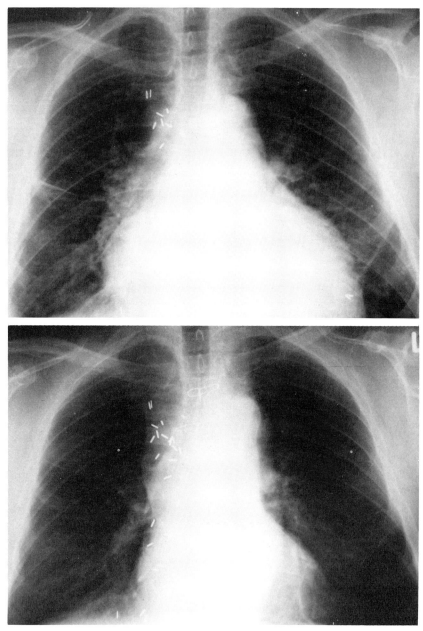

Fig. 1. (*Top*) Pre-transplant x-ray appearance of patient with clips marking site of previous surgery. (*Bottom*) X-ray appearance of same patient two years after cardiac transplant.

pathy). One patient underwent vein graft and aneurysmectomy followed by implantation of a carotid sinus stimulator. The remainder underwent a variety of Vineberg or vein graft procedures.

In 5 patients operated upon as above for congestive heart failure as a consequence of coronary artery disease, none received relief in the sense of decreased symptoms or increased exercise tolerance. The mean time between the operation to the transplant was approximately 10 months. In 2 further patients, the initial complaint was angina and the first operation caused relief of symptoms for 2 and 6 months. In one patient the angina returned and a subsequent implantation of a carotid sinus stimulator was ineffective. In the other patient, continued angina and the appearance of congestive heart failure forced the patient to transplantation 22 months later. Thus, the mean time of relief for 7 patients with coronary disease was only 1.2 months and the average time to transplant was 12 months.

Nine of 10 patients had pronounced cardiomegaly. The mean cardiothoracic ratio was 0.60 before transplant and 0.48 from 9 to 24 months after transplant. Figure 1 (*top*) illustrates one patient from this group with a cardiothoracic ratio of 0.6, pleural effusion, and clips marking the site of previous surgery. Figure 1 (*bottom*) illustrates the decreased heart size and pulmonary vascularity in the same patient 2 years after the transplant.

The survival statistics for the group with a previous cardiac operation is markedly different from the group as a whole, being 100%, 87%, and 87% at 6, 12, and 24 months respectively. There is a decreased severity of the reversible rejection episodes. The rejection grade on a scale of 0–4 in this group of 10 patients was 1.6; the nonoperated group mean rejection grade was 2.4.

In this group hospitalization utilization was documented. The average length of stay in the hospital was 110 days in the year before transplant. After discharge following transplantation, 8 patients returned for an average of 20 days with a range of 0 to 70 days. Five of these patients have gone into the second year with an average stay of 5 hospital days.

DISCUSSION

Clinical transplantation of the heart followed a relatively prolonged period of direct experimental investigation combined with several years of clinical experience in renal transplantation. Basic and applied immunological investigations continue. It is unfortunate that the clinical introduction of this procedure should have been attended with such a confusion of high hopes combined with controversy. The immunological processes in rodents and canines did not appear to be significantly different for heart or kidney. However, the physiological and clinical problems are quite entirely different and require clinical experience to work out in some detail. Those details continue to be evaluated. In addition, a level of nonscientific mystique exists among renal transplantation groups which those involved in heart transplants need to sort out from their real and important contributions.

Our evaluation of the current status of heart transplantation is that it is a therapeutically useful procedure in patients with far advanced heart disease. The physiological response and function is excellent for long periods of time. Social and vocational rehabilitation is gratifying. The problems to concentrate on in the future are: 1) more specific immunosuppression and 2) the supply of cardiac donors.

The control of rejection is still a major problem area. Use of currently available immunosuppression will control rejection in the great majority of instances, but is associated with the onset of infection. Drug-resistant acute rejection was responsible only for 14% of the deaths, whereas infection was responsible for 50%.

The other vexing problem is the control of chronic rejection/graft atherosclerosis. In contrast to the acute rejection, recognition of this state requires stress testing, or invasive procedures to visualize the coronary arteries. Control of the process is uncertain.

While it may appear that the solution to these aspects of cardiac transplantation is elusive, those working in the area find past and future encouragement. First, from the past clinical experience, there is a year-by-year improvement in the one year survival statistics, even using standard immunosuppressives. Second, use of rabbit antithymocyte globulin has recently been associated with a high survival rate in human cadaver renal transplant. Third, the association of previous cardiac surgery and prior exposure to blood with a high cardiac transplant survival suggests the possibility of pretransplant modification of the immune status of the potential recipient. Finally, significant experimental work is appearing that points to the possibility of using donor specific enhancing sera; thus the immune state of the recipient may be left intact except towards the donor organ.

All in all, we conclude that the risks of cardiac transplantation are now well defined, although the biological mechanisms are still unclear. To the clinician, the course consists of careful evaluation of the potential candidate for cardiac transplant and a judgment of whether or not he has a better than 50% chance of surviving one year without this procedure. From the physiological viewpoint, there is no comparison; these patients achieve a remarkable state of recovery, subjectively and objectively documented for periods so far up to four years.

Basically then, cardiac transplantation is neither a panacea for cardiac disease nor a therapeutic nostrum. It is the recommended therapy for a specific group of terminally ill cardiac patients.

REFERENCES CITED

1. Shumway, N. E., Dong, E., Jr., and Stinson, E. B. 1969. Surgical aspects of cardiac transplantation in man. Bull. N.Y. Acad. Med. 45:387.
2. Stinson, E. B., Dong, E., Jr., Iben, A. B., and Shumway, N. E. 1969. Cardiac transplantation in man. III. Surgical aspects. Amer. J. Surg. 118:182.
3. Stinson, E. B., Dong, E., Jr., and Shumway, N. E. 1969. Experimental and clinical cardiac transplantation. Postgrad. Med. 46:199.
4. Stinson, E. B., Dong, E., Jr., Bieber, C. P., Popp, R. L., and Shumway, N. E. 1969. Cardiac transplantation in man. II. Immunosuppressive therapy. J. Thorac. Cardiov. Surg. 58:326.
5. Stinson, E. B., Dong, E., Jr., Angell, W. W., and Shumway, N. E. 1970. Myocardial hypothermia for cardiac transplantation. Lav. Med. 41:195.
6. Griepp, R. B., Stinson, E. B., Dong, E., Jr., Philips, R. C., Morrell, R. M., and Shumway, N. E. 1972. The use of antithymocyte globulin in human heart transplantation. Circ. 45 (CV Suppl. I):I–147.
7. Lower, R. R., and Shumway, N. E. 1960. Studies on orthotopic homotransplantation of the canine heart. Surg. Forum 11:18.
8. Dong, E., Jr., Griepp, R. B., Stinson, E. B., and Shumway, N. E. 1972. Clinical transplantation of the heart. 176:503.
9. Stinson, E. B., Griepp, R. B., Payne, R., Dong, E., Jr., and Shumway, N. E. 1971. Correlation of histocompatibility matching with graft rejection and survival after cardiac transplantation in man. Lancet ii:459.
10. Caves, P. K., Billingham, M. E., Schulz, W. P., Dong, E., Jr., and Shumway, N. E. 1973. Transvenous biopsy of canine orthotopic heart allografts. Amer. Heart J. 85:525.

NUCLEAR-FUELED CIRCULATORY SUPPORT SYSTEMS III.

JOHN C. NORMAN and FRED N. HUFFMAN

Artificial organs, both as assist and replacement devices, have a history almost as ancient as that recorded of man. Before Western Civilization began its ascendancy with Socrates and Hippocrates, devices were being fashioned in Asia, India, and the Middle East to replace portions of the body. The available records do not suggest that these modalities of treatment were considered to be different in any way from others then available (1). Acceptability and utilization have increased with the passage of time. Today, nonetheless, there is a certain mystique regarding the possibility of implanting *fissionable* materials in man to power artificial internal organs. Our laboratories have been involved for nearly a decade in exploring these possibilities and their physiologic, engineering, economic, and social implications (2–4). Because these investigations are multidisciplinary, the reporting of significant progress, major problems, successes, and failures has been difficult. Moreover, because much of what has been accomplished is predicated on continual problem solving in a series of critical areas in widely disparate disciplines, reporting has been to a large degree intradisciplinary.

The objectives of this report then are to: 1) review the rationale for the development of artificial circulatory assist and replacement devices; 2) reiterate the evolving rationale and continuing coordinating role of federal agencies involved in these activities; 3) describe and briefly define implantable circulatory support systems currently being investigated; 4) focus on two implantable nuclear-fueled circulatory support systems which utilize miniature implantable thermal engines of unique design; 5) give a glossary of terms particular to these latter evolving systems.

THE CONCEPT

The heart is essentially a pump. The notion of building an artificial heart should therefore not be new. Nearly four decades ago, John Gibbon initiated studies to bring this idea to reality by beginning work on an artificial pump-oxygenator (5). This temporary method of bypassing the heart and lungs not only proved to be successful in animals but also in the first human patient to undergo successful

This work is supported in part by U.S.P.H.A. Grants HL 14291, Contracts PH 43-66-982, PH 43-68-455, the John & Mary R. Markle Foundation, the Charles E. Merrill Trust, and the Kelsey and Leary Foundation.

J. C. Norman and F. N. Huffman

cardiopulmonary bypass in 1953. By the late 1950's there was widespread use of cardiopulmonary bypass to support patients during intracardiac surgery. Moreover, workable intracardiac valves and blood vessel prostheses were developed. These prostheses supported the notion that small mechanical pumps might be designed for implantation within the chest as a substitute for the irreparably damaged human heart.

THE MANDATE

When investigations on implantable circulatory support or replacement devices began, there was ample reason to doubt that a workable device could be developed. At present, the idea is no longer far-fetched and families of systems have been evolved. Pneumatically driven implantable left ventricular assist devices have undergone federal review and approval for pre-clinical trials. Nuclear systems (this report) have been implanted in animals to demonstrate short-term feasibility. This change in outlook over a period of only ten years is largely a consequence of programs supported by the National Heart and Lung Institute.

More specifically, in 1963 the National Advisory Heart Council decided to give priority to the development of an artificial heart; the West German and Russian Ministries of Health followed suit in 1970–72. In 1964, after clarifying the needs for materials, driving mechanisms, and control systems, coordinated investigations in the areas of implantable circulatory assist and replacement systems were initiated. In 1966, a systems analysis approach was adopted to direct and coordinate the programs in order to make feasible the optimal utilization of resources from medicine, the basic sciences, engineering, industry, and systems management to implement and give impetus to these endeavors (6).

These activities have evolved and continue to mature, initially under the aegis of: 1) the Artificial Heart Program; 2) the Medical Devices Applications Program and, most recently, as NHLI achieved Bureau Status; 3) the Division of Technological Applications.

The most recent statement of the long range objectives can be summarized as follows: 1) to develop emergency cardiac systems and techniques which may be effectively applied outside, as well as inside the hospital for the emergency treatment of cardiac lesions, cardiogenic shock, and circulatory insufficiency; 2) to develop temporary cardiac assist systems—both implanted and external—for periods of hours to months until the clinical condition can be reversed, stabilized, or until more effective treatment can be instituted; 3) to develop permanent left or right ventricular assist devices capable of assuming significant physiologic loads for the remainder of the patient's life; 4) to develop totally implantable artificial hearts with internal controls and energy sources for replacement of the irreparably damaged heart.

Until 1969, the programs focused on the separate development of each component of circulatory support or replacement devices. That year, the direction shifted somewhat in that efforts were initiated to integrate devices and techniques, developed and developing, in order to evolve a complete, fully implantable left ventricular assist device in order to create experimental models and a data base for the development of subsequent, more advanced prototypes.

CURRENT CIRCULATORY SUPPORT SYSTEMS

The term "artificial heart" is somewhat imprecise and frequently a misnomer. The generic terms "implantable circulatory support systems" are better suited to define current developments. The genealogy of such systems and designs currently undergoing active development is shown in Figure 1. The essential components are: 1) an energy source; 2) a means of energy storage; 3) a means of energy conversion; 4) a control unit; 5) a blood pump(s).

The three primary energy sources are: 1) biologic fuel cells (7,8) (glucose oxidation); 2) electromagnetic transmission (9–11) (electrical); and 3) nuclear energy (12–14). A biologic fuel cell which oxidizes glucose from the circulating

IMPLANTABLE CIRCULATORY SUPPORT SYSTEMS GENEALOGY

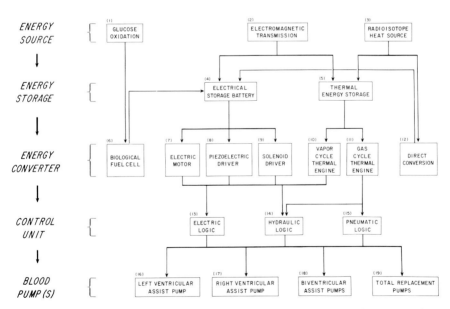

Fig. 1. Circulatory support systems genealogy (numbers indicate subsystem options integrated in the last five columns of Table 1).

blood of the host would seem to be an ideal solution. However, extrapolations from current technology indicate the required power density will be difficult to achieve. Electromagnetic transmission systems (15) appear to require less development than the nuclear option. Electromagnetic energy systems, however, require frequent recharging. The nuclear option involves the use of implantable plutonium-238 heat capsules which can provide an essentially unlimited energy source, i.e. the fuel requires the passage of 89 years to decay to one-half of its initial value.

Energy from any of these primary sources (biologic, electromagnetic, or nuclear) can be stored in a battery (16,17) or in the heat of fusion (18). Energy conversion can be accomplished with a fuel cell (19) or an electromechanical actuator, e.g. an electric motor (20–22), a piezoelectric driver (23,24), a pulse solenoid (25), or direct thermoelectric conversion (26,27).

Thermal engines can usually be characterized as either vapor (28–30) or gas cycle (31–34). Much of our effort has been in this area and the status of this segment of these studies will be detailed. The control units can utilize either electronic, pneumatic, or hydraulic logic (35). The last two have been utilized in initial in vivo testing.

The blood pump can be an assist device–left ventricular (36) or right ventricular (37), separately or in combination (38)–as well as a total replacement. Because the left ventricle performs approximately 80% of the total work of the heart (39), major efforts have been focused on implantable left ventricular assist devices. Right ventricular assist pumps have also been developed; biventricular systems utilizing a combination of left ventricular and right ventricular assist pumps can function as total replacements with the biologic heart in situ functioning as a conduit. In comparison, total replacement cardiac prostheses define devices which replace the excised biologic heart.

Left and right ventricular assist pumps can be either temporary or permanent. Biventricular and total replacements are permanent. It is evident that many combinations and permutations of their component options are possible (Fig. 1). Although implantable nuclear systems should provide recipients with a degree of freedom impossible with rechargeable systems, they raise the questions of the possible effects of chronic intracorporeal radiation (40 43), radiologic safety (44), and the economics of fuel production.

A reasonably comprehensive summary of totally implantable circulatory support systems currently being investigated in the United States is presented in Table 1. The component subsystem options utilized in these systems (energy source, energy storage, energy converter, controls, and blood pump) are listed in the last five columns and refer to the interrelated options on the left in Figure 1. The first five systems utilize nuclear heat sources. Rotary electric motors, pulse solenoids, and piezoelectric power sources are included. All the nuclear-fueled systems utilize the concept wherein a fraction of the heat of radioisotopic decay

Table 1. Totally Implantable Circulatory Support Systems

Power source identification	Agency	Engineering developer	Location	Thermodynamic cycle	Heat source temp. °F	SUBSYSTEM OPTIONS				
						Energy source	Energy storage	Energy convt.	Control unit	Blood pump(s)
Tidal Regenerator	NIH	Thermo Electron	Waltham Mass.	Huffman	930	3	5	10	13	16
Modified Stirling	NIH	McDonnell Douglas	Richland, Wash.	Modified Stirling	1,200	3	5	11	15	16
Thermo-Compressor	NIH	Aerojet	Sacramento, Cal.	Modified Stirling	1,200	3	5	11	14	16
Modified Rankine	NIH	Atlantic Richfield	Apollo, Pa.	Modified Rankine	1,594	3	5	10	13	16
Rotary Stirling	AEC	Westinghouse	Pittsburgh, Pa.	Classical Stirling	1,550	3	5	11	--	19
Rotary Electric Motor	NIH	Thermo Electron, Statham, Stanford Res. Inst.	Waltham, Mass. Oxnard, Cal. Palo Alto, Cal.	— — —	—	2	4	7	13	19
Pulse Solenoid	NIH	ANDROS	Berkeley Cal.	—	—	2	4	9	13	16
Piezoelectric	NIH	Physics Int.	San Leandro, Cal.	—	—	2	4	8	13	16

from plutonium-238 is converted into hydraulic power for driving a left ventricular assist device via a miniature implantable thermal engine.

Figure 2 depicts the basic elements of the first system to undergo in vivo
testing for seven hours (2). Reduced to essentials, it is an implantable tidal
regenerator thermal engine fueled with a 52 watt plutonium-238 nuclear heat
source; it has an innovative thermodynamic cycle, an electronic control system,
and an advanced pusher-plate left ventricular assist pump. The essential elements, e.g. working fluid, condenser, boiler, hot-cold junctions, isotope heat
source, superheater, interface piston, and blood pump are illustrated.

Figures 3 and 4 are block and idealized diagrams of this system in vitro and in
vivo. The left ventricular assist pump accepts a portion of the stroke volume
from the apex of the left ventricle at low pressure (20–30 mm Hg) and elevates
it in pressure to perfuse the systemic circulation via the descending thoracic
aorta.

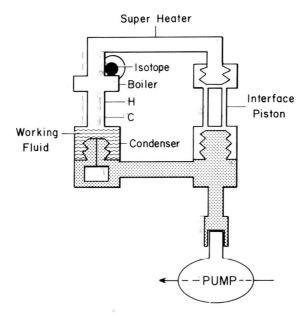

Fig. 2. The nuclear fueled tidal regenerator engine is a cyclic pressure generator in which
the engine pressure is established by the temperature of the coldest point of the enclosure.
The configuration of the engine is arranged so that this point is the interface between the
working fluid and its vapor. The temperature of the interface equilibrates to that of the
adjacent structures (the condenser, boiler, and liquid regenerator). When the liquid level is
in the condenser, the engine pressure is the saturation pressure corresponding to the
condenser temperature. The engine is pressurized by displacing the liquid level into the
boiler so that the engine pressure becomes the saturation pressure corresponding to the
boiler temperature. As a consequence of this pressure differential, energy is extracted from
the engine by the pump via the interface piston.

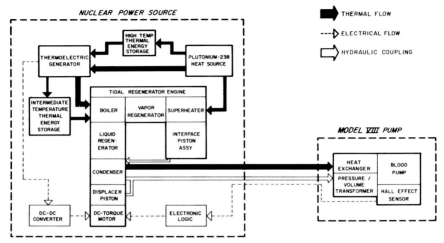

Fig. 3. Block diagram of the nuclear fueled left ventricular tidal regenerator circulatory assist system.

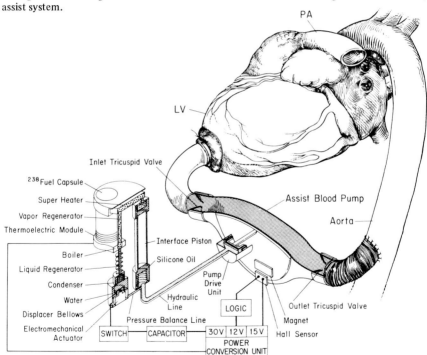

Fig. 4. Idealized diagram of the nuclear fueled left ventricular assist system. Pressurization of the implantable thermal engine is controlled by a displacer which is coupled to an electromechanical actuator. The electrical power for the displacement transducer, electronic logic, and electromechanical actuator is provided by a thermoelectric module interposed between the superheater and the boiler. A power conditioning unit converts the low voltage thermoelectric output to the proper potential levels. The engine is hydraulically coupled to the pusher-plate left ventricular assist pump.

PUSHER-PLATE LEFT VENTRICULAR ASSIST PUMP

The pusher-plate left ventricular assist pump is designed for coupling to nuclear-fueled power sources. It also functions as a blood-cooled heat exchanger, as a sensor for the control logic, and as an integral pressure-volume transformer. The entire surface of the pump which comes in contact with the blood is flocked with Dacron fibrils to promote the growth of a blood-compatible neointimal lining. The pumping chamber is pancake-shaped. The upper surface of the bladder rolls under the action of the pusher-plate, attached to the integral pressure-volume transformer to propel the blood through the outlet tricuspid valve to the descending thoracic aorta. The bladder is designed to minimize stress and compliance as it is collapsed by the pusher-plate; it is fabricated from 0.040-inch thick Dacron-reinforced silicone rubber.

The nonflexing common wall between the blood and the plenum (filled with hydraulic fluid) is used to transfer heat, rejected from the nuclear energy system, from the hydraulic drive fluid to the blood. Thus the bladder is not subjected to significant temperature rises. In this design, the parallel thermal path transfers most of the heat through a metal wall to the blood instead of through the elastomer bladder. Polyurethane foam is used to insulate thermally the heat exchanger plenum from the biologic left hemidiaphragm. A pressure-volume transformer is contained within the pump in such a manner that the volume swept by the transformer is common with that displaced by the collapsing bladder of the blood pump.

In addition, a Hall-effect sensor is mounted on the drive unit. Its signal is proportional to the magnetic field from a small permanent magnet mounted on the pusher-plate. Position as a function of time constitutes sufficient information for counterpulsation control.

ENGINEERING SPECIFICS

The Tidal Regenerator Engine

The tidal regenerator, a mechanically simple engine, contains neither valves nor sliding seals. It is a vapor cycle analog of the regenerative gas cycle engine which has characteristics in common with the Rankine and Stirling engines; e.g., the tidal regenerator engine has a boiler, condenser, and superheater similar to the Rankine engine. It also has a displacer, vapor regenerator, and power piston similar to the Stirling engine. In addition, it has unique components; e.g., a liquid regenerator and an interface piston. Specifically for left ventricular assist application and as a consequence of miniaturization, the displacer and interface pistons are replaced by zero leakage pressure balance bellows. As in the Stirling engine, there are only small differential pressures throughout, regardless of wide pressure fluctuations. Unlike the Stirling engine, the tidal regenerator engine utilizes a liquid-to-vapor phase change which enables a small volume of working fluid to provide a high pressure differential output with a moderate heat source temperature. As in the Rankine engine, the pressure work is low. In addition to allowing control by a small energy expenditure, these factors enable this miniature engine to operate at biologic heart beat rates with moderate thermal losses. In this manner, the engine supplies power at nearly constant pressure as needed for driving the blood pump without an intermediate hydraulic accumulator. Moreover, it is also insensitive to position orientation. Other than the liquid regenerator and condenser, all the engine structures which contact the vapor are maintained above the saturation temperature corresponding to the maximum engine pressure. The pressure throughout the engine corresponds to the temperature at the coldest point in the engine, which is always at the interface between the liquid and vapor phases, i.e. pressure in the engine follows the temperature of the liquid-vapor interface which equilibrates to the temperature of the adjacent structures. Otherwise stated, this means that the engine can be controlled with the small energy required to displace a single drop of water from the condenser to the boiler. Since the engine utilizes a phase transition, less than 0.02 ml of water needs to be vaporized and condensed to vary the system pressure between 5 and 150 pounds per square inch, absolute (psia). Inasmuch as the engine is pressure balanced, only a modest energy expenditure is required to displace the working fluid. This important factor makes the engine particularly suitable for electronic actuation.

Electronic Logic Actuation

Electronic logic is utilized to enable this system to synchronize with the biologic heart in a counterpulsation mode regardless of biologic left ventricular rate and stroke volume. The Hall effect sensor mounted inside the pusher-plate left ventricular assist device gives an electric signal which is a function of pumping chamber position. The Hall signal is interrogated by complementary metal oxide semiconductor (MOS) logic to identify the times of pump filling and ejection. Flip-flop integrated circuits are used for logic and memory. In addition to counterpulsing the engine from a normal input from the Hall effect sensor, the electronic logic circuitry has the capability of maintaining engine function when these signals may be lost. In this event, an interval timer triggers the pulsing circuit if the position sensor does not provide the expected signal within an arbitrary time span. As a result, the system will operate at a nearly fixed beat rate if no signals are received from the position sensor. A capacitor discharge energizes the electromechanical actuator which may be either a binary solenoid or a miniature electric motor. Both have been used for in vivo and in vitro testing. The polarity of the current is reversed with each pulse by a solid-state reversing switch.

Thermoelectric Module*

The thermoelectric module is placed in thermal series with the superheater (900°F) and boiler (380°F) of the engine. The boiler heat, which is typically several times greater in magnitude than that of the superheater, would normally be degraded in temperature and in availability to perform work by the engine structure. In this system the boiler heat is degraded through the thermoelectric module, thus producing electricity to power the control logic virtually free from additional thermal input. That is, since the heat rejected from the cold junctions of the module is reused in the boiler, the additional heat required for the electrical requirements is less than one watt. On this basis the control logic efficiency is greater than 95%. The electrical output from the 39 bismuth telluride thermocouples of the thermoelectric unit is approximately 300 milliwatts at design temperature.

The Hall effect sensor requires approximately 15 milliwatts at 1.5 volts; the metal oxide semiconductor logic consumes approximately 10 milliwatts at 12 volts. The logic power consumption, independent of the electromechanical actuation, is approximately 25 milliwatts. The actuator power is proportional to biologic left ventricular rate. The total electrical power requirements vary from approximately 125 milliwatts at 60 beats per minute to 225 milliwatts at 120 beats per minute. The thermoelectric module delivers approximately 300 milliwatts (electrical) and 25 watts (thermal) to the boiler.

Since the load potential of the thermoelectric module is 0.8 volt, a power conditioner unit must provide an output of 1.5 volts to the Hall effect sensor† and a 12 volt output to the MOS logic and torque motor. The required pulse polarity reversal is achieved by a solid-state switch.

Electromechanical Actuation

Binary pulse solenoids yielding linear displacement and torque motors yielding rotary displacement have been utilized as electromechanical actuators for displacing the water droplet for pressurization of the engine. In both instances, energy is utilized only during armature displacement. The direction of movement of the solenoid on the torque motor is dependent on polarity.

This tidal regenerator left ventricular circulatory assist system has been fueled with a 52 watt plutonium-238 nuclear heat source, as described previously, and implanted in two calves weighing 250 pounds each. These acute in vivo evaluations have demonstrated total system functional capability and counter synchronization with the biologic heart. Modifications are in progress to obtain increased efficiency, reliability, and function. The technical approaches in the

---

*Timonium, Maryland (Teledyne/Isotopes).
†Bell Laboratories, Columbus, Ohio.

Pu-238 VAPOR CYCLE ENERGY SYSTEM PROGRAM PLAN

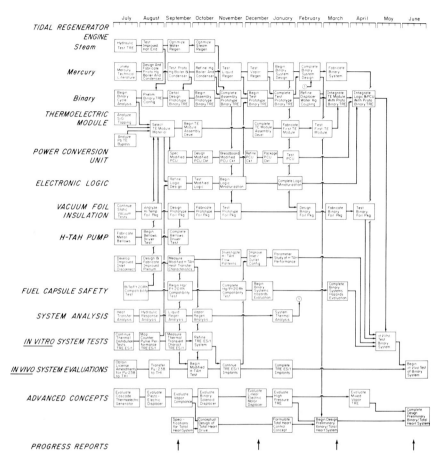

Fig. 5. As a result of current in vivo studies, system modifications have been implemented to improve efficiency, reliability, and control function. The technical approach to these problem areas is as indicated. The development of a binary tidal regenerator engine using a combination of mercury and water working fluids has the potential for significantly improving efficiency. The binary engine elevates the mean temperature of heat addition to the cycle, thus improving its efficiency. In vivo evaluations are planned in parallel with relevant improvements in system performance.

current developments of the tidal regenerator engine system are shown in Figure 5. These activities include refinement of the steam tidal regenerator engine in parallel with the initiation of a binary tidal regenerator engine utilizing both water and mercury as working fluids. The latter has the potential for significantly improving thermal to mechanical conversion efficiency.

THE MODIFIED STIRLING ENGINE SYSTEM

A related circulatory assist system utilizing a modified Stirling (32–34) engine has also undergone initial acute in vivo testing in the calf. Flow charts of the surgical and engineering subtasks for experimental implantation of the tidal regenerator engine system have been reported (2). A similar flow chart of the interrelated engineering and surgical subtasks we have utilized for implantation of the modified Stirling engine system is shown in Figure 6. This system utilizes a 52 watt plutonium-238 fuel capsule, the pusher-plate left ventricular assist pump, and vacuum foil thermal insulation. The modified Stirling engine extracts external work from a thermodynamic cycle in which a mixture of gases (helium-argon) is alternately compressed and expanded. The pressure varies between 200 and 230 psi during each cycle. This system runs at 10 to 15 times the biologic heart rate. In comparison, the tidal regenerator system runs at the same rate as the biologic heart. The modified Stirling system utilizes a hydraulic accumulator to store energy for utilization on a biologic heart rate basis. It operates essentially as a gas compressor.

An external gas regenerator allows heat stored during depressurization to be used during the next pressurization stroke. High pressure fluid is applied to the blood pump via a hydraulic control actuator. The position and speed of the actuator pistons are sensed for control purposes. Full pressure is applied to the actuator piston over a period of 25 milliseconds. A 40-millisecond holding period before and after pump ejection allows the momentum of the blood to assist in filling and emptying the pumping chamber.

NUCLEAR HEAT SOURCE

The 52 watt plutonium-238 fuel capsule compatible with both of these implantable thermal engines measures 1.28 inches in diameter and 2 inches in length and weighs 480 grams. Its maximum temperature in air varies between 750 and 1,000°F. The plutonium oxide fuel (120 grams) is enriched with oxygen-16 to minimize neutron production and is triply encapsulated in tantalum, a pressure vessel of T-111 (an alloy of tungsten, tantalum, and niobium), and an outer corrosion and oxidation resistant shell of platinum-rhodium (80–20%).

THERMAL ENERGY STORAGE

Thermal energy storage allows the fuel capsule to be structured for mean rather than peak power inputs with a resulting decrease in intracorporeal heat load, radiation exposure, and cost. Heat from the capsule is stored at high temperature (930°F in the tidal regenerator engine and 1,200°F in the modified Stirling

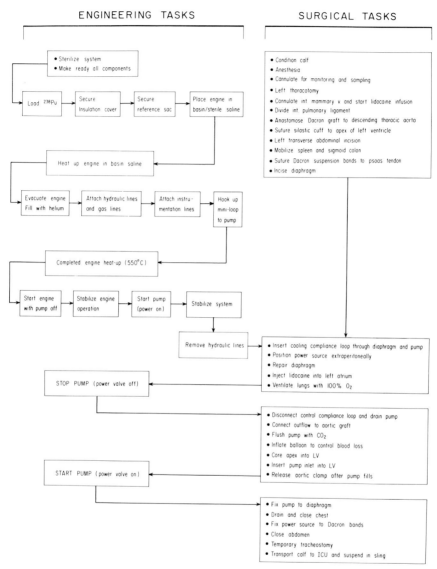

Fig. 6. Interrelated engineering and surgical tasks developed and utilized for implantation of the Modified Stirling Engine System.

engine) in the latent heat of fusion of the eutectic composition of lithium chloride/lithium fluoride* in the tidal regenerator engine system and sodium fluoride/lithium fluoride† in the modified Stirling system.

*Melting point: 930°F
†Melting point: 1,200°F

VACUUM FOIL INSULATION

Vacuum foil insulation is used in both systems to minimize thermal losses and protect the surrounding tissues. During in vivo testing the superheater temperatures were in the range of 900°F and the temperature at the surface of the power source was approximately 103°F. This is the result of the optimized coating of each of 80 layers of one-half mil thick titanium foils with zirconium oxide. At the design temperatures of 930°F for the tidal regenerator engine system, the measured heat loss through the vacuum foil insulation is approximately 6 watts.

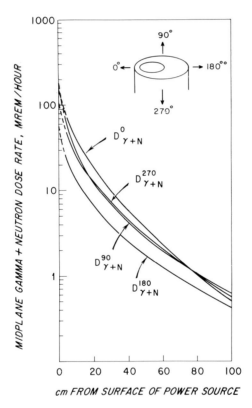

Fig. 7. The 52 watt nuclear heat source contains approximately 120 grams of plutonium-238 or 1,600 curies in a three-layer metal capsule designed to withstand corrosion, high impact and crush pressures, cremation, and the maximum credible accident temperature of 2,400°F. The isotope is primarily an emitter of alpha particles which have high energy but low penetrating power. The source also emits more penetrating gamma and neutron radiation which is rapidly attenuated by distance.

INTRACORPOREAL DOSE RATES

The dose rates in air from the implantable 52 watt plutonium-238 power source are shown in Figure 7. As indicated in the inset at the top of the illustration, insertion of the fuel capsule per se into the structure of the engine is eccentric. The measurements were taken through the midplane of the capsule along the indicated directions. The dose rates in tissue are slightly less. The neutron and gamma components are approximately equal. The maximum dose rate at the surface of the power source is approximately 175 mrem/hr.* The dose rate decreases sharply with distance as indicated (approximately an inverse square function). Previous analyses have indicated that the reduction in dose rate by shielding the high energy neutrons and gamma radiation is not practical because of excessive weight.

GLOSSARY

1. *Binary Solenoid*	A linear electromagnetic actuator whose armature is held in either of two positions by a permanent magnet after its translations.
2. *Boiler*	A heat exchanger for vaporizing the working fluid.
3. *Cold Junction*	The junction between the dissimilar legs of a thermocouple which is maintained at a low temperature relative to the hot junction.
4. *Compression Work*	The work which must be supplied to the engine at the end-of-stroke to return it to the beginning-of-stroke configuration.
5. *Displacer*	Device which transfers the position of a fluid volume.
6. *Electromechanical Actuator*	Unit which converts electrical energy to mechanical energy (e.g., solenoid or torque motor).
7. *Eutectic*	The composition of a mixture that has the lowest melting point.
8. *Flip Flops*	Binary integrated circuits whose output potentials are reversed by a pulse.

---

*Primates and canines subjected to sources which deliver 1,000 mrem/hr have survived in good condition for periods up to 4 years and continuing in our laboratories (43,45,46).

9.	*Flock*	A matted surface formed by attaching fibers with an adhesive.
10.	*Gas Cycle*	A thermodynamic engine in which power is extracted from a gas which is alternately heated and cooled.
11.	*Hall Sensor*	A sensor which provides a signal output proportional to the magnetic field.
12.	*Hydraulic Accumulator*	A compliant structure for reversibly storing and supplying hydraulic power.
13.	*Interface Piston*	High thermal impedance piston which isolates the hot vapor from the cold liquid.
14.	*Liquid Regenerator*	Structure for improving thermodynamic cycle efficiency by storing heat from the liquid during depressurization for reuse during pressurization.
15.	*MOS Logic*	Metal-Oxide-Semiconductor electronics which function at very low power levels.
16.	*Phase Transition*	A change of physical state (e.g., liquid-to-vapor).
17.	*Power Piston*	Piston for extracting the power output of the engine to a mechanical load.
18.	*Pressure Balanced*	A pneumatic/hydraulic configuration such that the pressure throughout the system is uniform.
19.	*Pressure-Volume-Transformer*	A mechanism for converting a high pressure, small displacement into a low pressure, large displacement.
20.	*Pt-20Rh*	An alloy of platinum and 20% rhodium.
21.	*Saturation Temperature*	The temperature at which a pure liquid in equilibrium with its vapor will have a given pressure.
22.	*Stirling*	A gas cycle engine invented by Robert Stirling in 1817.
23.	*Superheater*	A heat exchanger for heating a vapor above its saturation temperature.
24.	*T-111*	A high strength, high temperature alloy of tungsten, tantalum, and niobium.
25.	*Thermoelectric Module*	Converter of thermal-to-electrical energy using series connected thermocouples.
26.	*Thermal Series*	Sequential heat flow (as opposed to parallel flow) through stated components.

27. *Vapor Cycle*   A thermodynamic engine in which power is extracted from a working fluid which is alternately vaporized and condensed.

28. *Vapor Regenerator*   Structure for improving thermodynamic cycle efficiency by storing heat from the vapor during depressurization for reuse during pressurization.

29. *Working Fluid*   The fluid in the engine which undergoes cyclic vaporization and condensation.

ACKNOWLEDGMENTS

The authors gratefully acknowledge the continuing help, advice, parallel investigations, and assistance of Dr. Clarence Dennis, Dr. Lowell T. Harmison, Dr. William F. Bernhard, Dr. Walter J. Bornhorst, Dr. C. Grant LaFarge, Dr. William Martini, Dr. Benedict D. T. Daly, Dr. Joseph J. Migliore, Mr. William J. Robinson, Mr. Kenneth Hagen, Mr. James W. O'Brien, Mr. James Martin, Mr. Peter Riggle, Mr. Arthur Ruggles, Mr. Edward Murphy, Mr. David Lieb, Mr. Robert Lynch, Mr. Marvin Smith, Mr. Charles Doyle, Mr. Robert Whalen, Mr. John Fuqua, Mr. Everett Price, Mr. Gordon Dove, Mr. Leon Feigenbutz, Mr. Jess Oster, and Mr. Robert Faser. Special notes of thanks are due Ms. Carolyn Cox, Ms. Cynthia Murphy, Ms. Vivianne Baskins, Ms. Eugenia Campbell, Ms. Judy Salazar, Ms. Nellie Stephan, and Ms. Judy Reich for help in many essential areas.

REFERENCES CITED

1. Cooper, T., and Harmison, L. T. 1971. Cardiopulmonary support systems. Transplantation Proc. 3:1497–1501.
2. Norman, J. C., Sandberg, G. W., and Huffman, F. N. 1970. Implantable nuclear-powered cardiac pacemakers. New Engl. J. Med. 283:1203–1206.
3. Norman, J. C., Molokhia, F. A., Harmison, L. T., Whalen, R. L., and Huffman, F. N. 1972. An implantable nuclear-fueled circulatory support system I: Systems analysis of conception, design, fabrication and initial in vivo testing. Ann. Surg. 176:492–502.
4. Norman, J. C., Harmison, L. T., and Huffman, F. N. 1972. Nuclear-fueled circulatory support system II. Arch. Surg. 105:645–647.
5. Gibbon, J. H. 1954. The application of a mechanical heart and lung apparatus to cardiac surgery. Minnesota Med. 37:171–180.
6. A report by *ad hoc* task force on cardiac replacement, National Heart Institute: Cardiac replacement, medical, ethical, psychological, and economic implications. 1969. U.S. Government Printing Office, Washington, D.C.
7. Malachesky, P., Holleck, G., McGovern, F., and Devarakonda, R. 1972. Parametric studies of the implantable fuel cell. Seventh Intersociety Energy Conversion Engineering Conference Proceedings: 727–732.
8. Lahoda, J., Liu, C. C., and Wingard, L. B. 1972. Electrochemical evaluation of the activity of glucose oxidase immobilized by various methods. Seventh Intersociety Energy Conversion Engineering Conference Proceedings: 740–744.
9. Farim, F. W., and Huffman, F. N. 1971. Performance of a tuned ferrite core transcutaneous transformer. IEEE Trans. Biomed. Eng. 18:352–359.
10. Heimlich, L. A., and Christiansen, F. H. 1969. Energy transmission through the intact skin. Chapter 79 *in* R. J. Hegyeli, ed. Artificial Heart Program Conference Proceedings. U.S. Government Printing Office, Washington, D.C.

11. Newgard, P. M., and Eilers, G. J. 1969. Skin transformer and power conditioning components. Chapter 78 in R. J. Hegyeli, ed. Artificial Heart Program Conference Proceedings. U.S. Government Printing Office, Washington, D.C.
12. Norman, J. C., LaFarge, C. G., Harvey, R. J., Robinson, T. C., van Someren, L., and Bernhard, W. F. 1966. Heat dissipation: a common denominator of implantable power sources for cardiac prostheses. Surg. Forum 17:162–164.
13. Norman, J. C., Covelli, V. H., Bernhard, W. F., and Spira, J. 1968. An implantable nuclear fuel capsule for an artificial heart. Trans. Am. Soc. Artif. Intern. Organs 14:204–208.
14. Sandberg, G. W. 1970. Implantable nuclear power for an artificial heart: Studies of the effects of intracorporeal heat and radiation. Thesis, Harvard Medical School.
15. Powell, R. S. 1971. Electric energy systems for artificial hearts. Third National Conference on Electronics in Medicine, April 13-15, Boston.
16. Hamlen, R. P., Siwek, E. G., Rampel, G., and Wechsler, L. D. 1969. Internal energy storage for circulatory assist devices. Chapter 86 in R. J. Hegyeli, ed. Artificial Heart Program Conference Proceedings. U.S. Government Printing Office, Washington, D.C.
17. Miller, R. A., and Glanfield, E. J. 1969. Development of an electrical energy storage system for use with a circulatory assist device. Chapter 87 in R. J. Hegyeli, ed. Artificial Heart Program Conference Proceedings. U.S. Government Printing Office, Washington, D.C.
18. Bluestein, M., and Huffman, F. N. 1969. Development of a heat source for an implantable circulatory support power supply. Chapter 88 in R. J. Hegyeli, ed. Artificial Heart Program Conference Proceedings. U.S. Government Printing Office, Washington, D.C.
19. Giner, J., Holleck, G. L., Turchan, N., and Fragala, R. 1971. An implantable fuel cell to power an artificial heart. Sixth Intersociety Energy Conversion Engineering Conference Proceedings:256–266.
20. Newgard, P. M., Woodbury, J. R., and Harmison, L. T. 1972. Implantable electrical power and control system for artificial hearts. Seventh Intersociety Energy Conversion Engineering Conference Proceedings:799–805.
21. Griffith, N. J., and Burns, W. H. 1969. Development of an electrohydraulic energy source to power and control circulatory assist devices. Chapter 81 in R. J. Hegyeli, ed. Artificial Heart Program Conference Proceedings. U.S. Government Printing Office, Washington, D.C.
22. Chambers, J. 1969. Implantable energy system for a cardiac assist device. Chapter 80 in R. J. Hegyeli, ed. Artificial Heart Program Conference Proceedings. U.S. Government Printing Office, Washington, D.C.
23. Smiley, P., and O'Neill, C. G. 1972. Development of an implantable, low-frequency piezoelectric driver for an artificial heart. Seventh Intersociety Energy Conversion Engineering Conference Proceedings:778–783.
24. Benson, G. M., and Christie, J. W. 1969. Piezoelectric implantable energy converters. Chapter 84 in R. J. Hegyeli, ed. Artificial Heart Program Conference Proceedings. U.S. Government Printing Office, Washington, D.C.
25. Portner, P. M., Jassawalla, J. S., and LaForge, D. H. 1972. An implantable controlled solenoid energy system for driving an artificial heart. Seventh Intersociety Energy Conversion Engineering Conference Proceedings:784–791.
26. Raag, V. 1971. Review of thermoelectric conversion in micro/milliwatt power range for bio-medical applications. Sixth Intersociety Energy Conversion Engineering Conference Proceedings:245–255.
27. Altiere, F. D., and Judrick, J. A. 1970. Implantable electrical power source for an artificial heart system. Trans. Amer. Nuclear Soc. 13:505.
28. Huffman, F. N., Coleman, S. J., Bornhorst, W. J., and Harmison, L. T. 1971. A nuclear powered vapor cycle heart assist system. Sixth Intersociety Energy Conversion Engineering Conference Proceedings:277–287.
29. Huffman, F. N., Hagen, K. G., Ruggles, A. E., and Harmison, L. T. 1972. Performance of a nuclear-fueled circulatory assist system utilizing a tidal regenerator engine. Seventh Intersociety Energy Conversion Engineering Conference Proceedings:771–777.

30. Blair, M. G., and Purdy, D. L. 1971. Preliminary developments of an implanted Rankine steam conversion system for circulatory support. Sixth Intersociety Energy Conversion Engineering Conference Proceedings:299–309.
31. Riggle, P., Noble, J. E., Emigh, S. G., Martini, W. R., and Harmison, L. T. 1971. Development of a Stirling engine power source for artificial heart applications: A program review. Sixth Intersociety Energy Conversion Engineering Conference Proceedings:288–298.
32. Martini, W. R., Riggle, P., and Harmison, L. T. 1971. A radioisotope fueled Stirling engine artificial heart power system. McDonnell Douglas Astronautics Company (MDAC) Paper WD 1421. Richland, Washington.
33. Riggle, P., Noble, J., Emigh, S. G., and Martini, W. R. 1971. Development of a Stirling engine power source for artificial heart applications: A program review. McDonnell Douglas Astronautics Company (MDAC) Paper WD 1610.
34. Watrous, J. D., Smith, T. H., Greenborg, J., and Andelin, R. L. 1971. A radioisotope heat source for artificial heart heat engines. McDonnell Douglas Astronautics Company (MDAC) Paper WD 1883.
35. Peterson, G. H., Kessler, A. G., Thorne, G. H., Clark, R. R., and Wood, O. L. 1969. All fluid control system to couple a Stirling engine gas compressor to a left ventricular assist device. Chapter 92 in R. J. Hegyeli, ed. Artificial Heart Program Conference Proceedings. U.S. Government Printing Office, Washington, D.C.
36. Huffman, F. N., Harmison, L. T., Whalen, R. L., Bornhorst, W. J., Molokhia, F. A., and Norman, J. C. 1971. A direct actuation left ventricular assist device (LVAD) suitable for integrating into a totally implantable system. Clin. Research 19:710.
37. LaFarge, C. G., Bankole, M., Bernhard, W. F. 1971. Physiological evaluation of chronic right ventricular bypass. Circulation (Suppl.) 43 and 44:I-90 and I-95.
38. Bernhard, W. F., Bankole, M. A., LaFarge, C. G., Bornhorst, W., Frieze, S., and Curtis, G. W. 1971. Development of an experimental model for functional cardiac replacement. Surgery 70:205-214.
39. Robinson, T. C., Harvey, R. J., van Someren, L., LaFarge, C. G., Bernhard, W. F., and Norman, J. C. 1967. Determination of blood pumping power requirements for an artificial heart. Biomedical Engineering Symposium, 243–257.
40. Sandberg, G. W., Huffman, F. N., and Norman, J. C. 1970. Implantable nuclear power sources for artificial organs: I. Physiologic monitoring and pathologic effects. Trans. ASAIO 16:172–179.
41. Sandberg, G. W., Huffman, F. N., and Norman, J. C. 1970. Experimental observations of intracorporeal strontium 90-americium 241/beryllium sources simulating radiation fields from nuclear-powered artificial hearts. Ann. Thoracic Surg. 9:401–409.
42. Ponn, R. B., Molokhia, F. A., Huffman, F. N., Curtis, G. W., and Norman, J. C. 1971. Abdominal implants of strontium 90-americium 241/beryllium sources. Arch. Surg. 103:701–704.
43. Sandberg, G. W., Huffman, F. N., Molokhia, F. A., Ponn, R. B., and Norman, J. C. 1972. Studies of long-term effects of implanted discrete heat and radiation sources in dogs and primates. National Conference on Research Animals in Medicine Proceedings, National Heart and Lung Institute, Washington, D.C., January 28–30, 1972.
44. Smith, M. L., Greenborg, J., Smith, T. H., and Fuqua, P. A. 1972. Standards for prosthetic devices containing radionuclide power sources. Med. Research 10:9–13.
45. Norman, J. C., Covelli, V. H., McCandless, W. J. C., and Bernhard, W. F. 1967. Feasibility of implantable Pu 238 power sources for circulatory assist devices. Circulation (Suppl.) 36:200–201.
46. Molokhia, F. A., Robinson, W. J., Huffman, F. N., and Norman, J. C. 1972. Observations on chromosomal morphology during simulated intracorporeal radiation from nuclear powered artificial hearts. National Conference on Research Animals in Medicine Proceedings, National Heart and Lung Institute, Washington, D.C., January 28–30, 1972.

PANEL DISCUSSION

COMPARATIVE EFFECTS OF MEDICAL AND SURGICAL THERAPY ON THE PROGNOSIS OF THE PATIENT WITH CORONARY DISEASE

DWIGHT E. HARKEN, CHAIRMAN,

CHARLES P. BAILEY, GEORGE E. GREEN, W. DUDLEY JOHNSON,
EUGENE DONG FOR NORMAN E. SHUMWAY, and F. MASON SONES, JR.

HARKEN: [Dr. Harken had given the panelists warning that each should prepare a "three minute pearl" that would constitute his most important message for the audience.] We will start by saying: Charlie Bailey, you and I are the oldest cardiac surgeons in the world. What is your three-minute pearl on surgical progress?

BAILEY: I have listened to these three days of speeches with a great deal of interest and I think it is almost inevitable that we should be in the position in which we now find ourselves.

Bypass surgery is a new enterprise, a new effective method that can now be used. Coronary artery disease, however, is a metabolic disease with local overtones, and we have a local treatment to treat the local overtones and that is all. Common sense, or as we surgeons call it, "surgical judgment," should tell us that in those cases where the patient is not in any danger, where he is happy and getting along well, that even an operation with an operative risk of 2% should probably not be applied.

On the other hand, we should be able to identify those patients who are at great risk from their disease and who are probably going to die soon if something is not done. If the local lesions are suited to local surgical attack, then it would be worthwhile to consider such an approach.

Your clinical experience and that of others, together with the angiographic findings, should give us enough information to reach a logical conclusion and to do a fairly reasonable job, except in those cases that are quite controversial, such as after infarction, in the case of the stone heart, or in any of those other extreme situations.

HARKEN: To sum up Dr. Bailey's pearl, we may say that if a patient needs an operation very badly, he will do very well, and if he does not need it badly, do not operate. Dr. Sones, your three minutes.

SONES: This is not going to take three minutes. I hope that we do not let the Federal government, through the insistence of the National Heart and Lung Institute, con us into a prospective randomized study in institutions which now "enjoy" a 2–3% surgical mortality rate in an attempt to tell us whether we can do a good job prospectively. Write to your Congressman. That is my three minutes.

HARKEN: I think that is a lovely comment; it is tremendously important for us not to overtest the obvious, and I think that the scientific method can certainly overrun us. Yes, Dr. Sones, some institutions have excessive diagnostic and surgical death rates. Dr. Dudley Johnson.

JOHNSON: I think the data in our series and certainly those of Dr. Sones and their group are very strongly suggestive, at least, that with this type of surgery the patients do live longer.

If you look at the overall deaths from coronary disease, probably two out of three men who die with coronary disease have never had significant angina. Their only symptoms during the disease course are infarction or death.

To me, the biggest future here is to learn more about these groups without angina, to learn how to identify them, and to learn when they should have surgery so that we can apply the benefits of this approach to preserving ventricular function and myocardial tissue. We must strive to help this large group of patients in addition to those who are fortunate enough to develop angina as a nice warning factor.

HARKEN: Hear! Hear! We do agree! Dr. George Green.

GREEN: I had the good fortune to be with Dr. Sones last night, and the best pearls that I can come up with are to repeat some of the things that he said. He has emphasized that in what we are doing, the task is more important than any of the people who are doing it; and to do it well you have to have a proper environment, one that is devoted to a rigid scrutiny of all activities and results and that enlists a group of cardiologists and surgeons who are committed to that point of view.

HARKEN: Great. A very laudable view! Dr. Russek?

RUSSEK: I would only like to reiterate what I have already said. I would hope that the patients who are sent to the surgeons have had an adequate trial of intensive medical therapy. The surgeons are put on the spot when patients are referred who have not had this. Obviously, a bottle of nitroglycerin is not the total therapy of angina pectoris. Many surgeons naturally are reluctant to return patients to their referring physicians with the request that they be treated medically, more intensively, before considering them proper candidates for surgery. As a consequence, some patients are apt to be operated upon who really have not had an adequate trial of medical therapy and who perhaps do not need surgical intervention, at least in the present state of the art.

HARKEN: We must agree with Dr. Russek. The surgeon must be certain but the true test of good medicine is hard to assay in a transient. But a good surgeon must be rigid in his insistence on same. We must carefully classify and have subsets. It is axiomatic that when good surgery comes to a new field, it makes the medical men more critical, more sensitive, and more competent. This is no exception. Dr. Dong, will you comment for yourself and Dr. Shumway's group?

DONG: I think that prevention of myocardial disease is probably the most important feature of the discussions this morning. This may be accomplished either by medical means, by coronary bypass, or what have you. I believe that with the current technology that we can provide, it is very important that you consider transplantation for those patients with severe congestive heart failure and coronary artery disease or myopathies.

HARKEN: As the first and most vigorous antagonist of transplantation, I can only salute this group. I stressed at the outset that Dr. Shumway's group was the right one to carry on this experiment rather than we. This is in spite of the fact that transplantation of organs started at Peter Bent Brigham with kidney transplantation. Additionally, our colleagues had solid knowledge of rejection and its control.

Please convey the congratulations of this assemblage as well as my personal salute to your whole group, Dr. Dong, and specifically to Norman Shumway. Dr. Norman, now for your pearl.

NORMAN: Dr. Harken knows it has been difficult for me to reduce anything to three minutes. He also knows that we have been working in Houston as well as Boston for the past year. The series numbers some 1,400 patients in our clinic.

I am working with one of our medical students, Lloyd Youngblood, and have been impressed with the extent and severity of the disease in the young. We have recently finished a review of the 1,400-odd patients and have found about 100 between the ages of 28 and 39 years with significant disease. We are focusing on this area and will report our findings in the near future.

I would like to throw one counter-pearl at Dr. Sones—for whom I have the greatest respect. As the "Feds" are not here, I must speak because I feel myself to be some part of them. Dr. Russek is right, we need balance; we do need prospective studies. I am sure that the intent in Bethesda and NIH is to establish what Dr. Sones may well already know, but then again, large, monitored studies do have their value.

In general, it is an exciting area. I hope that the results continue to be as good as they seem to be now. We in Houston will be focusing on the young, relatively asymptomatic patient with triple-vessel disease.

HARKEN: Thank you, Dr. Norman. You in the audience have observed by now that Dr. Sones has worked out an ideal technique for offending editors, thereby keeping his papers from being accepted. He can expect to present his material independently in a publication financed by himself.

SONES: You have an amazing capacity to misunderstand the obvious.

HARKEN: Allright. Ready for a case presentation to the distinguished panel. A 57-year-old male executive had "his first manifestation of coronary artery disease as a minor diaphragmatic infarct." He makes an unusually good recovery; his enzymes become normal within a week; he is the head of an important business. What do we do? Does he have an angiogram to see if he has a silent "widow maker" in his left main coronary artery? Do we simply follow him to see if he develops symptoms? Do we tell him to forget it? Or do we tell him to resign from his important post and lead the life of an invalid?

This is a common problem, but I have a friend in mind. He is responsible. He is important. What do we do for or with him? We'll start with the medical man, Dr. Russek.

RUSSEK: I think that every patient is important and I think that if the patient in question made an uneventful recovery and had no symptoms, I would treat him by attempting to remove all of the risk factors that might prevail. If he had hypercholesterolemia, I would treat it intensively, see to it that he lost weight if necessary, and so on. Of course you cannot always get the cooperation of patients.

HARKEN: He is thin, has normal lipid levels, a normal glucose tolerance test, is a nonsmoker, and every factor in the predictive category is under control.

RUSSEK: I would treat this man conservatively by medical means.

HARKEN: Rightly or wrongly, we will use the word "conservative" as synonymous with "medical" means. Dr. Sones?

SONES: I am going to take Dr. Russek on here for just a moment. That amazing group of "good-risk" people that he sees die—what, 1% per year, was that it, Dr. Russek?

RUSSEK: 1.25% per year.

SONES: 1.25% per year. How many of those patients had the extent and severity of their disease defined? What were their angiographic characteristics?

RUSSEK: Only 32 of the 133 had selective cinecoronary angiography. Twenty-six of the 32 had severe triple coronary artery disease. Of these, 15 had good left ventricular function and were therefore classified as "good risk."

SONES: You characterized them as being people with triple-vessel disease and talked about a mortality rate of 1.2% per year. I deny that that is possible; that does not happen in Western civilization.

RUSSEK: It happens out in Staten Island. I can promise you that patients even with severe angina pectoris and good left ventricular function have a far better prognosis than is realized.

SONES: Well, the best thing we can make them do, then, is to make them all move out to Staten Island.

HARKEN: You have both defended your positions well. We have not come to grips with the problem of the case presented. Dr. Sones?

SONES: I would study him. Find out what is the matter with him and then behave accordingly. If he has 80%-plus obstruction in a dominant right coronary artery, and he managed to squeeze the vessel down to a point where he suffered a minor diaphragmatic infarct, and he does not have adequate compensation in terms of unjeopardized collateral channels from some other source, fix it before he has a big infarct or before he drops dead.

HARKEN: Right, that is what I wanted you to say, and I expected Dr. Russek to say exactly what he did. Yes, Dr. Johnson?

JOHNSON: As an *absolute minimum* he ought to have a maximal stress test, and if this is abnormal, I think he certainly ought to be studied. Personally, I should lean heavily towards studying him anyway.

Again, he had no symptoms before his first infarct; I think it is almost hallucination on his doctor's part to assume that he is going to develop a warning sign before his next and major infarct. If he has blocked off one branch of a coronary artery and it is totally occluded and is not going to get worse, then he does not need surgery. But if he is also sitting there with an 80 or 90% block in another artery, we would fix it.

HARKEN: Agreed. Now, Dr. Green?

GREEN: Half the patients who die of coronary artery disease die without previous symptoms. The ones who die probably could be picked by selective coronary angiography. I think he should be studied.

HARKEN: Well, of course all patients are important, but not all can have an ideal case. I said that he should have angiograms, and if it was a minor obstruction with otherwise excellent coronaries, he could be told he could more or less forget it. If there were other significant, nonoperable circumstances, he should be told to modify his life, and if he had a readily jumpable lesion, he should have surgery. In the illustrative case that you experts (save Dr. Russek) felt obviously should be studied, your judgment coincides precisely with mine. However, against my judgment, it was decided to have him ignore his warning.

Now a slight change in direction. Will Dr. Russek define the preinfarction syndrome? Is it definable? Are there too many subsets? In short, please give us your concept of the preinfarction syndrome.

RUSSEK: We spent about three-quarters of an hour yesterday trying to define it, and we did not get very far.

HARKEN: In that case I must try. Some of us believe that the preinfarction syndrome exists when a patient with previously stable angina suddenly develops a crescendo angina without provocation or with very slight exertion and does not respond to nitroglycerin and the usual methods of control.

RUSSEK: It was concluded that we are considering a probability rather than an actual determinable fact that the patient is indeed on the verge of developing an infarction.

HARKEN: Thank you. Would the other panelists agree with this definition of preinfarction syndrome? Dr. Sones?

SONES: Yes, you can only make the diagnosis really retrospectively. If the patient had the infarct, then what happened to him before was preinfarction angina. If, on the other hand, you dive in and fix the thing by doing a bypass at that stage of the game and you manage to do this effectively enough to protect him from myocardial injury, then semantically they will tell you he was not having preinfarction angina.

HARKEN: Well, that is not going to be very helpful to the person who has crescendo angina and is in a hospital 180 miles from Cleveland. What patients do you decide ought to be transferred at once to Cleveland?

SONES: If the doctor calls and tells me he is in trouble with a situation like this I say, "do you think we can move him?" And if he says he thinks we can, well we move him, and we study him that day or the next day. If he really has a tight situation he is on the schedule.

HARKEN: Can you, or Dr. Russek, or Dr. Green, or Dr. Johnson tell me which preinfarction syndromes are going to have an occlusion, and if so with what degree of accuracy? Starting with Dr. Sones.

SONES: No.

HARKEN: Dr. Russek?

RUSSEK: No, but I think we can tell from experience at the Massachusetts General Hospital and elsewhere that the overwhelming majority of the patients survive the attack with medical management alone.

HARKEN: I have been frustrated by the fact that we have polarized the preinfarction syndrome problem into two schools of thought, one in which it is believed that all patients should be treated medically, and the other in which it is equally vigorously contended that all should be treated with emergency angiography and, in many instances, bypass. I think this is the zone where we should give added thought to *counterpulsation*. Of course, every man believes in "his thing," but I think this is one special area where it may be of value. Dr. Bailey, does that seem rational to you?

BAILEY: I would incline to the active program, thinking of bypass surgery if the initial emergency studies showed an indication.

HARKEN: The next two questions have been asked several times. I believe them to be inappropriate. I do not see why we are faced with competitive bidding. However, if I am to maintain academic integrity as Chairman, I must ask them. First, Dr. Dong, the first question is, "What is the cost of transplantation?" and the second question is, "What is the cost of revascularization?" While allowing our panelists a chance to marshal their thoughts, I might throw out a few somewhat related comments.

It always costs too much, there is no question about that, but it always costs less as time goes on. There is no substitute for prevention, and happily we are entering the era of predictive medicine. There is no point in talking about prevention to people who have their disease. There will come a time when we can cut down on these problems appreciably. Then we will not worry about the cost so much.

Meanwhile, the greatest economy measure that you as fanciers and followers of the American College of Cardiology can institute is to spread the word about Heart House. There we will have a harvesting and delivery system that will help us to identify the people who need aid and to deliver protection before the fact and better treatment after the fact. However, cost is the question. Dr. Dong.

DONG: Obviously the cheapest thing for a patient is to die; then medicine and treatment do not cost him anything. But if we are going to make an attempt to restore him to his vocational livelihood, then I think that we have to make a major effort to do so.

I should point out the effect of inadequate or inappropriate surgery on hospitalization. The mean hospitalization *prior* to transplant in our eight patients was something like 100 days. That is, 100 days in hospitals as the result of repeated admissions for congestive heart failure or recurrent angina.

After that, it is 60 days of hospitalization for the transplant, and then after that, very little. Now we have calculated the cost of a heart transplant at Stanford, and this does not necessarily apply to any other institution. It costs $14,000 for the first hospitalization for a patient who has no complication. This includes 30 days of intensive care unit monitoring and 30 days in a clinical research center.

If you have a complication, such as a pulmonary infection, the average cost will go up about $10,000. Now this is not all patient care costs. We maintain our patients in the intensive care unit at approximately $200 or $250 a day for the monitoring, as we are engaged in a significant amount of data collection for research purposes. If we are aiming to reduce patient cost simply for care, I would venture the guess that it would run around $8,000.

HARKEN: On reflection, I am not going to ask Drs. Bailey, Green, Johnson, and Sones about the cost of revascularization. I think this would be improper; it would enter us into a kind of bidding situation that would be in poor taste.

DONG: Dr. Harken, I think that it is appropriate to discuss the cost of heart transplantation at this point because . . .

HARKEN: Oh yes, I asked the question about heart transplantation, but I did not allow the competitive question of revascularization. Dr. Dong.

DONG: And it is not because I think it is competitive with these other procedures, it is just that they are two different ball games.

HARKEN: I agree.

DONG: What I am trying to say is that the cost for a transplant today is considerably different from the so-called cost of a transplant in 1968. But before that, of course, there was no cost at all, because you could not do it.

HARKEN: I agree, and the same thing applied to Dr. Norman. There is no way for Jack Norman to answer a question like the cost of implanting his device.

Obviously, the expense for implantation of a nuclear-powered engine is astronomical, and that has no bearing on the problem of the future.

Now a question for Dr. Russek. Someone wants to know whether or not he can obtain Anginin, where it comes from, and whether it can be used.

RUSSEK: Pyridinolcarbamate or Anginin comes from Japan. It is currently being used on prescription all over Asia and in parts of Europe and South America. It is not at present being studied in this country because as far as I know there is no pharmaceutical company that has licensed it for investigation.

HARKEN: Two questions, the first to give you panelists a chance to organize your thoughts. What is the place for oxygen therapy in ischemic heart disease? The second is for Dr. Russek. Would you tell these gentlemen the contraindications to the use of propranolol?

RUSSEK: The major contraindication to the use of propranolol is incipient or frank congestive heart failure. However, this is not an absolute contraindication, for when these patients are digitalized and given an oral diuretic, one may often safely initiate or continue propranolol. Bronchial asthma is a contraindication because of the effect of propranolol on bronchial muscle; it may aggravate bronchial asthma as well as other allergic conditions, since epinephrine is essential as a protective mechanism against these conditions.

HARKEN: To those contraindications I should add bradyarrhythmias. There, a pacemaker might afford an opportunity to correct the rhythm and then to treat the patient's myocardium, be it with foxglove, diuretics, and/or propranolol.

Now did any of you have a chance to catch your breath a little on that question about oxygen? I do not know whether that question embraces hyperbaric oxygenation, but you say what you like. Dr. Green?

GREEN: I have never been impressed with the use of oxygen in coronary disease. I am concerned primarily with the postoperative period, and I do not really know about the preoperative period.

HARKEN: Dr. Sones?

SONES: Back in the old days I knew an internist who used to make house calls. He was a rare bird. We do not find many like that.

HARKEN: He is dead now.

SONES: No, he is still alive, but he used to do something that I thought was wonderful. If a patient had a stroke, he would insist on getting the patient on an ironing board on the floor. Then he would run the husband or wife around to boil water and do all sorts of busy things. Oxygen therapy in coronary disease is much like that; it keeps everybody happy because they think they are doing something, but it does not really help the patient very much.

HARKEN: Dr. Dong.

DONG: I think oxygen is indicated when there is a clear need for it, and you cannot tell this without blood gas studies. If the patient has arterial hypoxia for whatever reason, he may need oxygen.

JOHNSON: In our flow studies on vein grafts, we uniformly and consistently have demonstrated that oxygen increases coronary constriction. For example, if you do a PO_2 analysis and find it in the normal physiologic range of around 100 and demonstrate a flow through the graft of 100 cc a minute, by switching the anesthetic and raising the PO_2 to 300 or 400 there is uniformly a decrease of about 30% in the coronary flow, and this to me could be potentially far more significant in terms of myocardial perfusion than the mild increase in saturation which occurs by raising the PO_2 to that degree. So I think that oxygen could be potentially deleterious. If there is a normal physiologic arterial PO_2, I think that there is very little indication for added oxygen therapy.

BAILEY: I would give oxygen if the venous return blood were low in oxygen saturation. I think that we are missing a point that has been emphasized for me by Roy Clauss. He stresses that in the postoperative management of surgical patients, the most fundamental study that we can do is to note trends in simultaneous PO_2 of venous and arterial blood. I think we should do that kind of study on our hospitalized patients. In general, if the arterial PO_2 is normal and the venous PO_2 is rising, the cardiac output is rising. If the venous PO_2 is falling, the cardiac output is falling. I do not have any use for oxygen in the home.

HARKEN: Yes, Roy Clauss taught me the same lesson, and we must give him credit. Dr. Russek?

RUSSEK: About 25 years ago, we did a study on patients with angina pectoris employing exercise-electrocardiography. We recorded the ischemic patterns of the electrocardiogram and found that there was no difference in the response whether they breathed with a mask 100% oxygen or room air. So we have lost our confidence in the use of oxygen in high concentrations in patients who have a normal oxygen saturation of the blood.

HARKEN: Yes, Dr. Russek, you mean if they have a normal arterial PO_2. Dr. Norman?

NORMAN: I would think at perhaps a more cellular level. Oxygen in high concentrations is bad and in low concentrations is also bad. With a monitor for PAO_2's, we try to monitor our patients and hold them between 80 and 120 mm Hg. When we go below that, we are concerned. When we go above that, we are concerned.

HARKEN: I am amazed that a panel of this distinction would not have said if the patient's angina is relieved by oxygen, give him oxygen. If it is not, do not give him oxygen. Charlie Bailey has emphasized Roy Clauss' thesis, and that is not only very important, but too-little emphasized. However, it is appropriate only in the hospital where blood gas studies can be done. I hope all hospitals will soon be in this category. You must have more than one set of arterial and venous oxygen measurements. I run a series of simultaneous determinations. When these values are coming together with the arterial level remaining normal in range, the patient's cardiac output is probably rising. When the venous PO_2 is falling, the cardiac output is probably falling. This is a very good "seat of the pants" technique here, available to all of us to recognize relative changes in cardiac output.

Is there anybody at that panel table who would deny that some patients who have angina get relief when they are given oxygen? Would anybody take the oxygen away from the patient so relieved?

BAILEY: I would not take the oxygen away, Dr. Harken, but I fail to see how oxygen could relieve angina in the ordinary sense. Angina is a self-limiting thing that will last for one to two minutes or thereabout. I believe you are referring to the patient who at bedrest has recurrent episodes of angina. Is this type of patient one with acute coronary insufficiency?

HARKEN: Yes, the patient with angina is presumably the one who has heart pain from myocardial ischemia. We see it in various conditions when the oxygen supply fails to meet the myocardial demand, be it coronary artery disease, aortic stenosis, etc. I have an 85-year-old woman scheduled for surgery tomorrow morning with aortic valve disease, and she can be comfortable only with oxygen running.

RUSSEK: I would agree certainly to give it to her.

HARKEN: I should like to have you agree, thank you. Now, what is the status of anticoagulant therapy in ischemic heart disease? This question has been asked by many in the audience, so will somebody deal with it? . . . There seem to be no volunteers in answering that tired old question, so I will try to frame it in special situations, specifically in the context of the person who is having pain, first, though, in the context of the preinfarction syndrome. However, I do not see any useful purpose in going over this old haggle about whether it is good or bad. I respond to the questions from the audience. Dr. Russek, please take a crack at the general question while Dr. Sones reflects on the preinfarction specific a little while.

RUSSEK: I have a long-standing opinion that anticoagulants are of no value on the arterial side of the circulation. They are excellent to prevent venous thrombosis and thromboembolism. I have no confidence in their use to prevent subsequent infarction after a first myocardial infarction. Finally, I do not think that anticoagulants benefit the patient with acute myocardial infarction who is not in congestive failure or having an arrhythmia or other condition.

HARKEN: All right. Would you extend that to the platelet antiadhesive agents dipyridamole and/or aspirin, or a combination of warfarin with the antiadhesive agents? Have I made that too complex?

RUSSEK: I think I follow you. I would certainly prefer the latter agents to the oral anticoagulants or even heparin in the uncomplicated case and certainly for the patient who is ambulatory and in whom you are trying to prevent a recurrence of myocardial infarction or coronary occlusion.

HARKEN: Dr. Green and Dr. Johnson? Would you feel that there is any useful purpose served by antiadhesive agents in connection with bypass grafts or the basic disease itself?

GREEN: In a number of the patients I have operated on with impending infarction, when the arteriotomy was extended proximally to allow a look at the stenosis, I have noticed aggregates of amorphous material at the site of the stenosis. This would suggest that in the patient with impending infarction, perhaps platelet antiadhesive agents might be worthwhile.

In terms of maintaining patency in a bypass graft, I do not believe they are of value.

JOHNSON: I think our knowledge of controlling platelet function is very deficient, but this may well be an extremely fruitful area in the future for helping these patients. I do not think there is enough knowledge now to understand it.

Well, we did place every other person on Persantine (dipyridamole) for one year, 1969 . . .

HARKEN: In what doses?

JOHNSON: It was either 50 or 100 mg Q.I.D.; I think it was 100.

HARKEN: It has to be at least 100 mg Q.I.D. or it will not affect the platelets very much, Dr. Johnson; I can tell you because I know something about that subject.

JOHNSON: At any rate, we were not able to demonstrate any change in patency rate in these patients.

SONES: I would like to ask a question. How about aspirin? What about the dose of aspirin as it relates to platelet aggregability?

HARKEN: I can answer that. Salicylates vary from man to man as a platelet antiadhesive agent, and they vary in the same man from month to month. However, there is substantial evidence that a combination of dipyridamole or Persantine (which is too expensive for most people) and Coumadin may be valuable in prophylaxis. If a patient has a thrombogenic valve in place and takes 400 mg of Persantine (that is 16 of those miserable little tablets), and is anticoagulated with Coumadin, he is almost completely protected against thromboembolism. This is a fact; Sullivan, Gorlin, and I studied 100 randomized patients for a year and confirmed that.

Second, since this program is too expensive for the average patient, the group at the University of Washington Medical School in Seattle looked into our work in the laboratory and then in man. They discovered that salicylates, 5 grains with each meal, plus 100 mg of dipyridamole (that is only four of those little tablets of Persantine) plus Coumadin had a hematologic effect similar to the big, expensive doses of Persantine combined with Coumadin.

However, we now have a series going, the Seattle program we call it, in which we are comparing three groups: first, all three drugs; second, just Coumadin; and third, aspirin and Persantine without Coumadin. Probably the patients with specific valves of the nonthrombogenic aortic variety that I demonstrated are better off with no anticoagulants. On the other hand, if a thrombogenic valve is used and you can stabilize your patient with the aspirin, Persantine, and Coumadin, that is the safest procedure.

Back to our questions, here is a dandy. How do you feel about vitamin C in ischemic heart disease? If the patient has scurvy, I am certainly for it, how about you, Dr. Russek?

RUSSEK: If he also has a cold I am for it.

HARKEN: All right now, one of you authorities must answer with firmness and finality for it has been asked over and over. "What about vitamin E, doctor?" Okay, Dr. Russek.

RUSSEK: I, too, am asked this question every day in the week by my patients. I believe that there is more vitamin E being sold than any other drug that I know of in this country. One of the representatives of a pharmaceutical company said to me one day, "This drug has nutritional value." I asked, "What do you mean?" He replied, "Well, if I sell it, I will eat." But as far as vitamin E is concerned, I have never seen any benefits from it. The controlled studies in this country done many years ago proved that vitamin E was of no value in ischemic heart disease. If anybody is a believer, I should ask him to read the book on vitamin E that has been published in two or three editions by its advocates. If you are a believer and read the testimonials in this book you will become a nonbeliever, as I did.

HARKEN: Absolutely, and if there is a dissenter among the panelists let him hold up his hand. I hope we can present a united front against this absurdity.

Sadly, time is running out and there are several additional questions to be answered. Prominent among them: "Is surgery prolonging life?" We can hardly expect to deal with that question in the few remaining minutes. I might generalize. Angina pectoris presents a series of subsets; there are people with disease patterns who without doubt are having their lives prolonged. There are patients that do not need to have coronary bypass to have their lives prolonged. There are those who only, but importantly, require surgery to relieve their pain. I do not know how we can go much further in these closing seconds of discussion. Can any of the panel offer a take-home pearl in this area?

GREEN: Yes. In regard to subsets, I know that Dr. Gorlin has said that in his patients with left main coronary artery disease, the mortality is 25% per year. I am sure that Dr. Johnson and the other surgeons in the audience have operated on many patients with left main coronary artery disease, and there is no question in my mind that following operation, the mortality is greatly reduced.

HARKEN: Yes, I think that is an important point. I am glad you picked that up, Dr. Green. I should have stressed it in my introductory comment. This is the "widow maker," and I think that there is no question that 80% or more obstruction of the left main coronary artery has a very high mortality and ought to be prophylactically bypassed. Is that a fair statement, in the opinion of all?

RUSSEK: I can only refer to Dr. Corday's remarks the other day; he quotes a follow-up study in which the mortality rate of the so-called widow maker was about 14% per year.

GREEN: Correction, Dr. Russek. He was talking about left anterior descending obstructions! We're talking specifically about 80% left main coronary artery obstruction.

SONES: Yes, he was talking about *isolated* anterior descending lesions.

HARKEN: I hope we all got that straight. What I talked about was left main coronary artery, 80% obstructed. That is the "widow maker," not LAD.

Now, I do not believe the next question is answerable, because it is the whole subject of rejection. Dr. Dong, is there any pearl you want to leave, over and above the fact that these people have to be followed like kidney transplants?

DONG: Yes, I think that is true. Using current technology, the survival for heart transplants is equivalent to the cadaver kidney transplant, 50% per year.

HARKEN: Thank you very much. You, the panel have entertained while edifying. We are greatly in your debt.

SUBJECT INDEX

A

Acetaminophen, anticoagulant uses of, 224
Actinomycin D, cardiac transplant rejection therapy with, 467–468
Adrenal corticoids, myocardial necrosis role of, 394–395
α-Adrenergic agonist, synergistic effects with nitroglycerin, 116, 118
α-Adrenergic blocking agents
  action mechanisms of, 255
  use in cardiogenic shock, 151
β-Adrenergic blocking agents
  action mechanisms as antihypertensive drugs, 255
  avoidance of side-effects with, 90
  use in cardiogenic shock, 151
Afterload, nitroglycerin potential to alter, 116
Age
  as factor in increased mortality in myocardial infarction, 190–191
  influence on survival after heart transplant, 469
Alcohol
  abstinence from and management of cardiomyopathy, 229-230
  effect on cardiac arrhythmia, 130
Aldosterone
  interrelationship between plasma renin activity and excretion of, 288–289
  patterns of excretion in hypertension, 285–286
  renal sodium reabsorption, effect on, 20
Aldosterone antagonists, diuretic value of, 23–24
Allopurinol
  anticoagulant actions of, 224
  use in cardiogenic shock, 151
Alpha-adrenergic. *See under* Adrenergic
Anastomosis, internal mammary-coronary artery, 437–443
Anemia, anginal intractibility caused by, 91
Angina pectoris
  accelerated, 92
  drug-caused intractibility, 91

effective drug use for, 88–91
ileal bypass surgery effect on, 54
intractibility, causes of, 91
medical therapy for, 87, 453–462
normal arteriograms with, 219–222
post-anastomosis recurrence of, 440–441
precipitating and contributing factors in, 87–88
prognosis with normal arteriograms, 221
propranolol and isosorbide dinitrate use in, 88–89, 90, 92
pyridinolcarbamate therapy in, 398, 400–401
risk factors in, 454–455
therapeutic management of, 92, 456–457
Angina pectoris, disabling, as indication for bypass surgery, 197
Angina pectoris, preinfarction, as indication for surgery, 196
Angiotensin II, platelet aggregability effect of, 379
Anticoagulants, use of, 223–228
Anticoagulation therapy, oral
  contraindications for, 224
  indications for, 224
Antihypertensive agents
  action mechanisms of, 249–261
  effectiveness of, 269–280
  plasma volume effect of, 259–261
  side effects of, 273–274
  planning, 278–279
  results of, 278–279
Antilymphocyte globulin, heart transplant immunosuppressive use of, 467–468
Antithymocyte globulin, heart transplant immunosuppressive use of, 467–468
Anxiety. *See also* Emotional stress
  myocardial infarction and, 58
Aorta, atherosclerosis in, 1
Aortic stenosis, role in anginal intractibility, 91
Aortic valve. *See also* Heart valves
  prosthesis and repair of, 407–408
Arterial occlusion, potassium loss and, 178
Arteriography, coronary, risks in, 69